DR. WILLARD CARDWELL
GREENSBORO, N. C.

ELECTROCARDIOGRAPHY
IN PRACTICE

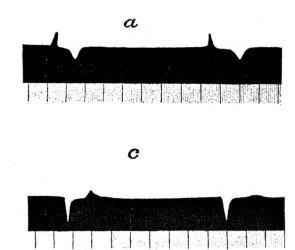

Electrogram from the fly-catching leaf *Dionaea*. Time signal: each heavy black line = 0.5 second.*

In the pursuit of knowledge of the modern techniques in electrocardiography, it is well not to lose sight of the remarkable accomplishments of early investigators. At the same time, while one's attention must be concentrated on the electrical properties of heart muscle, it should not be forgotten that other tissues have electrical properties of interest and importance.

The two strips illustrated in this tracing are curves obtained by leading from the under surface of the fly-catching leaf *Dionaea*. They were recorded with the capillary electrometer by J. S. Burdon-Sanderson in 1888.

Two lead points were secured on the under surface of the leaf, one on the left side, the other on the right. Each complex shows an initial rapid and a slow final deflection corresponding to *QRS* and *T* complexes of the human electrocardiogram. Lead "a" was obtained by mechanical stimulation (stroking) of the right side of the leaf, while lead "c" was recorded after similar stimulation of the left side. Each *QRS–T* complex represents response to a single stimulus.

* From Burdon-Sanderson, J. S.: On the Electromotive Properties of the Leaf of *Dionaea* in the Excited and Unexcited States. Philos. Trans. 179B, 1888, pp. 417–419. By permission of the publishers, Royal Society, Burlington House, London.

Electrocardiography
in Practice

ASHTON GRAYBIEL, M.D.

Captain, Medical Corps, United States Navy;
Director of Research, United States Naval
School of Aviation Medicine, Pensacola, Florida

PAUL D. WHITE, M.D.

Executive Director, National Advisory Heart Council;
Consultant in Medicine, Massachusetts General Hospital

LOUISE WHEELER, A.M.

Executive Secretary, the Cardiac Laboratory,
Massachusetts General Hospital

CONGER WILLIAMS, M.D.

Instructor in Medicine, Harvard Medical School;
Associate Physician, Massachusetts General Hospital

THIRD EDITION WITH 294 FIGURES

W . B . S A U N D E R S C O M P A N Y

PHILADELPHIA · LONDON · 1952

Preface

Six years of ever increasing interest and investigation in the field of electrocardiography, both clinical and theoretical, have elapsed since the publication of the second edition of this book. That fact and the constant demands for a volume such as this by the medical practitioner, be he specialist or not, have caused us to prepare a new edition.

The book has been entirely rewritten and amplified as needed, to include not only the current status of the so-called unipolar leads, both limb and precordial, but also an account of the early trials which have been in progress now for a number of years in attempts to apply vectorcardiography to clinical practice. It is true that the electrocardiogram as we have known it has been a limited record of the heart beat, restricted to one plane only; its expansion to the three dimensions of space where it truly belongs is at last laboriously under way. Although herein we briefly discuss and present illustrations of these studies in progress, we describe in greater detail the significant number of practical advances recently registered in clinical electrocardiography. The book continues to have as its main purpose the production of an atlas containing many electrocardiograms primarily for the practitioner of medicine; it is not intended to be a textbook.

Despite this primary aim, we are pleased to call attention to a novel, indeed almost unique, feature of the present edition. This is Part I, which consists of a comprehensive, albeit concise, historical account of the slow evolution of the physical and physiologic concepts of electrocardiography from the days of its pioneers over one hundred years ago. We have ourselves found this helpful, and we hope that others may too, in the understanding of the gradual and belated development of electrocardiographic theory which has in the past constantly lagged behind empirical advances in the field. There is some reason to hope that the situation may be reversed in the not far distant future to permit more enlightened theory to direct advances in the practice of electrocardiography.

The book is divided into eight parts. Part I, an introduction to physiologic principles, presents the history and summarizes the development of clinical electrocardiography, and describes the operation of the galvanometer. Part II deals with methodology. Part III is a consideration of the various electrocardiographic leads and the variations in the curves obtained from healthy persons. Part IV is devoted to a discussion of the means of identifying the disorders of rhythm, including bundle branch block. Part V deals with changes produced by drugs and certain other chemical agents. Part VI is concerned with the description and illustration of electrocardiographic patterns, in particular atrial enlargement, ventricular enlargement, and myocardial and pericardial disease. Part VII is the longest in the book, illustrating the records obtained in the different etiologic types of heart disease and their subdivisions. Finally, Part VIII contains "unknowns" for practice.

Because of the need of supplying ample illustrations of the normal and abnormal electrocardiogram and at the same time of keeping the book within the bounds of an atlas of this sort, it has been necessary to reduce the number of "unknowns," but because of the value of this part of the volume in previous editions, a carefully selected smaller group of new ones will be found here.

We take pleasure in acknowledging the help and advice of our colleagues at the U.S. Naval School of Aviation Medicine at Pensacola, Florida, especially Lts. John M. Packard and John S. Graettinger, MC, USN, for furnishing many of the electrocardiograms used as illustrations; C. S. Ezell, HMC, USN, for photographing and mounting those illustrations; Mrs. Mary L. D. Ranlett for typing manuscript; and Miss Vivian P. Payne for many of the sketches and drawings. We wish also to express our appreciation to Dr. Edward F. Bland, Chief of the Cardiac Clinics and Laboratory, Massachusetts General Hospital, for the use of the facilities of the Cardiac Laboratory and for the illustrations drawn from his personal files; to

Drs. Edwin O. Wheeler, Gordon S. Myers and Ernest Craige, for their continued cooperation and practical help in assembling many of the cases; to the Cardiac Research Fellows and the laboratory technicians for their interest and assistance; and to Mrs. Paul Mannix for her help in the typing of manuscript and the mounting of some of the electrocardiograms. We are particularly grateful to our publishers for their patience and cooperation.

Pensacola, Florida
Boston, Massachusetts
October, 1952

ASHTON GRAYBIEL
PAUL D. WHITE
LOUISE WHEELER
CONGER WILLIAMS

Table of Contents

PART I

Introduction

CHAPTER 1

Physiologic Principles

The history of the development of knowledge in the field of electrocardiography has many parallels in other branches of medicine, in which useful techniques for measuring biologic events have evolved without precise understanding of the underlying mechanisms. Among the factors responsible for increased usefulness of electrocardiography in clinical medicine are improvement in instrument design, routine use of multiple leads over the precordium, and special investigations, including those utilizing intracardiac leads. These contributions have also thrown some light on the theories which attempt to explain electrical activity in heart muscle.

It must be emphasized that understanding of the electrical activity of heart muscle is still in an imperfect state, with differences of opinion not only as to the mechanism of production of electrical activity in the muscle unit, but also as to the manner in which countless individual units are joined to produce the total effect recorded by the electrocardiogram. Even the pathway of transmission of potential variations from the surface of the heart to remote points on the body surface is disputed. Nevertheless, the situation in clinical electrocardiography, so far as theory is concerned, is far from hopeless. Good working hypotheses continue to evolve, modifying the art of electrocardiographic interpretation in the direction of a somewhat more enlightened empiricism.

It is far beyond the scope of this book to present a detailed critical evaluation of the enormous mass of literature contributing to modern theory of the genesis of the electrocardiogram, nor can full justice be done to dissenting schools of thought in a brief presentation. It is, however, essential that the student of this subject be provided with some background of theory, leading to more thoughtful, less rigid interpretation of tracings and easier understanding of the current literature.

In modern texts most explanations of the genesis of the electrocardiogram begin with a description of the electrical wave of activation, described as the equivalent of a traveling dipole, with the positive portion preceding, the negative portion following. It is the chief purpose of this chapter to trace the development of the hypothesis on which this explanation is based. When one tries to follow through the literature the evolution of this concept which forms the basis for the most widely accepted theory, he encounters considerable difficulty. The following pages have been prepared because of our failure to find such a historical approach in other publications.

In 1790 Galvani's observation that electrical stimulation applied to the exposed spinal cord of a frog produced contraction of skeletal muscle laid the groundwork for important discoveries in the fields of physiology and electrophysics. The further observation that skeletal muscle in turn is a source of electric current was not made until the experiments of Matteucci in 1838. He discovered that current could be made to flow between the cut end of an isolated muscle strip and its uncut surface when these points were connected through a galvanometer. In 1843 and the years following, these observations were extended by duBois-Reymond, who added much to the knowledge of electrical phenomena in living tissue during a lifetime of work devoted to the study of that subject. He believed that muscle tissue was composed of electrical particles or molecules which were active with the tissue in the resting state. This was later disputed by Ludimar Hermann (1877), who maintained that muscle at rest was isoelectric and that electrical changes were manifest at the time of muscle activity or injury. He showed that current flow in excised muscle was the direct result of injury at the cut end (current of injury). Hermann also believed that the measurable electrical events did not issue from special molecules in muscle, but could be explained on the basis of internal molecular change in tissue architecture.

The fact that contraction of *heart* muscle is accompanied by electrical activity originating in the muscle was not demonstrated, however, until 1858, years before the development of adequate instruments for measuring minute, rapidly changing electrical potentials. In that year Kölliker and Müller showed that a frog's heart produced two electrical discharges with each systole. This was observed with a crude apparatus—a frog nerve-muscle preparation. When the nerve from this preparation was connected directly with a frog's heart, each systole produced two contractions of the skeletal muscle. It is of interest to note that these investigators reported that the skeletal muscle preparation contracted "a scarcely perceptible time before systole of the ventricle."

These basic observations made in the middle part of the nineteenth century stimulated further investigations, which were essentially an attempt to explain why electrical effects were produced in living muscle tissue and which involved some study of the curves recorded by the inadequate instruments then available. During the latter part of the nineteenth century, observations were confined mostly to the hearts of cold-blooded animals, but considerable progress was made toward an understanding of muscle electricity. An important related observation was made by Bernstein, who showed in 1871 that transmission of impulse in nerves took the form of a negative wave.

After the work of Müller and Kölliker in 1858, little was done to define the duration and time relations of the double electrical discharge they had described until Marchand's first publication in 1872. Using a crude measuring device called "Bernstein's differential rheotome" connected with a galvanometer, he was able to quantitate the electrical variations of a frog's heart at given intervals from the time of stimulation, producing what would correspond to isolated points on the curves we now get with the string galvanometer. From this he concluded that the electrical variation has two phases (later labeled *QRS* and *T*), the expression of "progress of a wave of negative tension from the seat of excitation." He also showed that the wave of excitation precedes that of contraction, an important discovery.

Engleman had begun the study of electrical variations in heart muscle before the first published work of Marchand (1872), and in an article which appeared later he contributed numerous detailed analyses of frog heart muscle potentials measured with the rheotome. Paired electrodes were placed on the isolated ventricle, one on the apex, the other on the base. By using these data, curves were constructed which showed two phases of electrical activity for each heart beat: the first deflection was of brief duration and relatively high potential (*QRS*); the second of lesser potential, longer duration, and usually of opposite sign (*T*). The nearer the proximal electrode was placed to the site of excitation, the earlier the beginning of the first deflection, further proof that activity spread in wave form through muscle. Since galvanometer deflection occurred in a direction best explained by the assumption that the proximal electrode became negative first, electrical activity was thought to take the form of a wave of negativity proceeding from the point of stimulation.

An outstanding contribution during this era of investigation was made by Burdon-Sanderson, working with an improved rheotome and with the capillary electrometer. The latter instrument depended for its operation upon oscillation of a narrow column of mercury in contact with acid, and represented a real advance in that movements of the mercury column with appropriate magnification could be photographed on a moving light-sensitive plate. Thus curves could be recorded directly, although the inertia of the instrument introduced errors which had to be corrected by calculation.

Burdon-Sanderson studied in considerable detail the electrical changes in frog and tortoise ventricles, presenting evidence of the effects of temperature variations on duration of electrical events and on the "second phase" (*T*) of the curves obtained (1879). He believed that the electrical change traveled in the form of a wave from base to apex.

Other investigators had established the fact that two separate electrical effects could be observed in excised cardiac and skeletal muscle (see Hermann, p. 3). One, the current of action, could be recorded during contraction of intact muscle; while the other, the current of injury, arose from surfaces injured by burning or cutting.

Injury effects were described in a paper published in 1878, and actual curves were published in 1883. It was shown that after injury the usual curve of action having "initial" and "terminal" phases (*QRS* and *T*) was supplanted by a monophasic curve. Figure 1, *A*, is a curve of the action current recorded with the capillary electrometer from a frog's heart, with electrodes on the base and apex. The stimulus was applied to the atrium and appears as an interruption in the narrow black line. Figure 1, *B*, is a curve recorded with electrodes in the same position,

tion from the atrium along a nerve network from base to apex of the ventricle to explain their experimental results only a short time after histologists had found evidence of such a network. Although Lewis showed later that this concept was incorrect in detail, it represented

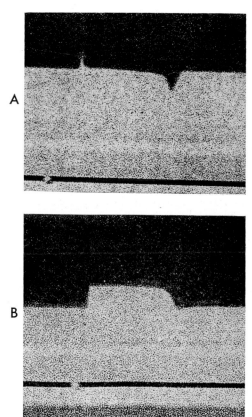

Fig. 1. *A*, Curve of action current (*QRS* and *T* waves) recorded from a frog's heart, with electrodes on apex and base (capillary electrometer). Stimulus applied to atrium is shown by interruption in black line.

B, Curve recorded from frog's heart with electrodes in the same position. The curve shows one large upward deflection—the injury effect—corresponding to what is now called *S-T* segment shift.

(Burdon-Sanderson, J., and Page, F. J. M.: On the Electrical Phenomena of the Excitatory Process in the Heart of the Frog and of the Tortoise, as Investigated Photographically. J. Physiol., *4:* 327, 1883. Courtesy of The Cambridge University Press.)

after injury to the apex with a hot wire. It will be seen that this alteration is produced by what is now called "*S–T* segment shift" in an upward direction.

Until 1887 little work was done on electrical activity of the mammalian heart. This was begun by Waller, using the capillary electrometer; his best known contribution was the recording of the first electrocardiogram in man (Fig. 2). Bayliss and Starling (1892), using dogs as subjects in a series of significant experiments on the heart in situ, showed that, in general, curves of action and injury effects in mammals were similar to those obtained from cold-blooded animals. They postulated conduction of excita-

an important advance at the time. They also recorded a lead from the intact human chest corresponding to the modern lead CR_4.

By the end of the nineteenth century considerable progress had been made in the study and definition of electrical phenomena in the hearts of animals, without formulation of detailed theory to explain the origin of the potential differences known to be present in muscle tissue. It was obvious to the early investigators that muscular contraction per se did not give rise to the observed phenomena, nor could simple transmission of the stimulating current through muscle account for the curves already described. It was also evident that the stimulus

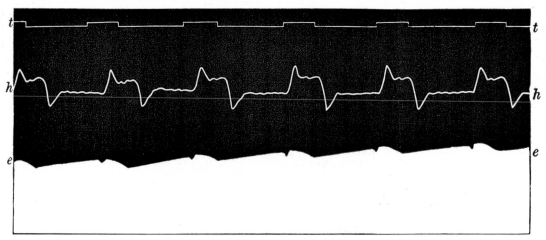

Fig. 2. First electrocardiogram of man, as recorded by Waller in 1887.

t-t = time in seconds
h-h = cardiograph (tracing of apex beat)
e-e = electrometer

(Waller, A. D.: A Demonstration on Man of Electromotive Changes Accompanying the Heart's Beat. J. Physiol., 8: 231, 1887. Courtesy of The Cambridge University Press.)

served only as a detonator or "trigger" mechanism to release much greater potentials produced by the tissues themselves taking the form of wavelike electrical activity of two phases in intact muscle, one phase in injured muscle.

Meanwhile, there had been by 1900 much progress in the study of general cell chemistry and electricity. It was known that potential difference developed across membranes permeable to only one ion of an electrolyte. In 1902 Bernstein proposed and later (1912) elaborated a hypothesis which combined the knowledge in related fields to explain electrical properties in muscle on the basis of potentials developed across cell membranes (membrane hypothesis).

This concept, later modified, is the basis of all textbook diagrams which represent the muscle unit as a block having a row of positive charges on its outer surface, negative charges on the inner surface (Fig. 3). Space does not permit

detailed discussion of the evolution of this concept, but those who are interested will find a review of the subject in Bayliss' textbook.[1]

Given a situation in which the site of electrical energy production is stated to be a membrane, which from its property of being permeable to only positively charged components (cations) of an electrolyte can exist in a state of equilibrium as pictured in the diagram (polarization), it is then necessary to explain known characteristics of the recorded curves on such a basis.

The activity in intact muscle covers a considerable time interval (as great as 0.5 second in the human heart) and has two phases. If the membrane becomes permeable as the result of an applied stimulus at the beginning of activity, migration of the positive charges across the membrane might then give rise to an electrical potential. This would end in a period of inactivity with no charge existing across the

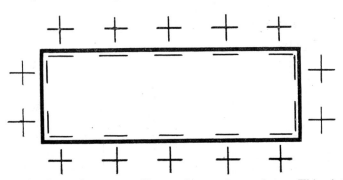

Fig. 3. Concept of polarized cell membrane according to the membrane theory. This pictures the state of balance known as polarization, in which positive charges on the outside of the membrane balance negative charges on the inside.

membrane (depolarized state). Such initial activity is thought to give rise to the *QRS* deflection. Toward the end of systole, with the membrane again becoming impermeable to positive charges, realignment of ions on both sides gives rise to another potential (*T*) and finally ends in the state of equilibrium which existed prior to excitation (polarized state). It should be stressed that this concept is still hypothetical, but it does explain why the action potential has two phases, and, granting that more time might be required for re-establishment of equilibrium (*T*) than for its destruction (*QRS*), the longer duration and greater variability of the former can thus be explained. Such a source of electrical energy, dependent upon movements of ions, could also produce the more sustained potentials seen as the result of injury, in which there is a state of altered equilibrium between normal and damaged tissue.

When Bernstein's concept was introduced, it formed the basis for a more detailed explanation of the origin of electrical potentials in heart muscle, which with certain important modifications is still acceptable. It is of some interest, however, to observe that his ideas of the next step in the production of recorded curves—that is, the manner in which distribution of potential through muscle operates to produce the curves—were accepted for only a few years.

The contributions of duBois-Reymond, Hermann, Engleman, Marchand, Burdon-Sanderson, and others suggested that excited muscle becomes electrically negative to unexcited muscle. This conclusion was based on the fact that a galvanometer connected to a muscle strip or exposed heart with the two electrodes placed directly on the tissue always moved in a certain way. Its direction of deflection could then be explained by the assumption that the active tissue is negative with respect to resting tissue.

This concept was elaborated by Bernstein in connection with his views on the behavior of electrolytes in cell membranes, as the "nega-

tivity hypothesis." In it was embodied the idea that excited muscle tissue becomes negative *en masse* with reference to the remaining muscle about to be activated (Fig. 4). The curves were then explained on a basis of waxing and waning negativity.

The introduction of the string galvanometer electrocardiograph by Einthoven in 1903 provided great stimulus to further research. For the first time it was possible to record directly accurate time curves of electrical phenomena in tissues, eliminating the necessity for the laborious corrections applied to curves made with instruments of greater inertia (capillary electrometer). Within a few years Einthoven himself had made many important contributions as a result of the use of his electrocardiograph, but much detailed information and the formulation of a new theory came from the work of another investigator of that period, Sir Thomas Lewis.

Historical accounts of the early work of Lewis often omit reference to one crucially important factor relative to the value of his contribution to electrocardiographic theory. He used a galvanometer having two strings in place of the conventional single string suspended in a magnetic field. Thus he could record two curves from different pairs of electrodes (leads) on the same strip of film, and, in his words, "our apparatus permits us to obtain simultaneous electrocardiograms, and to examine the relation of any point in the one to any point in the other in precise fashion."[2]

Using the special two-string instrument, Lewis performed many precise experiments on the hearts of dogs, leading directly from the surface of the atrium and from electrodes placed within the heart. Curves thus obtained formed the basis for new and important deductions. From these data most of our present knowledge of the sequence of activation of the heart chambers has been derived. Also, his studies established another concept which had great influence on later investigations. In direct cardiac leads, his observations led him to the

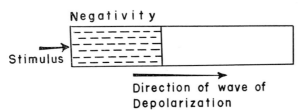

Fig. 4. Depolarization of a muscle strip according to the "negativity" hypothesis. The depolarized muscle is shown as a large block of negative charges, while inactive muscle remains electrically inert.

conclusion that the sharp spike of the initial deflection represented the passing of the wave of activation beneath the proximal electrode. This was termed the "intrinsic deflection."

One proof of the validity of this concept is to be found in Figure 5, from the 1914 article cited.[2] In this experiment, electrodes were placed on the tip of the right atrial appendage, and the recorded curve is shown in the left upper section (Fig. 5, A). The lower curve is

Figure 5, A, the Q wave was believed to represent the time taken for the "excitation wave" to travel from the pacemaker in the sinoatrial node to the atrial appendage. From this it is apparent that a direct lead from a muscle is a mixture of effects arising from the area beneath the electrode and from more remote points. Before Lewis' work, the possibility of remote effects was hardly considered.

As a result of his precise studies on time

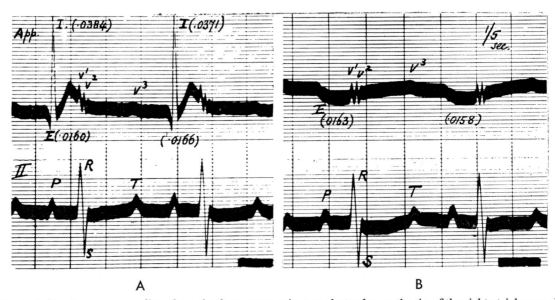

Fig. 5. A, Simultaneous recordings from the dog: upper strip, two electrodes on the tip of the right atrial appendage; lower strip, Lead II.

B, Electrodes in same position after crushing of the base of the atrial appendage. See text.

(Lewis, T., et al.: On the Excitatory Process in the Dog's Heart. Philosophical Transactions, *205B:* 420, 1914. Courtesy of The Royal Society, London, Publishers.)

Lead II recorded simultaneously. With direct leads on the atrium, the first upward deflection is large, as it is in ventricular curves. It occurs about the same time as the appearance of the P wave in Lead II. After the base of the atrial appendage had been crushed in a thin ring to destroy muscle continuity, another curve was obtained (Fig. 5, B). This shows that the large initial spike (intrinsic deflection) was no longer present, although the limb lead II was unchanged. This was achieved by preventing transmission of the wave of activation to the atrial appendage, without interfering with simple conduction to that area.

In addition to the sharp spikes, most initial deflections of direct leads showed slower components, such as the small Q wave in the upper curve of Figure 5, A, which were thought to arise in distant parts of the muscle and were termed "extrinsic deflections." In the curve in

relationships in ventricular activation,[3] Lewis began to challenge the negativity hypothesis. He found that, contrary to the beliefs of many supporters of the negativity theory, the ventricular base was not the first part of the heart to be activated. This was a serious objection to the theory, because its proponents explained their curves obtained from base-apex leads on the assumption that negativity began at the apex and progressed to the base. Figure 6 is a curve (only QRS is shown) obtained by leading from the mouth and abdomen of an intact toad in the long axis of the heart. It is a diphasic curve which cannot be produced by a wave of negativity progressing from base to apex.

This experiment, along with many others, led to the formulation of the "hypothesis of limited potential differences." In this concept, excitation produces a double electrical effect, with the excited tissue relatively negative and the arrow (vector) shown in Figure 8 could represent the potential difference developed between two adjacent points at the center of the triangle.

It should be emphasized that this concept was offered only as a schematic representation of electrical forces present in the heart, working backward from values actually obtained in the

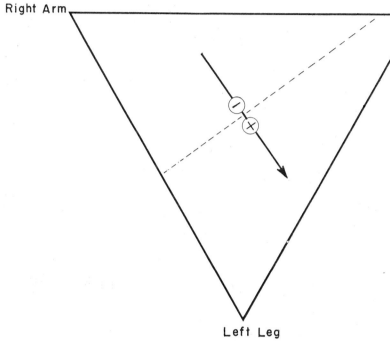

Right Arm

Left Leg

Fig. 8. Representation of cardiac action current as a vector—a force having direction [a]
thoven triangle hypothesis, the body is represented as a triangle formed by the right s[houlder]
symphysis pubis. The force is considered to arise from difference in potential between two [poles in the center of the]
triangle. Actually, Einthoven did not represent these as positive and negative poles in his [hypothesis, although they are usually]
so considered.

curves from limb leads. Thus the heart in the Einthoven triangle hypothesis is represented as two electrical poles lying close together in the center of a triangle formed by the right shoulder, left shoulder, and symphysis pubis. An electrical field exists with the two poles as its center (dipole).

An oversimplified but similar system can be constructed artificially by introducing two insulated electrodes with open tips into a tank of saline solution. If one electrode is attached to the positive pole of a battery, the other to a negative pole, an electrical field will be set up in the saline solution with the dipole as its center (Fig. 9). Analyses of such fields have been made by measuring the potential of many points in the saline solution. The diagram shows that the field around a doublet has positive and negative halves, with the perpendicular between

the dipoles indicating [the boundary between] positive and negative [portions. On the side of each] other, the line of zero p[otential . . .]

The potential of any [point in a] saline volume conducto[r depends on several] factors, including the fo[rce of the dipole . . .] determined by position [in relation to the posi-] tive portion of the field; [. . .]

upon the distance from [. . .] tivity of the medium, [. . .] between a line from the [. . .] the line connecting the t[wo . . .]

These relationships [are illustrated sche-] matically in the case of [. . .] they are the basis for t[he . . .] Einthoven triangle hypo[thesis. It must be re-] membered that leads in [Einthoven's . . .] time were obtained from [. . . express-] ing potential on the bo[dy . . .] representation the pote[ntial . . .] registered by the galva[nometer at a given] instant bears a simple ge[ometric relation to] the potential in the hea[rt . . .] of the angle between the [. . .] and the line representing [the direction of the] potential. Whether or n[ot the various] postulates of this hypo[thesis . . .]

the tissue immediately distal from the point of excitation relatively positive. The wave of excitation therefore has two components, a positive wave preceding and a negative wave following.

Figure 7 is the diagram produced by Lewis in terms of his theory to explain the curve of Figure 6 (QRS portion). The wave with a positive front as it travels toward the apex explains the upward deflection, while the final progress in reverse direction toward the base explains the terminal negative deflection. It is this concept, modified later by others, which is used now to explain the deflections of the electrocardiogram.

In his Mellon lecture (1922) Lewis[4] outlined his concept of the sequence of ventricular activation based on the work just mentioned. It is well worth quoting because it remains the most widely accepted explanation. "The excitation wave is found by observation to start in the septum of the ventricles; it is traced down the septum to the apex and from the latter up the lateral wall to the base. . . . But in moving along this semicircular path the wave does not proceed in a direction parallel to the borders of the muscular track, it is penetrating the wall in successive segments of its course; it moves always from within outwards along centrifugal paths; each part of the wave moves from the endocardial to the pericardial surface."[4]

In this same paper, Lewis also points out some of the fallacies inherent in leading from two contacts placed directly on the heart. In essence this may be stated as follows: while direct leads consist of intrinsic and extrinsic effects, they nevertheless record chiefly the potential variations of small areas. Leads at a distance from the heart (as in Figure 5 and in clinical practice) express the electrical changes from a much greater mass of cardiac muscle. This fact had been known by Waller and by Einthoven long before, but many investigators working with muscle strips and isolated heart had failed to appreciate its significance.

It is fitting at this point to say something about the influence of conducting media around the heart. In clinical practice and in much research, the recorded curves are modified by the presence of tissues which act as a conductor in three dimensions. This is termed a volume conductor. Since curves representing electrical activity in the heart may be recorded at distant points in the body, it is at once apparent that the electrical forces, however small, arising in the

heart create a "sphere of influence" extending through all body tissues. The presence of such a system in relation to a source of electrical energy is in no way unusual. The concept of a field of influence in relation to a magnet, to a wire or coil carrying current, is familiar to all. However, in attempting to apply this reasoning to the heart, which is placed in a conducting medium of tissues of varying conductivity, investigators have met with many difficulties. The problem is obviously complex and still far from precise resolution, although good working approximations have evolved.

Waller and Einthoven were aware of the importance of the concept of the electrical field in the study of the electrocardiogram. Waller (1913) produced a diagrammatic concept of the electrical field around the heart in which the apex and base were represented as positive and negative poles respectively. However, the first field hypothesis of clinical significance was presented by Einthoven in two papers (1912, 1913)* and has been known since as the Einthoven triangle hypothesis. It is well to remark at this point that Einthoven regarded his concept as only an approximation of the truth, limited by many factors which he carefully enumerated.

In his work on the human electrocardiogram, Einthoven was concerned with the form of curves obtained by leads from distant points on the body—right arm, left arm, and left leg. By leading from various combinations of these points, two at a time, he obtained the classical leads 1, 2 and 3 (see Fig. 15, a diagram of a galvanometer hook-up). He then became interested in variations produced in these leads by respiration, and it became apparent that the variations could be explained if the cardiac potential at a given instant were represented as a force having direction and magnitude (Fig. 8).

Details of the hypothesis need not be considered here, but understanding of its implications is important. The form of the curves in Leads 1, 2 and 3 not only indicated different values of potential for distant points in the field, but suggested also a certain orientation of positive and negative parts of the field with relation to the long axis of the heart, determined by the general direction of movement of the electrical activity responsible for QRS and T deflections. Such a force as that represented by

* These are now available in English in the current literature. See Am. Heart J.: *40:* 163, 195, 1950.

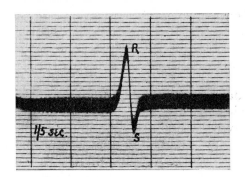

Fig. 6. Curve obtained by leading from the mouth and abdomen of the intact †
QRS is shown.

(Lewis, T.: Interpretations of the Initial Phases of the Electrocardiogram with S
'Limited Potential Differences.' Arch. Int. Med., *30:* 282, 1922. Courtesy of Th
Publishers.)

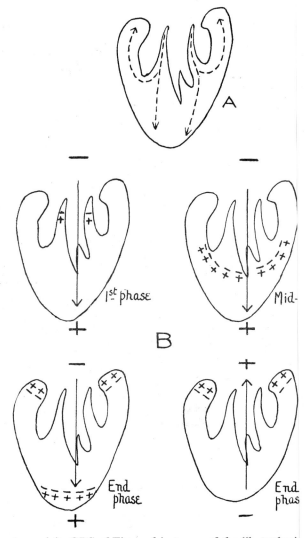

Fig. 7. Lewis' diagram to explain *QRS* of Figure 6 in terms of the "hypothesis
Toad heart.

(Lewis, T.: Interpretations of the Initial Phases of the Electrocardiogram with S
'Limited Potential Differences.' Arch. Int. Med., *30:* 281, 1922. Courtesy of Th
Publishers.)

In any case it has influenced the thinking of many investigators from the time of Einthoven to the present by focusing attention on the importance of the electrical field concept.

A significant step in the study of electrical changes in heart muscle suspended in a volume conductor was carried out by Craib in 1927.[5] He believed that if the dipole or "doublet" concept of the origin of the cardiac electrical field were valid, it should be possible to prove its validity by a comparison between a field

postulates of the old "negativity" hypothesis (see p. 7), but were consistent with a new concept of Craib's which he called the doublet hypothesis. This may be summarized as follows: to explain the orientation of electrical forces as shown by curves obtained from muscle strips, several phenomena must be accounted for in a consistent manner. First consider the complexes obtained from stimulation of a muscle strip suspended in a volume conductor (Fig. 10). Inscription of the first deflection (*QRS*) is a

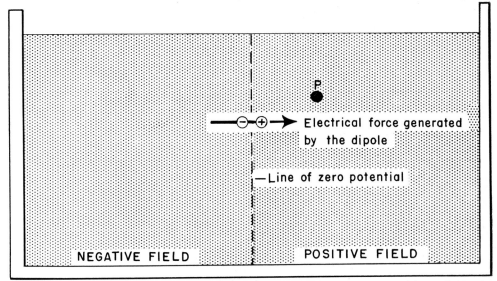

Fig. 9. Artificial dipole set up in a tank of conducting fluid. The poles are connected to positive and negative terminals of a battery (connections not shown).

established by placing active heart muscle in Ringer's solution, and an artificial field set up by inserting positive and negative electrodes in the same conducting medium. This was done, using a glass sphere filled with Ringer's solution and containing a number of lead points set along a rigid axis at an angle to the axis of an artificial doublet consisting of positive and negative electrodes at the center of the sphere. The experiment was repeated, using a terrapin heart with its long axis in the same position as that of the artificial dipole. It was found that the fields, as measured by deflections from the lead points, were similar in general characteristics.

Craib also studied the curves produced by stimulation of strips of cardiac muscle suspended in the same volume conductor. Curves were registered through two lead points placed near, but not on, the strips, and each set of curves showed *QRS* and *T* deflections. The curves thus obtained from electrodes placed in a volume conductor could not be explained on the

single rapid upward deflection. Because of the way in which the galvanometer is connected, this means that the left-hand electrode must remain in the negative part of the field during the first phase of electrical activity. It is well established that activation of the muscle takes the form of a wave moving from the point of stimulation to the distal end. Craib believed that the excitation wave gave rise to a series of doublets, each of brief duration, with positive and negative portions located as shown in the figure. The recovery wave *T* was then formed by a series of doublets of longer duration with charges reversed, producing a curve of opposite polarity and longer duration.

No attempt was made to correlate the doublet hypothesis with Bernstein's membrane theory, and in details Craib's concept has been superseded by the work of Wilson and others. Nevertheless it marked an important step in the development of electrocardiographic theory, and it embodied many concepts emphasized in the work of Wilson, begun independently before the publication of Craib's paper in 1927.

The next significant development in electrocardiographic investigation was in essence a move toward simplifying the form of curves obtained with leads placed on the heart or close to it. The experimental procedures previously outlined in this chapter utilized two lead points equally distant from the heart. In his work on the exposed heart of the dog, Lewis[3] found that curves from two points on the ventricular surface were unsatisfactory because in many instances the intrinsic deflection could not be clearly distinguished. When the behavior of the galvanometer is clearly understood (see p. 19), the reason for this is at once apparent. The galvanometer is an instrument which registers only the potential *difference* between two lead points. Thus, when it is connected to two points on the ventricular surface, each of considerable potential, rapidly fluctuating, the resulting curve represents only the difference between these two points, and its form is practically meaningless in its relation to the curves of potential variation present at either point.

Lewis obtained better intrinsic deflections by moving one electrode to a more distant point on the chest wall with the other placed directly on the exposed dog heart as an exploring electrode. It is now known that leads from the chest wall also show considerable potential variation, although of less magnitude than those directly from the ventricle. Nevertheless, the *principle* involved was of the greatest importance and is now utilized in all clinical electrocardiography. By placing one electrode at a

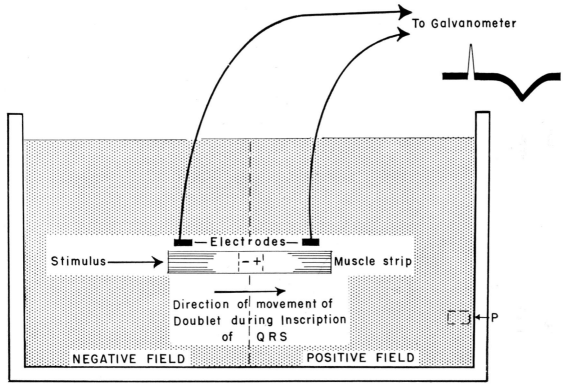

Fig. 10. Curve obtained from muscle strip suspended in volume conductor with electrodes placed as shown. (Modified from Craib,[5] p. 84.)

more remote point on the body, where potential variations are small, the variations of the other point nearer the heart, which are much greater, will be only slightly modified in recording a curve. Thus the curve will represent, for practical purposes, the changes under the "exploring" electrode. This fact now seems quite obvious, yet electrophysiologic research had been going on for more than fifty years before its application, and in clinical electrocardiography the principle was not widely used until about 1940.

A simple analogy may be drawn by using a muscle strip suspended in a liquid volume conductor (Fig. 10). By moving one of the electrodes to the position indicated by the dotted rectangle, a similar situation is created. The galvanometer close to the muscle will then record curves which represent variations at a single point because influence of the distant electrode is negligible. According to Groedel,[6] Nicolai (1909) was the first to suggest a method for obtaining chest leads representing potentials from different parts of the heart with one electrode far from the heart ("indifferent" electrode).

Techniques now in use are explained elsewhere in this book. Recent work of the greatest importance in formulating theory to explain the genesis of the electrocardiogram has been done by

through a conduction system and thick walls were avoided. Recordings were made on a double galvanometer, with simultaneous registering of another lead to serve as a base reference for comparing time units in the various curves obtained. These curves represented potential variations, both intrinsic and extrinsic, of a small area of atrial surface.

The initial complex of one of their curves obtained with the exploring electrode halfway between the upper end of the sulcus terminalis

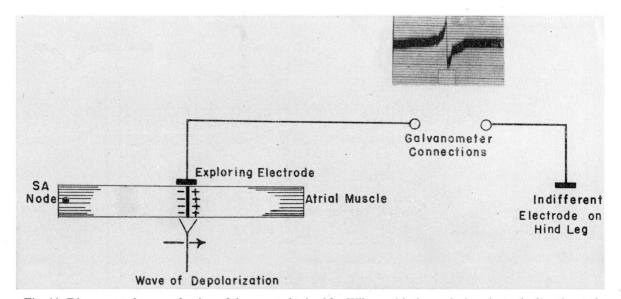

Fig. 11. Diagram to show production of the curve obtained by Wilson with the exploring electrode directly on the right atrium of the dog, and the indifferent electrode on the left hind leg. The wave of depolarization with its positive and negative components is shown at the point where it passes beneath the exploring electrode. This corresponds to the rapid downswing of the curve (intrinsic deflection).

(This is a portion of the curve from the figure published by Wilson, F. N.: Distribution of Currents of Action and of Injury Displayed by Heart Muscle, University of Michigan Press, with polarity reversed to conform to present usage. Courtesy of The University of Michigan Press.)

Wilson, who made use of the principles outlined earlier relating to flow of electricity in volume conductors and to the use of a remote or indifferent lead point paired with an exploring electrode.

In a monograph published in 1933, Wilson and co-workers[7] laid the groundwork for what is now the most widely accepted explanation of the genesis of the electrocardiogram. To obtain curves of the current of action from the atrium, they used an exposed dog heart. The "indifferent" electrode was placed on the left hind leg, the exploring electrode on various points of the external surface of the right atrium. The atrium was selected because it is a thin muscle sheet with radial spread of action current from the sinus node. Thus the complexities of spread of ventricular activation

and the tip of the right atrial appendage is shown in Figure 11. This curve is simple in form, consisting of a slow positive (upward) deflection, a rapid negative (downswing) deflection, and a slow return to the baseline. Curves from other points on the atrium at varying distances from the sinus node showed different times of onset and different over-all pattern, but the rapid downstroke remained and its duration was relatively constant. This rapid deflection, called the "intrinsic" deflection by Lewis, is obviously produced by a quick change from positive to negative potential of the explored area. In the summary of his monograph Wilson says: "The shape of these curves indicates that the electrical phenomena associated with the excitatory process are similar to those that would occur if the crest of the wave of excitation were immediately preceded by a positive pole, or source, and immediately followed by a negative pole, or 'sink.' It is the rapid passage of this double charge beneath the exploring electrode which accounts for rapid swing of the galvanometer from positive to negative, producing the intrinsic deflection" (Figure 11).

Having recorded curves which represented fluctuation in potential from a small area of

"monophasic" response is similar in form to that obtained by Burdon-Sanderson with two electrodes placed on the injured frog ventricle (see Fig. 1, *B*), Wilson's experiment differed in one important respect from the work of previous investigators dealing with currents of injury. His method of leading, using an "indifferent" electrode for each lead, permitted observation of the injury effect from within the area and outside it simultaneously. In the older

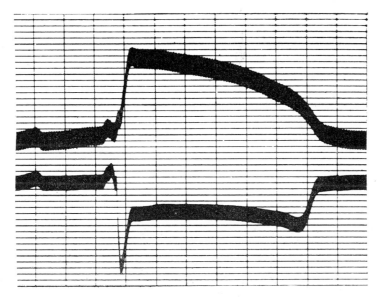

Fig. 12. Curves obtained from injured surface of a turtle's ventricle: top curve, exploring electrode within the area of injury; bottom curve, exploring electrode 5 mm. from the margin of the burned area. Polarity reversed to conform to present usage. Indifferent electrodes were placed on left and right hind legs.

(Wilson, F. N.: Distribution of Currents of Action and of Injury Displayed by Heart Muscle. University of Michigan Press. Courtesy of The University of Michigan Press.)

atrial muscle, Wilson, in the same monograph, proceeded to mathematical analysis of a theoretical wave of excitation involving a thin, flat sheet of muscle. His curves, produced by calculation, were similar in form to the actual recorded tracings.

Injury effects were studied in the exposed turtle heart, using two galvanometers recording simultaneously (Fig. 12). It was then possible to register potential variations from injured and intact muscle at the same time by placing one exploring electrode on the injured ventricular surface (top curve), the other on intact muscle near the injured tissue. Each of the exploring electrodes was paired with an indifferent electrode on the right and left legs.

Reference to Figure 12 will show that each of the curves is practically "monophasic" in form, in that it consists of deviation from the baseline through most of systole. Although this

experiments, the curves obtained were of complex form, representing the difference between two points on the heart, each having considerable potential variation. Also many investigators had been in error in assuming that the burned area carried no potential.

The curves in Figure 12 permit certain important deductions concerning the injury effect. Obviously one electrical force is producing the galvanometer deflections in opposite directions during systole (one positive, the other negative), and it is equally obvious that the zone producing this force must lie between the electrodes.

This zone is considered to be a band of injured muscle lying between dead muscle in the center of the burned zone, and active muscle outside it. Thus an electrical field is set up in the injured but living muscle, so oriented that an electrode within the injured zone is positive during systole while an electrode outside it has the opposite polarity. Dead tissue in the center of the burned area is not itself active, but serves as a conductor and lies within the electrical field produced by the injured muscle. (Actually, the neutralizing current used to center the string in the recording instrument introduces a complication which need not be considered in detail at this time.) During diastole the forces produced by the electrical disturbance of injury are so directed that the inner part of the injured zone is negative, the outer portion positive. During systole these relationships appear to be reversed. The significance of this lies not in its detail, but in the fact that destruction of a portion of cardiac muscle produces an electrical imbalance between injured and whole tissue, which in turn gives rise to an electrical field. This is a valuable clue to the origin of electrical force in muscle. Obviously such injury does not "introduce" electrical potential into muscle, but alters muscle structure so that forces already present are released. Wilson stated that the electrical field produced by muscle injury could be explained by polarization of the surface lying between injured and uninjured tissue. Thus the widespread effects arise within a narrow band.

The same concept of a narrow band of activity is used in Wilson's explanation of the wave of excitation. Here the conditions are somewhat different (see Fig. 11) in that the boundary zone lies between muscle which has been depolarized and that which is about to be depolarized. Thus the wave of excitation may be visualized as a traveling zone of activity, with positive charges on the advancing edge, negative charges on the following edge. The electrical field in this case results from the imbalance produced by depolarization.

In both injury and action currents the electrical activity results from loss of balance of electrical charges, and, as Wilson clearly pointed out, the exact manner of its production is immaterial so long as the concept represents a reasonable symbolization of the site of its origin and distribution of its force. Wilson thought that his explanation for the origin of action and injury currents could be integrated with the membrane theory, and a section of his monograph was devoted to consideration of this problem. Again it is unnecessary to present the details here, but it should be remembered that the concept of electrical force arising within a narrow band of tissue is a simplification of the actual situation. Stated in his own words: "The membrane theory has the important advantage that it explains the current of action and the current of injury on the same basis. According to its postulates, the effective electric forces responsible for the current which accompanies excitation do not actually arise within the transitional zones referred to, but only appear to do so because of the disturbance within these regions of a previously existing equilibrium."[7]

It will be seen that the theories of Craib and of Wilson were not greatly different in their end result. Wilson's work, however, was conceived in harmony with accepted theories of cell chemistry.

It is not within the scope of this chapter to develop in detail the application of basic concepts of muscle electricity to the form of curves found in clinical electrocardiography. This has been done very well in many current publications in electrocardiography. An excellent article in the periodical literature explaining the form of the QRS complex was published by Gardberg and Ashman in 1943.[8]

Most of the discussion in this chapter has been confined to the QRS wave, which repre-

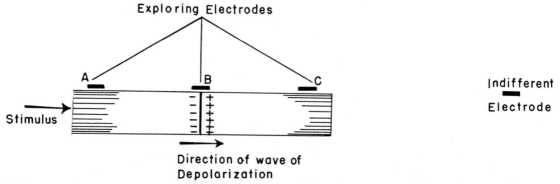

Fig. 13. Passage of a wave of depolarization through a muscle strip suspended in a volume conductor with three electrodes, A, B and C, and one indifferent electrode at a distance. See text.

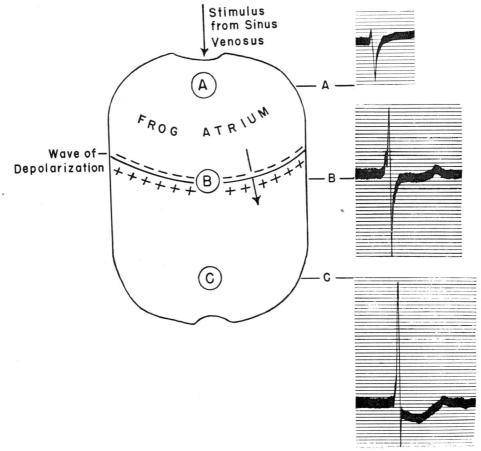

Fig. 14. Curves obtained experimentally with exploring electrodes on the atrium of a bullfrog, indifferent electrode on left hind leg. Conditions essentially similar to those seen in Figure 13. Polarity reversed to conform to present usage.

(Macleod, A. G.: The Electrogram of Cardiac Muscle: An Analysis Which Explains the Regression of T-Deflection. Am. Heart J., *15:* 181, 183, 185, 1938. Courtesy of C. V. Mosby Company, Publishers.)

sents the depolarization of the ventricular muscle. This same process takes place also in the atria in a well established sequence. It measures the forces released by destruction of a pre-existing equilibrium. Thus *QRS* tends to be constant, as many authors have pointed out, and is altered only by rather potent factors such as disease.

For our purpose here it is sufficient to summarize the electrical effects of the wave of depolarization in a general way as follows: the wave of depolarization may be considered the equivalent of a dipole, or collection of dipoles, moving along muscle from the point of stimulation. The polarity of an exploring electrode at any given instant will depend upon its position with relation to the dipole at that instant. Figure 13 illustrates these factors. It shows a segment of muscle lying in a volume conductor. At the instant shown, the wave of depolarization has traveled halfway along the muscle segment from the point of stimulation. At this instant, point

"A" is negative because it lies in the negative field set up by the dipole, while point "C" is positive because it lies in the positive field. Point "B" is at the point where these two influences cancel each other, and therefore is zero.

Next, consider the potential fluctuations of each exploring electrode during the whole cycle of depolarization, which lasts until the wave ends at the termination of the muscle strip on the right. It is obvious that point "A" will be positive for only a short time, until the wave passes beneath it; point "B" will be positive for the first half of the cycle, negative for the second half; while "C" will be positive for most of the cycle and will become negative only at the very end, when the wave finally passes beyond it.

A series of such curves has been obtained in many experiments. Figure 14 shows curves obtained by Macleod[9] from the atrium of a giant Louisiana bullfrog. The curves are labeled "A," "B," "C," to correspond with the points illustrated in Figure 13. Only *QRS* complexes are to be considered at this time. Macleod used these curves to illustrate a somewhat more complex modification of Wilson's theory, but the principle remains the same.

On the other hand, the process of reconstruction of the equilibrium, or repolarization, manifested as the T wave, does not take place in any established sequence, and is easily altered by minor factors such as temperature. Thus no complete explanation of T wave variation is available. It is true that concepts such as the ventricular gradient express relationship between QRS and T, but much is yet to be done in elucidating T wave forms. Craib and Wilson thought that the wave of repolarization consisted of positive and negative components arranged in reverse relationship to those existing during inscription of QRS, that is, with the negative portion preceding the positive, and with a greater distance separating the components; this would explain the longer duration of T and the absence of intrinsic deflections.

References

1. Bayliss, W. M.: Principles of General Physiology. 2d ed., revised. New York, Longmans, Green, and Co., 1918.
2. Lewis, T., Meakins, J., and White, P. D.: The Excitatory Process in the Dog's Heart. Phil. Tr. Roy. Soc., *205B:* 375, 1914.
3. Lewis, T., and Rothschild, M. A.: The Excitatory Process in the Dog's Heart. II. The Ventricles. Phil. Tr. Roy. Soc., *206B:* 181, 1915.
4. Lewis, T.: Interpretations of the Initial Phases of the Electrocardiogram with Special Reference to the Theory of 'Limited Potential Differences.' Arch. Int. Med., *30:* 284, 1922.
5. Craib, W. H.: Study of Electrical Field Surrounding Active Heart Muscle. Heart, *14:* 71, 1927.
6. Groedel, F. M., and Borchardt, P. R.: Direct Electrocardiography of the Human Heart. New York, Brooklyn Medical Press, Inc., 1948, p. 14.
7. Wilson, F. N., Macleod, A. G., and Barker, P. S.: The Distribution of the Currents of Action and of Injury Displayed by Heart Muscle and Other Excitable Tissues. Ann Arbor, Michigan, University of Michigan Press, Scientific Series, volume 10, 1933.
8. Gardberg M. and Ashman R.: The QRS Complex of the Electrocardiogram. Arch. Int. Med., *72:* 210, 1943.
9. Macleod, A. G.: The Electrogram of Cardiac Muscle: An Analysis Which Explains the Regression or T-Deflection. Am. Heart J., *15:* 165, 1938.

CHAPTER 2

Principles of Operation of the Galvanometer

At this point it is fitting to discuss the operation of the galvanometer without considering mechanical detail. Understanding of the simple basic principles involved is an essential background to electrocardiography, yet many who use the electrocardiograph do so without knowledge of these principles. Many kinds of galvanometers are manufactured commercially which provide tracings adequate for clinical practice. The movements of a string, rotating coil, or electron beam may be utilized to produce the recorded curve, but in every case the underlying operation is the same.

The whole situation is summarized simply in Figure 15. The instrument is pictured as having only two essential connections to the body

HOOK–UP FOR CLASSICAL LEADS

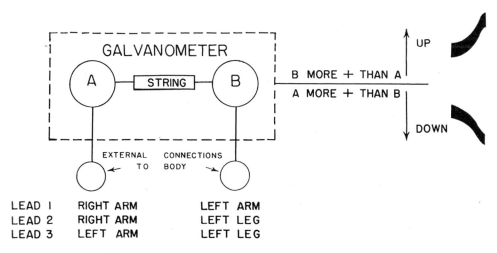

LEAD 1	RIGHT ARM	LEFT ARM
LEAD 2	RIGHT ARM	LEFT LEG
LEAD 3	LEFT ARM	LEFT LEG

HOOK–UP FOR UNIPOLAR LEADS

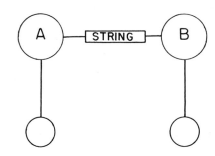

"INDIFFERENT" OR
"ZERO" ELECTRODE

EXPLORING ELECTRODE
FOR
ESOPHAGEAL LEADS
CHEST LEADS
EXTREMITY LEADS
INTRACARDIAC LEADS

Fig. 15.

Page 19

which can be altered in various combinations by the lead selector switch. Two important properties of the galvanometer must be kept in mind: (1) Movement of the string (or coil) either up or down depends upon direction of current flow through the string (or coil). This, of course, is determined by the relationship to one another of the potentials at A and B as follows: If B is *relatively* more positive than A, the string deflection is up; if A is *relatively* more positive than B, the string deflection is down. (2) The galvanometer measures only difference in potential between two lead points. Thus a potential of plus 20 millivolts at terminal A and plus 25 millivolts at terminal B will produce a galvanometer deflection of plus 5.

This simplicity in action of the instrument also imposes certain limitations. When it is used to measure the difference between two points of fluctuating potential (as in the classical leads 1, 2, 3), the recorded curve in any lead gives no indication of its components, that is, the curve of potential change at each lead point on the body. Thus one cannot predict by looking at Lead 1 what the curve at the right arm or the left arm should look like. Limitations of the instrument were an important stimulus to the development of unipolar leads. By the establishment of zero, or near zero, potential at one terminal the galvanometer is enabled to record fluctuations at the other terminal directly.

The working of the galvanometer, with particular reference to precordial leads, is illustrated as follows: each of the V chest leads represents fluctuations in potential at a given point on the chest with little distortion produced by minute fluctuations of the indifferent electrode, in this instance the Wilson central terminal. In this manner the V chest leads record curves which represent the potential variation at each one of the six standard points on the chest. By the recording of such curves and by the combining of two of the points of known potential variation at poles A and B of the galvanometer, the *difference* between the two known curves is expressed. Inspection of such a resultant curve and its two known components tells us much about the operation of the instrument at a glance. Figure 16 is an application of this method.

A. In the first horizontal row it will be seen that one electrode was placed in the V_1 position, the other in the V_2 position. The resultant curve, shown on the right-hand side, has a small up-

right QRS deflection and a larger upright T deflection. In effect, the galvanometer subtracts potentials at V_1 (terminal A) from those at V_2 (terminal B) to produce the final curve. The initial small positive deflection of this curve represents the difference between the larger R wave of V_2 and the small R wave of V_1. The S waves of V_1 and V_2 are rather similar. Therefore the galvanometer registers only a small deflection, just before the beginning of the S–T segment. It must be emphasized that, inasmuch as we do not have simultaneous recordings, only general statements can be made about the time relationships of these curves. Peaks of waves in different leads do not necessarily occur at the same time. The sizable T wave in the right-hand curve represents the difference between the large T of V_2 and the small T of V_1.

B. It is of interest here to observe that the QRS complex in the right-hand tracing begins with a small downward deflection, Q, in spite of the fact that neither V_3 nor V_2 shows negativity in the early part of the QRS complex. This occurs probably because V_2 becomes more positive than V_3 at the very beginning of QRS, although V_3 eventually becomes more positive. By consulting the diagram, it will be seen that when terminal A is more positive than B, movement of the string is in a downward direction. This explains why the galvanometer may record a negative deflection when its terminals are connected to two points of positive potential. Many Q waves in Lead 3 of normal persons are explained in this way. Also of interest is the tall R wave in the resultant curve, which is taller by 6 mm. than that of V_3. This is so because it is a measure of the difference between a positive quantity of 17 (peak of the R wave in V_3) and a negative quantity of 6 (nadir of the S wave in V_2). Expressed as a numerical relationship: RV_3 minus SV_2 = final positive deflection; 17 minus -6 = plus 23. The T wave is slightly inverted because the T in V_2 is slightly more positive than that in V_3. (See diagram, p. 19, summarizing rules for string movement.) It is small because the amplitude of T waves in V_3 and V_2 is almost the same, or, to express it in another way, their difference is small.

C. The resultant complex on the right shows a small R and slightly inverted T. It is of interest to see the large components responsible for the small resultant deflections. T is negative for the same reason that it is negative in B.

D. Here again the resultant deflections are small

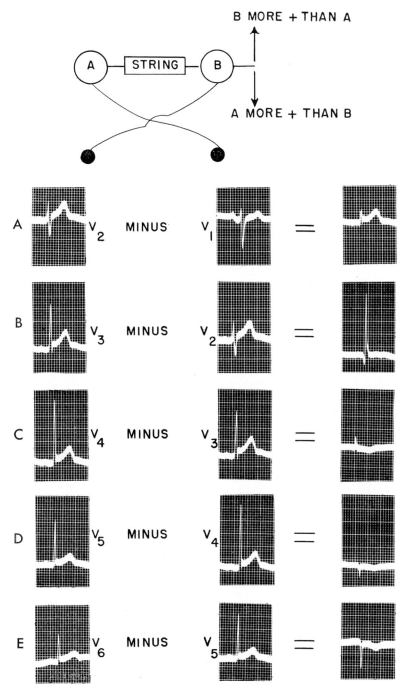

Fig. 16. Operation of the galvanometer, using paired points on the chest.

and negative in spite of the fact that the compo-nents (V_5 and V_4) are large and positive.
E. Here resultant deflections are negative, with the QRS rather large because of the considerable difference between R in V_6 and R in V_5.

These leads as shown have, of course, no practical value in electrocardiography, but they serve to demonstrate a few points about the galvanometer, especially its limitations in the taking of bipolar chest leads.

One point about the use of chest leads in following serial patterns of any kind should be kept in mind. The use of V chest leads rather than "bipolar" chest leads is to be recommended because the Wilson central terminal minimizes the effect of potential variations of the so-called "indifferent" electrode upon the curve produced at the chest lead point. If one of the extremities is used as the "indifferent" point (as in chest leads CR, CL or CF), the potential variations of that point may produce significant distortion of the final curve. Reference to the section on properties of the galvanometer (p. 20) will call to mind the fact that the galvanometer measures only differences in potential. Thus a tracing taken with lead CF, for example, will be distorted by left foot potentials; the distortion in a positive or negative direction is equivalent to the value of the potential present at that extremity.

It is often forgotten that in serial tracings of fluctuating patterns the values of potential at the extremities change along with the alterations taking place in the chest leads. Thus a second precordial electrocardiogram taken with leads CF in a changing situation will be distorted by a *new* factor. It is evident that the bipolar chest leads introduce a complex and misleading set of variables in the evolution of serial patterns. While it is not claimed that the Wilson central terminal is zero, it at least introduces the *mean* of the individual distorting values to be found in the left arm, left leg and right arm, and is therefore a much better indifferent point, especially in the study of changing patterns.

PART II

Methodology

CHAPTER 3

Methodology

Part II is concerned with the procedure used in obtaining electrocardiograms and the routine to be followed in interpreting them.

Electrocardiographs

The principle of the electrocardiograph has already been presented, and little need be said concerning the actual operation of the many different instruments available. This information is contained in the instruction booklets furnished by the manufacturers. Suffice it to say here that all are easy to operate, and the choice of instrument depends mainly on other factors such as cost, weight, recording method, servicing features, and so forth. If the lead selector switch is inadequate for readily obtaining unipolar and augmented unipolar leads, as is the case with older equipment, it is worth while to obtain an auxiliary lead selector switch box. This can be easily incorporated into the circuit between the patient and galvanometer and will greatly facilitate the obtaining of unipolar leads.

Electrocardiographic Leads

The word "lead" is used to denote both the particular connection of the subject to the galvanometer, and the curve obtained. The distinction is usually clear from the context, and in this book the word "lead" is capitalized when referring to a specific electrocardiographic curve.

In obtaining an electrocardiogram the form of the curve is determined, among other things, by the location of the electrodes placed on the body and the manner in which the connection is made between the subject and the instrument. In taking bipolar leads a direct connection is made between electrodes at two points on the body and the galvanometer; the resulting curve is a record of the differences in electrical potential between the two lead points. In taking unipolar leads according to the method of Wilson, the exploring electrode is paired with a central terminal connected to both arms and to the left leg through 5000-ohm resistors. The attachments to the electrocardiograph are such that positivity at the exploring electrode is declared by an upward deflection in the curve. This curve is an expression of the potential differences between a point of near-zero potential representing the center of the heart and the point where the exploring electrode makes contact with the body. Strictly speaking, it is a bipolar lead, although the form of the curve is determined almost entirely by the potential variations of the exploring electrode.

In taking unipolar limb leads Wilson's central terminal electrode should be used,* but with a modification suggested by Goldberger, namely, that the central terminal should not be connected to the extremity to which the exploring electrode is attached. This results in a 50 per cent increase in the amplitude of the curve, which is usually desirable, and is termed an augmented unipolar limb lead.

Bipolar ("Classical") Limb Leads

In the case of the three bipolar limb leads the two arms and the left leg are used as the points of contact (see Fig. 15, p. 19). Lead 1 represents the potential variations between the two arms; relative positivity at the left arm is declared by an upward deflection in the curve. Lead 2 represents the potential variations between the right arm and the left leg; relative positivity at the left leg is declared by an upward deflection. Lead 3 represents the potential variations between the left arm and the left leg; relative positivity at the left leg is declared by an upward deflection.

Augmented Unipolar Limb Leads

The arms and the left leg are also used in obtaining the augmented unipolar limb leads

* This procedure is followed wherever switch boxes are provided.

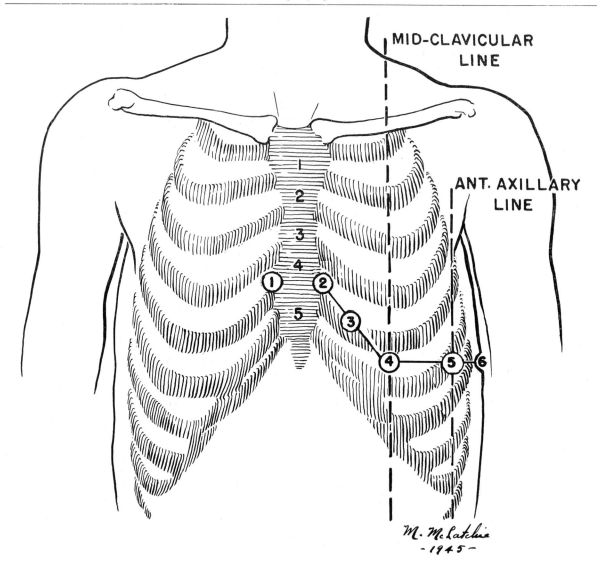

MID-CLAVICULAR
LINE

ANT. AXILLARY
LINE

M. McLatchie
- 1945 -

Fig. 17. Locations of electrodes in precordial electrocardiography.

which, for convenience, are designated Lead aV_R (right arm), Lead aV_L (left arm) and Lead aV_F (left leg`.

Chest Leads

The procedure to be used in obtaining precordial leads has been standardized by a committee appointed by the American Heart Association,* † and may be summarized as follows: Two letters and a subscript number define the position of the chest electrode and choice of indifferent electrode when a single extremity is used as an indifferent point. The first letter "C"

* Standardization of Precordial Leads. Supplementary Report. Am. Heart J., *15:* 235, 1938.
   † Second Supplementary Report by the Committee of the American Heart Association for the Standardization of Precordial Leads. Am. Heart J., *25:* 535, 1943.

refers to the chest, while the following letter designates the location of the indifferent electrode. Thus CR denotes chest-right arm; CL denotes chest-left arm; CF denotes chest-left leg (foot). The letter "V" refers to the combination of a chest electrode with a special indifferent point suggested by Wilson, a central terminal connected to the three extremities through 5000-ohm resistances. By convention only a single letter is used; the letter C is dropped. In every instance a following subscript (number) refers to the position of the electrode upon the chest.

There are six standard points on the chest, located as follows (see Fig. 17): Positions 1 and 2 are in the fourth interspace at the right and left sternal borders respectively. Position 4 is located at the intersection of the midclavicular line with the fifth interspace. Position 3 is a point on a straight line connecting positions 2 and 4, midway between them. A horizontal line passing through position 4 determines position 5 at the point of intersection with the anterior axillary line, position 6 at the intersection with the midaxillary line.

When in the past a single precordial lead was used, the electrode was placed at the outer border of the apex beat or, if the apex was not palpable, at the intersection of the fifth interspace and midclavicular line. This lead was called 4_R, 4_L or 4_F, depending upon which extremity was used as the indifferent point. However, this single precordial lead has been a source of confusion and is now essentially obsolete.

Additional lead points may be designated as follows: V_7, left posterior axilla at the same level as V_6; V_8, tip of the left scapula; positions on the right side of the chest comparable to V_3 through V_6 may be designated V_{3R}, V_{4R}, V_{5R} and V_{6R}; V_E refers to a position just to the right of the ensiform process.

Esophageal Leads

Electrocardiographic leads from the posterior aspect of the heart may be obtained by placing electrodes in the esophagus. These electrodes are in the shape of narrow metal bands closely applied along a duodenal tube with the lead wires carried inside. The tip of this tube is readily passed into the stomach, and lead points are then established along the entire course of the esophagus. Localization of a particular electrode can be accomplished with the aid of fluoroscopy or by introducing it a measured distance beyond the nares or the incisor teeth. If a series of tracings is obtained, localization in terms of the atrial deflection is also possible. The esophageal electrodes should be paired with Wilson's central terminal electrode, thus obtaining unipolar esophageal leads.

Terminology has not been standardized for the esophageal leads. We have used "EV" to designate the esophageal unipolar lead and the subscript a to indicate the lead obtained at the atrial level. Electrode positions above or below this level are easily indicated by a figure which represents the distance in centimeters. Thus EV_{a+10} would indicate that the electrode was 10 cm. above this point, and EV_{a-5} that the electrode was 5 cm. below atrial level.

Endocardial Leads

The introduction of cardiac catheterization technique has provided an opportunity to obtain electrocardiograms from within the chamber of the heart. These are of much interest, but have little place as yet in clinical electrocardiography.

The Choice of Leads

For routine use it is best to obtain bipolar and augmented unipolar limb leads and precordial leads V_1 through V_6. Only the experience which comes with great familiarity will allow the physician to interpret them with confidence. Occasionally it will be necessary to obtain curves using additional lead points over the chest or from within the esophagus.

Obtaining Standard Electrocardiograms

A number of factors may influence the shape of the electrocardiographic curve, including body position, the effects of recent exercise, anxiety, overventilation, and the effects of drugs. The position of choice is supine recumbency; if the patient is in some other position it should be noted on the record, inasmuch as position of body and of diaphragm may greatly alter the electrocardiogram. Sufficient time should be given to allow the patient to recover from the effects of exercise. Fear or anxiety may cause electrocardiographic changes, because of increase in the work of the heart, respiratory alkalosis, and nervous or hormonal influences. Some of the variables cannot be controlled, but should be noted. These include the age and sex of the patient, body build, peculiarities of chest and thorax, excessive fat or breast tissue.

In taking the electrocardiogram a standardization deflection should be introduced in every lead. If the voltage of QRS is great, the sensitivity may be reduced by one half. Care should be taken in developing, labeling, mounting and filing the records, and the services of an alert, experienced technician are invaluable.

Interpretation Routine

In examining an electrocardiogram it is helpful to follow some sort of routine procedure. The following points have proved of benefit in our experience:

1. It is essential to determine first which leads are present, and whether they have been correctly taken, labeled and mounted.

2. The calibration,* which should always be recorded, is then observed in order to ascertain that a deflection of 1 cm. was obtained when 1 millivolt was introduced into the circuit.

3. Any artifacts present should be noted; oscillations due to contractions of skeletal muscle and interfering extraneous currents are the commonest types of artifacts.

4. The fundamental ventricular rhythm and rate are then determined, together with the relationship between atrial and ventricular rhythms. Any arrhythmia should be specifically named.

5. The form, amplitude and duration of the P waves are determined.

6. The P–R interval is measured.

* The word "standardization" is often used instead of calibration.

7. The amplitude, form, electrical axis and duration of the QRS complexes are observed.

8. The form and displacement of the RS–T segments are determined.

9. The form, amplitude and electrical axis of the T waves are determined.

10. The duration of systole, as indicated by the Q–T duration, can be quickly estimated, but should be measured accurately if obviously abnormal, and corrected for differences in heart rate.

11. The relationship between the electrical axis of QRS and T should be determined.

12. Finally, the examiner is ready to consider side by side the electrocardiographic and the other clinical findings. The latter should of course be used as an aid in interpreting the electrocardiogram, as well as in coordination with the electrocardiographic findings for the final evaluation of the cardiovascular status.

PART III

The Typical Normal Electrocardiogram and Its Variations

This part is divided into five short chapters. The first deals with the electrical orientation of the heart; the next two are devoted to a discussion of the electrocardiographic variations observed in records obtained from healthy persons at rest; the fourth contains a description of electrocardiographic variations due to certain physiologic factors; and the fifth consists of a brief discussion of artifacts and technical errors.

CHAPTER 4

Electrical Orientation of the Heart

In this chapter electrocardiography will be discussed from the standpoint of the cardiac electrical field. Procedures for estimating the mean frontal plane vector, that is, the "electrical axis" of the electrocardiogram, and the mean spatial vector will be presented, and illustrations will be given of the use of these derived data in electrocardiographic interpretation. This presentation will also serve as a basis for pointing out certain relationships among the several electrocardiographic leads.

Electromotive Force of the Heart

In Part II the electrophysical principles underlying the electromotive force generated by the heart were discussed. For our purpose now it is sufficient to point out that the cardiac electrical field may be represented by a vector which has magnitude, direction and sense. The length is proportional to the electromotive force of the heart, the direction indicates the orientation of the electrical field, and the head of the vector points away from the negative and toward the positive half of the field. A plane separating the two halves of the field has zero potential and is called the transitional zone. The vector representing the cardiac electrical field at any instant is termed "the instantaneous cardiac vector." The length and direction of the instantaneous vectors vary throughout the cardiac cycle and traverse a complex pathway through space. If their heads are connected by a line, it will

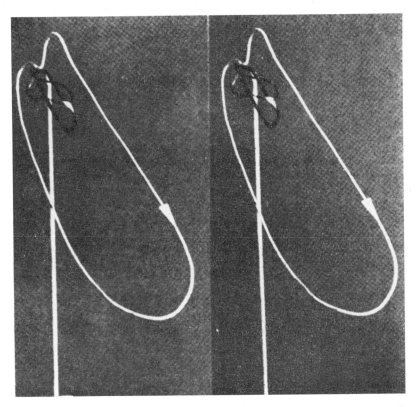

Fig. 18. Stereoscopic photographs of a wire model representing a typically normal vectorcardiogram. Stereoscopic effects may be obtained by placing a card between the two pictures. The *QRS* loop is in white.
(We are grateful for permission to reproduce this figure from an article entitled "Observations on the Spatial Vectorcardiogram in Man" by J. P. Conway, J. A. Cronvich and G. E. Burch in Am. Heart J., *38:* 537, 1949.)

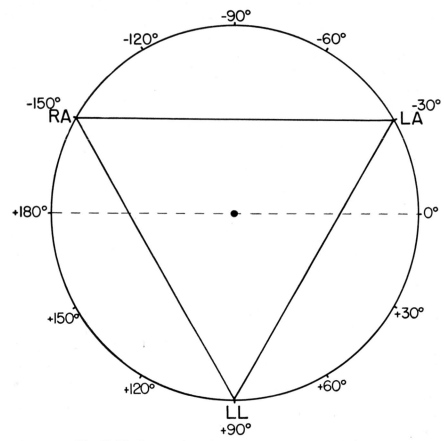

Fig. 19. Einthoven triangular reference system. See text.

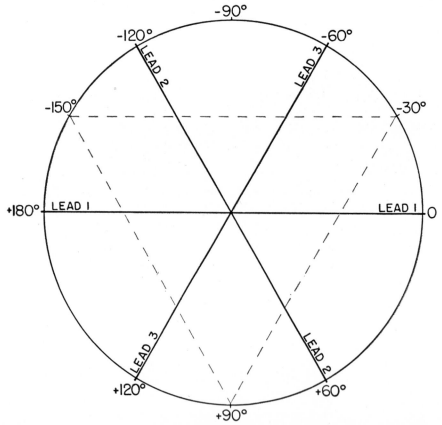

Fig. 20. Bailey's triaxial reference system superimposed on the Einthoven triangle. See text.

describe a series of "loops." These loops are called vectorcardiograms, and *P, QRS* and *T* loops are distinguishable (Fig. 18). ·

Unfortunately, at the present time, vectorcardiography is not a practical procedure for clinical use. However, it is possible from simple inspection of the usual electrocardiographic

and that all points are in a frontal plane bisecting the body. He further assumed that the body tissues act as a uniform volume conductor and that the electrical potential is distributed according to well known laws.

Einthoven devised the familiar triangular reference system (Fig. 19). The apices of the

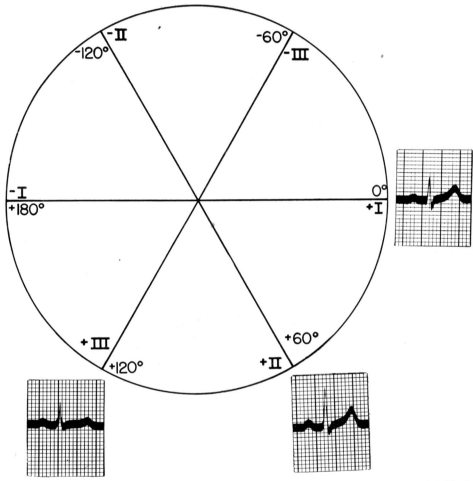

Fig. 21. The three bipolar limb lead electrocardiograms in their proper relation to the electrical field of the heart in the frontal plane. See text.

leads to make rough but worthwhile approximations of the changes in orientation of the cardiac electrical field throughout the heart cycle. For reasons which will soon be made clear these estimations are more reliable when limited to orientation in the frontal plane than for orientation in space.

Orientation in the Frontal Plane

This is based on Einthoven's hypothesis. He assumed that the heart is a point source of electromotive force located in the center of the body; that the three extremity lead points are equidistant from the heart and from each other;

triangle indicate the three lead points, the two arms and the left leg. The point in the center of the triangle represents a dipole which is the source of the cardiac electromotive force. The triangle is surrounded by a circle with a horizontal line forming a convenient diameter. By convention the intersection of the circle on the right side is designated 0 degrees, and on the left, 180. Degrees in the upper half are assigned negative and those in the lower half positive values.

A modification of the triangular reference system suggested by Bailey is more convenient for our use and is termed the triaxial reference system. In Figure 20 the two systems are super-imposed. It will be noted that both the direction of the lead axes and the angles between them remain the same. In Figure 21 the three bipolar limb lead electrocardiograms are shown in their proper position within this reference system. The asymmetry is due to the fact that the polarity is reversed in obtaining Lead 2 (+ 60 degrees); otherwise it would appear "inverted" at the opposite end of this axis (− 120 degrees). Einthoven made this change in order to deal with upright waves in Lead 2. It may be pointed out in passing that if this were done in the case of aV_F the curve would be more readily interpretable and the limb leads more meaningful.

The unipolar limb leads obtained by the use of Wilson's central terminal method are in reality bipolar leads, the axes represented by the medians in Einthoven's triangle (Fig. 22). The lead axis in each case lies between the dipole in the center of the heart and the point of application of the electrode. The unipolar limb leads differ from the bipolar leads in only two respects. First, the axes of the unipolar leads lie *between* the bipolar lead axes. Second, they differ in magnitude; this is indicated by the respective differences in length of the median and the side of the Einthoven triangle. However, augmented unipolar limb leads differ only slightly (−14 per cent) in magnitude from the bipolar limb leads. A triaxial system based on the unipolar limb lead axes is shown in Figure 23, with *augmented* unipolar limb leads properly placed in this reference system. The leads are symmetrically located around the field. If Einthoven's argument in regard to reversing the polarity of Lead 2 were followed, the polarity would be reversed in obtaining aV_R (−150 degrees) and a curve with upright waves would be placed at + 30 degrees.

In Figure 24 the two triaxial systems are superimposed to form the useful hexaxial system suggested by Sodi Pallares. The bipolar and unipolar limb leads do not bear the same proportionality to the electromotive force of the heart which is declared by the slightly smaller (14 per cent) amplitude of the augmented unipolar leads. This difference, however, does not influence the form of the curve. Hence all six leads are similar in that the form of the curve is determined by their relation to the cardiac electrical field.

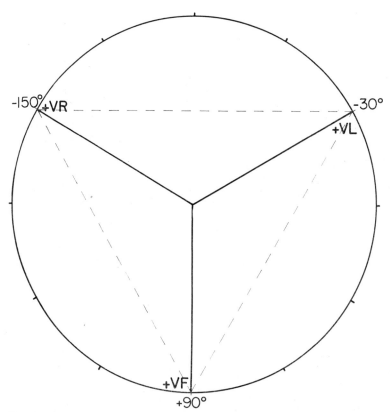

Fig. 22. The "unipolar" limb lead axes shown in relation to Einthoven's triangle. See text.

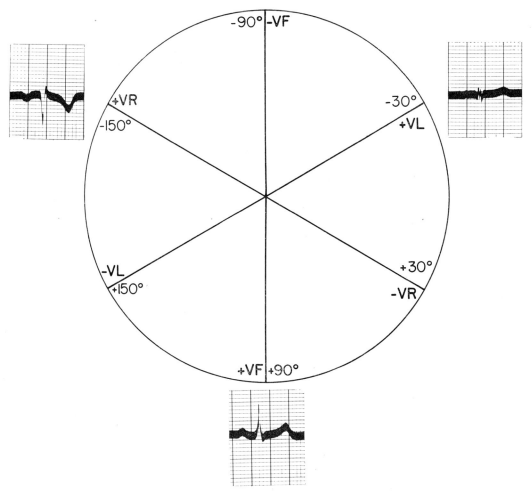

Fig. 23. The augmented unipolar limb leads shown in their proper relation to the electrical field of the heart in the frontal plane. See text.

If the polarity is reversed in taking the limb leads, six additional curves are obtained which complete the pattern around the cardiac electrical field in the frontal plane (Fig. 25). Note the steplike transitions in form of *P, QRS* and *T* around the field.

This presentation is helpful in several respects. First, it demonstrates the relationship between the augmented unipolar and the bipolar limb leads; second, it provides a means for illustrating a simple procedure for the estimation of *P, QRS* and *T* vectors; and third, this arrangement of the leads helps in visualizing the changing orientation of the electrical field in the frontal plane within a fixed reference system.

Relationship between the Bipolar and Augmented Unipolar Limb Leads

It is customary, at this time, to regard these two sets of leads as being fundamentally different in nature. This is declared by the different criteria used in their interpretation and also by the fact that some electrocardiographers regard one set as being superior to the other. Actually, they represent slightly different "views" of the cardiac electrical field in the frontal plane. They may and should be interpreted together.

Electrical Axis of the Electrocardiogram

The mean vectors or electrical axes of *P, QRS* and *T* can be determined from a consideration of their *areas* in two limb leads, using either a formula devised for this purpose or geometrical projection. This is time-consuming and needlessly exact for clinical use. The magnitude and direction of the electrical axis of *P, QRS* and *T* in the frontal plane can also be obtained by referring to tables compiled by Jackson and Windsor.*

* Jackson, C. E. and Windsor, T.: Aids for Determining Magnitude and Direction of Electric Axes of the Electrocardiogram. *Circulation*, 2: 975, 1950.

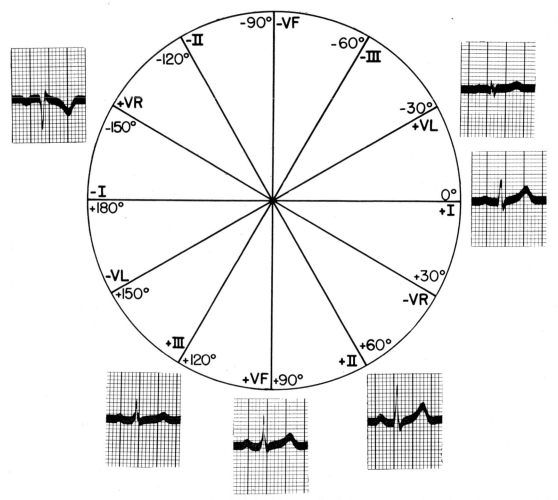

Fig. 24. The bipolar and augmented unipolar limb leads shown in their proper relationship to the electrical field of the heart in the frontal plane. Here the two triaxial reference systems have been superimposed to form the hexaxial reference system. See text.

Magnitude of the Electrical Axis

Both the magnitude and direction of the electrical axis can be readily estimated by *simple inspection* of the limb leads. The magnitude can be estimated for *P*, *QRS* or *T*, using Leads 1 and 3. If a wave has the *same sign* in both Leads 1 and 3, the magnitude is equal to their sum; in other words, it is equal to the amplitude* of that wave in Lead 2. If a wave is of *opposite sign* in Leads 1 and 3, the magnitude is equal to, or approximately equal to, the amplitude of the wave with the greater value. For example, in the electrocardiogram shown in Figure 26 the net value of *QRS* is +5 in Lead 1 and +2 in Lead 3. Inasmuch as *QRS* is of the same sign in Leads 1 and 3, the magnitude is approximately 7 (the net value in Lead 2). In the same

* Actually, net amplitude: this is determined by subtracting the sum of the amplitude of *Q* and *S* from the amplitude of *R*.

electrocardiogram the amplitude of *T* is $+2\frac{1}{2}$ in Lead 1 and $+1\frac{1}{2}$ in Lead 3. Inasmuch as *T* has the same sign in Leads 1 and 3, the magnitude of the vector is +4, or the amplitude of *T* in Lead 2.

In electrocardiograms obtained from healthy persons the magnitude of the *QRS* axis varies from about 0.4 to 2.5 millivolts. A small value merely indicates that the major component of the mean spatial vector does not lie in the frontal plane. In these instances the direction of the electrical axis does not have its usual significance because it does not indicate the principal electrical orientation of the heart.

Direction of the Electrical Axis

A simple method for estimating the *direction* of the electrical axis is based on two facts directly related to each other: namely, that the electrical axis of a wave *lies* 90 degrees away

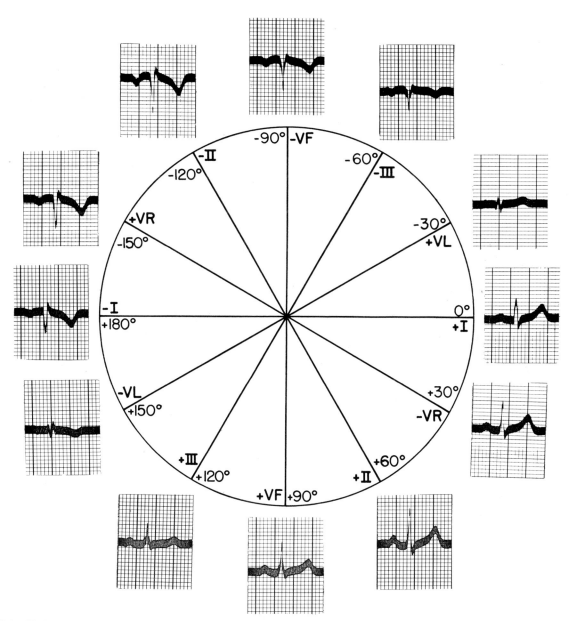

Fig. 25. The bipolar and augmented unipolar limb leads in their proper relationship to the entire electrical field of the heart in the frontal plane. In addition to the standard limb leads, six additional leads were obtained by reversing the polarity of the connections between patient and galvanometer. See text.

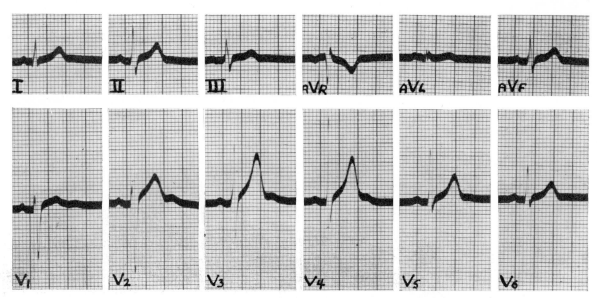

Fig. 26. Normal electrocardiogram. See text.

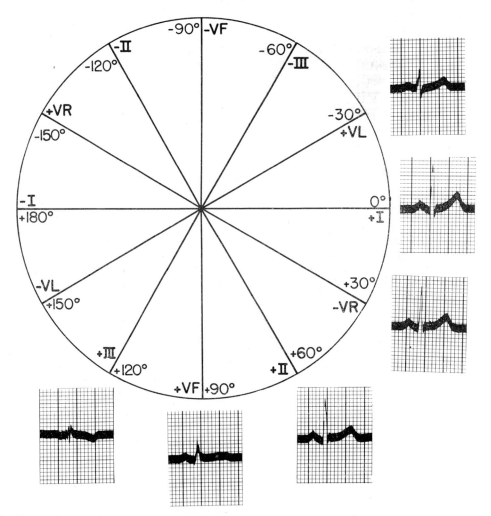

Fig. 27. The bipolar limb leads and the augmented unipolar limb leads (aV_R obtained with polarity reversed) properly arranged in relation to the cardiac electrical field in the frontal plane.

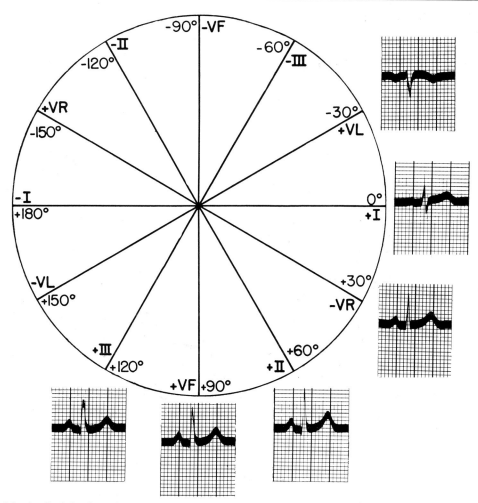

Fig. 28. The bipolar limb leads and the augmented unipolar limb leads (aV_R obtained with polarity reversed) **properly arranged in relation to the cardiac electrical field in the frontal plane.**

from the point where that wave has a transitional form* and *points* in the direction in which this wave is positive. For example, in Figure 25 a transitional QRS complex is found in Lead aV$_L$ (−30 degrees). The electrical axis of QRS must lie 90 degrees away from this point in the direction in which this wave is positive, namely, Lead 2 (+60 degrees). This corresponds with the fact that the maximal upright QRS deflection is seen in this lead. Locating the transitional T wave or point where it would be found is even easier than in the case of QRS because the T waves are usually monophasic. Thus in Figure 25 the transitional point must lie between aV$_L$ (−30 degrees) and Lead 3 ↓ †

---

* A transitional complex is one with a net amplitude of zero and defines a point on the line which divides the mean vector representing the electrical field into positive and negative halves.

† The arrow ↓ indicates that the usual polarity was reversed in obtaining the curve.

(−60 degrees), or approximately at −45 degrees. The electrical axis of T must point toward +45 degrees as indicated by the arrow in the figure. The P wave is nearly isoelectric in Lead aV$_L$ (−30 degrees); hence the electrical axis must point toward +60 degrees, or in the direction of Lead 2.

The electrocardiogram in Figure 27 has been arranged in proper order from above downward to depict the changes around the electrical field from −30 degrees to +120 degrees. To do this it was necessary to reverse the polarity in obtaining aV$_R$. A transitional QRS complex is seen in Lead 3 (+120 degrees); hence the electrical axis must point toward +30 degrees of Lead aV$_R$ ↓ with polarity reversed. The transitional point for the T wave must lie near Lead aV$_F$ (+90 degrees); hence the electrical axis points toward Lead 1 (0 degrees).

Another example is shown in Figure 28. A transitional QRS complex is seen in Lead 1

(0 degrees); hence the electrical axis must point toward aV_F (+90 degrees). The transitional point for the T wave must lie between aV_L (−30 degrees) and Lead 1 (0 degrees), at approximately −20 degrees; hence the electrical axis of the T must lie at about +50 degrees. The transitional point for P lies at about −10 degrees; hence the axis points toward +80 degrees. Usually a perfectly transitional complex is not observed in any lead, particularly if only three leads are available. It is often necessary to extrapolate, but this is easily done if six leads are available.

Relationship of the Electrical Axis of QRS to the Anatomic Axis of the Heart

Anatomically, the heart may be considered from different points of view. It is usually visualized as a space-filling organ with definite relationships to the thorax and to the various contiguous structures in the chest. Its position may be defined by a longitudinal axis running from base to apex through the center of the heart, and by coordinate axes in the other two planes in space.

The electrocardiographer in regarding the heart as a generator of electrical force must think in terms of the spread of the depolarization and repolarization processes throughout the muscle mass. The general direction taken by the depolarization process in the ventricles, i.e., the direction of the QRS axis, is determined by the specialized conduction tissue and the location of the main muscle mass. In the adult the "center of gravity" of the heart is considerably to the left of the geometrical center, slightly lower down, and posteriorly. Thus the electrical axis of QRS indicates the anatomic orientation of the main muscle mass of the heart in the frontal plane. If the magnitude of QRS is small, it may indicate that the orientation of the main muscle mass lies in other than the frontal plane. In such instances the QRS in the frontal plane does not have much significance.

The depolarization process in the ventricles is not readily affected except in the presence of conduction defects or after severe damage to the muscle cells. However, the heart is, within limits, free to rotate, and the changing relation of the cardiac electrical field within the reference system produces changes in QRS. The change in position of the heart is thus declared by a shift in the electrical axis of QRS. Consequently the electrical axis of QRS, although relatively stable for a given heart position, readily shifts with a change in heart position.

Repolarization, in contrast to depolarization, is easily affected by many physiologic factors, drugs, toxemia and disease. Hence the T waves and the electrical axis of T shift readily, for many reasons other than a change in heart position. Thus, if the electrical axes of QRS and T shift together, it may be due to shift in position of the heart; but if T shifts alone, it is due to some factor other than change in position of the heart. QRS is to be regarded as the stable reference and T as the variable factor. There will be reference to the importance of this fact in the discussions to follow.

The electrical axis of T usually points in the same general direction as the QRS axis, but there are exceptions to this. The difference in direction is readily expressed by the angle formed between them. This angle is a function of the ventricular gradient, which will now be discussed.

Ventricular Gradient

It might be reasoned that upon stimulation of the ventricular musculature the cells which were the first to be involved in the depolarization process would be the first to regain their charge during repolarization, in which case the T vector representing the electromotive forces of repolarization would be equal to but opposite the QRS vector representing depolarization. However, for reasons which are not fully understood, such is not the case. Indeed, it has been seen that in the electrocardiograms obtained from healthy persons the QRS and T waves tend to have a similar direction. This can only mean that the cells which were among the first to be stimulated are among the last to regain their charge. This disturbance in the time-course of repolarization is termed the ventricular gradient and can be expressed by a vector which represents the *difference* between the actual T vector and a hypothetical T vector which is equal to but opposite the QRS vector.

It follows that the same quantitative relationship is expressed by a vector which is the *resultant* of the T and QRS vectors, inasmuch as the QRS vector is equal to but opposite the hypothetical T vector. Thus the ventricular gradient can be determined for the frontal plane from the measurements of the mean QRS and T vectors in this plane and, in space,

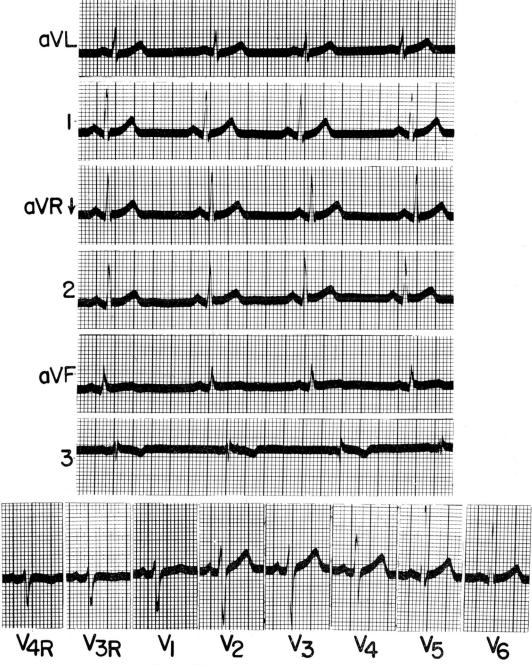

Fig. 29. Normal electrocardiogram. See text.

from the measurement of the mean spatial *QRS* and *T* vectors.

The determination of the ventricular gradient by this method is impractical for clinical purposes, but it is relatively easy to estimate the angle between *QRS* and *T* vectors. The magnitude of this angle is a function of the ventricular gradient; it is obvious that the smaller the angle, the greater the gradient.

Ordinarily the angle between the electrical axis of *QRS* and *T* in the frontal plane is 50 degrees or less. So long as this angle remains small, relative differences in magnitude of *QRS* and *T* are unlikely to be due to pathologic causes. If the angle is large, the reasons for it should be found if possible. One cause for a large angle is the fact that only a small component of the electromotive force is recorded in the frontal plane. This is a good possibility when the voltage of *QRS* or *T* is small in the

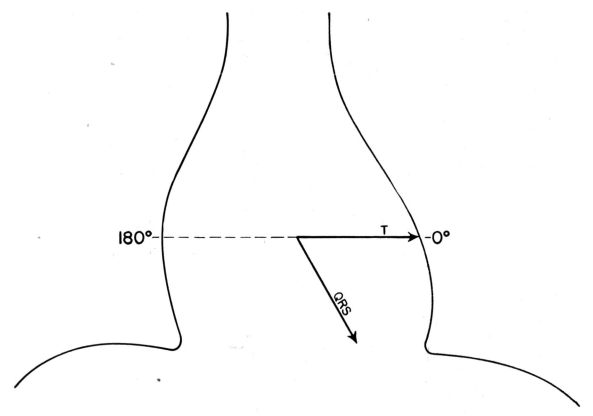

Fig. 30. The direction of *QRS* and *T* axes of the electrocardiogram in Figure 29 shown in relation to the frontal plane.

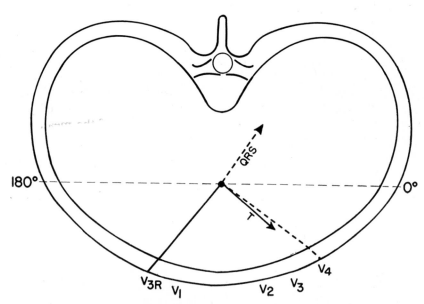

Fig. 31. The direction of *QRS* and *T* axes of the electrocardiogram in Figure 29 shown in relation to the transverse plane.

limb leads; in this case it is necessary to estimate the angle between the *spatial QRS* and *T* vectors.

Mean Spatial Vectors

The approximate *direction* of the mean spatial vector of either *QRS* or *T* can be readily determined by using Grant's method. In the case

must lie at right angles to this, as shown in Figure 31. A transitional *T* wave is seen in V_{3R}, and the electrical axis must lie at right angles.

The direction of the mean spatial *QRS* vector may be visualized as a backward displacement of the mean vector in the frontal plane until it coincides with the mean *QRS* vector in the

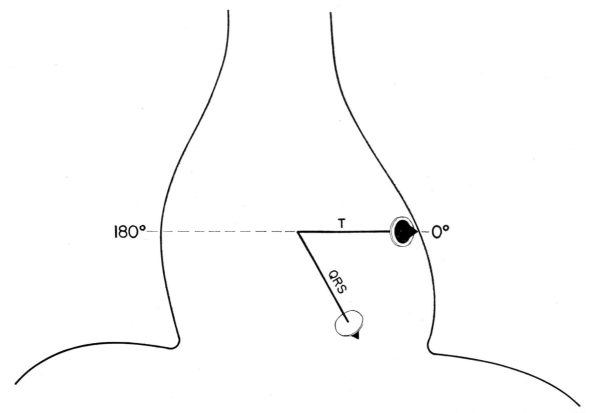

Fig. 32. The direction of *QRS* and *T* axes of the electrocardiogram in Figure 29 shown in their spatial relationship.

of *QRS* the procedure is as follows: first, estimate the direction of the mean *QRS* vector in the frontal plane; second, determine the axis of the V lead on the chest with the transitional *QRS* complex (this is simply an imaginary line running from the electrode to the center of the heart). The mean spatial vector must lie at *right angles* to this axis, thus defining its position in the horizontal plane. This procedure may be illustrated as follows: in the limb leads shown in Figure 29 a transitional *QRS* complex is seen in Lead 3; hence the electrical axis points to +60 degrees (Fig. 30). The transitional point for the *T* wave is approximately +90 degrees; hence the electrical axis points toward 0 degrees.

In the precordial leads a transitional *QRS* complex is seen in V_4; hence the electrical axis

transverse plane (Fig. 32). The mean spatial *T* vector may be visualized as a slight forward displacement of the mean vector in the frontal plane until it coincides with the mean vector in the transverse plane.

The same procedure is followed in determining the direction of the mean spatial vector of *P*.

To overcome the difficulties in recording the direction of the mean spatial vectors, it is only necessary to indicate the angle or electrical axis in the frontal plane and note the V lead containing the transitional complex: thus, *QRS* +65 degrees, V_4; *T* −10 degrees, V_2.

It is important to emphasize that this procedure gives only an approximation of the direction of the mean spatial vectors. Also, the procedure is based on assumptions not all of which are universally accepted as valid. Furthermore, the magnitude of the mean spatial vector cannot be calculated because of the difference in scale of the precordial leads, which are near the heart, and the limb leads, which are remote.

This is, nevertheless, a valuable procedure and an important forward step in the direction which clinical electrocardiography is certain to take in the future. With practice this procedure can be carried out in the absence of any visual aid and without referring to any tables or figures.

CHAPTER 5

Chest and Esophageal Leads

Unipolar Chest Leads

The procedure to be followed in obtaining chest leads is described in Chapter 3. Each lead records the potential variations at the point where the exploring electrode comes in contact with the chest wall. The form of the curve is determined by (1) the electrical forces generated by the heart, (2) the lead axis, (3) the distance between the heart and the electrode, and (4) the size of the electrode. Precordial Leads V_1 through V_6 should always be obtained. Additional lead points should also be used if, for any reason, it is desirable to extend the "electrocardiographic coverage" of the heart. The chest leads are very important, and later it will be shown how they aid in the detection of infarcts or areas of injury and in the diagnosis of bundle branch block and ventricular hypertrophy.

Over the precordium the heart is in close proximity to the chest wall. Indeed, the electrode is so close to the heart that Wilson and his followers believe that the resulting curve is similar to the curve which would be obtained if the electrode were placed directly on the subjacent portion of the ventricle. For this reason they term precordial leads "*semidirect leads*" and interpret them in the light of the results of experiments on dogs in which precordial and direct leads were compared. In a *direct lead* the form of QRS is explained by Wilson and his associates[*] as follows:

When the excitatory process reaches the muscle in contact with an epicardial electrode, the boundary between resting and active muscle disappears from that part of the ventricular wall upon which the electrode rests. The potential of the electrode then becomes the potential of the adjacent part of the ventricular cavity. The sudden drop in the potential of the electrode when the electromotive force across the wall beneath it disappears is responsible for the intrinsic deflection. The total length of this deflection (the downward deflection beginning with the peak of R) is an approximate measure of the voltage across the ventricular wall when the cardiac

[*] Wilson F. N. et al.: The Precordial Electrocardiogram. Am. Heart J., *27:* 19, 1944.

impulse arrives at the epicardial surface. If the excitatory process is still spreading through some part of the ventricular wall when the intrinsic deflection occurs the negativity of the ventricular cavity outlasts this deflection and an S wave is inscribed. If the subendocardial muscle of some part of the ventricular wall passes into the active state earlier than the subendocardial muscle which lies between the exploring electrode and the ventricular cavity, the initial negativity of the cavity is transmitted to this electrode and a Q deflection occurs.

In *precordial leads*, Wilson termed the deflection caused by the arrival of the excitation wave the "*intrinsicoid deflection*." The peak of R or R', which marks the arrival of the excitation wave on the surface of the ventricle beneath the electrode, was used as a means of mapping the order of excitation of different portions of the heart.[*] Thus it was found that the epicardium over the right ventricle is activated earlier than the epicardium over the relatively thicker left ventricular wall. It was obvious that the temporal position of R in the QRS complex was a chief determinant of its form. If R occurred early, it was usually rather small and was followed by a prominent S wave. If R was late, it was usually prominent and might be preceded by a Q wave and followed by a small S wave.

In using Wilson's central terminal method, the axis of the precordial lead may be regarded as lying between the dipole representing the center of the heart and the point of application of the electrode, just as in the case of the unipolar limb leads. A curve obtained from the diametrically opposite point on the body should have the same contour, though smaller amplitude because of the greater distance from the heart. In practice the general characteristics of these two curves are the same, but they may differ in detail, indicating that the precordial electrodes are not "satisfactorily remote" from

[*] Wilson and Sodi Pallares now think that the apex of the R wave does not mark the exact time of arrival of the depolarizing process at the epicardial surface in semidirect leads. Nevertheless the concept is still a useful one.

all parts of the heart. The vectorial point of view* has already been considered in Chapter 4 (p. 31). This viewpoint differs from Wilson's in that it regards the main features of the precordial electrocardiogram as representing simply the potential variations of a particular component of the entire electrical field and ascribes only a minor role to the effect of local influences occurring in the subjacent ventricular wall.

Normal Precordial "V" Leads

Typical changes in the form of the curve as the electrode is moved from right to left across the chest are shown in Figure 33. The P waves

LEAD V_1. P may be upright, diphasic (Fig. 34, D) and occasionally inverted. A Q wave is not seen normally, but the initial ventricular deflection may consist of a QS wave (Fig. 34, A). The R wave is usually small, but may be 10 mm. or more tall. Occasionally rsr' is seen (Fig. 34, D). The S wave is usually prominent and may be over 20 mm. in amplitude. The T wave may be upright, diphasic or inverted.

LEAD V_2. P is upright with a few exceptions, when it is diphasic (Fig. 34, D). Q is not observed. Rarely, R is absent and the entire complex consists of QS. An rsr' complex may be seen (Fig. 34, D). The R wave is usually tall

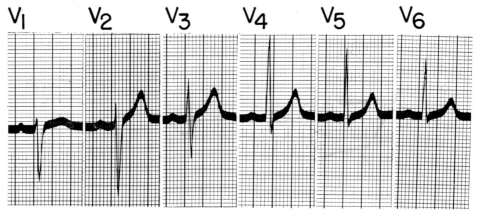

Fig. 33. Typical normal precordial leads.

are low but upright in all leads. The QRS† complex in Lead V_1 consists of a small R and prominent S wave, whereas the reciprocal is true in Lead V_6. Progressive changes between these extremes are shown in Leads V_2 through V_5. A transitional QRS complex is seen in Lead V_3. The RS–T junctions are characteristically elevated in Leads V_2 through V_4. The T waves are upright in all leads, and the waxing and waning of T in proceeding from the right to the left is typical.

Some of the variations encountered in the six precordial leads are illustrated in Figures 34 and 35. These electrocardiograms were obtained from young healthy persons.

* Duchosal, P. W., and Sulzer, R.: *Vectocardiographie*. Basle, Switzerland, Karger, 1949; Grant, R. P., and Estes, E. H.: *The Interpretation of the Electrocardiogram by Vector Methods*. Emory University, 1949.

† It is convenient to use small and capital letters to indicate the relative size of Q, R and S deflections; thus qRs would describe a complex consisting of a prominent R wave preceded by a small Q and followed by a small S wave.

and may be over 20 mm. in amplitude. S is usually greater in amplitude than R, and the range is from 3 to over 30 mm. T is usually upright, but may be inverted (Fig. 35, E), especially in children.

LEAD V_3. The P wave is usually upright. An R wave is always present and may vary from 1 to 30 mm. in amplitude. A tall R wave may be preceded by a small Q wave and is usually followed by an S wave. A transitional QRS pattern is frequently seen. T is usually upright and often very tall (Fig. 35, B), but may be inverted (Fig. 35, E), especially in women and children.

LEAD V_4. The P wave is always upright. The R wave is usually tall, may be preceded by a Q wave, and is nearly always followed by a prominent S wave. A transitional QRS pattern is frequently seen (Fig. 34, A). The T wave is usually tall, but rarely it may be low, diphasic (Fig. 35, F) or even inverted.*

* In children and young adults the T waves in precordial Leads V_4 and V_5 may be inverted; the cause is unknown.

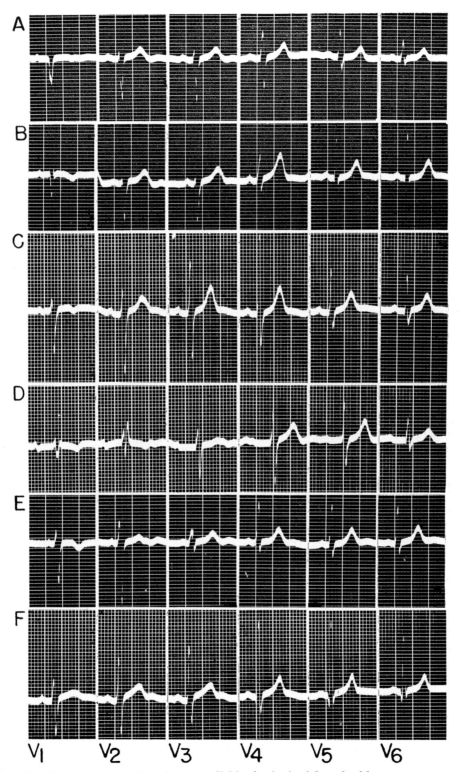

Fig. 34. Normal variations in precordial leads obtained from healthy young persons.

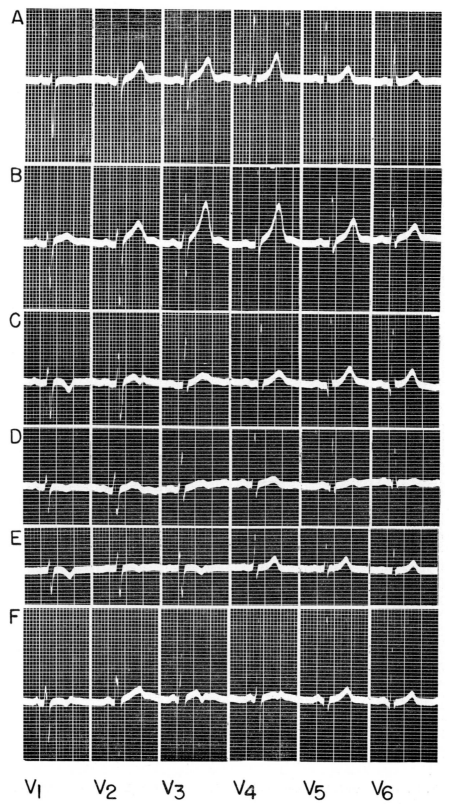

Fig. 35. Normal variations in precordial leads obtained from healthy young persons.

LEAD V₅. The *P* waves are nearly always upright. The *R* wave is usually tall and may be tallest in this lead. Sometimes it comprises the entire *QRS* complex (Fig. 35, *A*), but frequently it is preceded by a small *Q* and followed by an *S* wave which may be nearly as large as the *R* wave (Fig. 34, *D*). Lead V₅ sometimes resembles Leads 1, 2, or aV_F.

LEAD V₆. This lead usually resembles Lead V₅, but the amplitude of the waves is smaller, partly because the distance from the heart is greater. The *P* wave is never inverted. The *R*

as shown in Lead V₃ in Figure 34, *E*. Low voltage of *QRS* is present if the sum of *R* and *S* is less than 5 mm. in V₁, 7 mm. in V₂, 9 mm. in V₃ or V₄, 7 mm. in V₅ and 5 mm. in V₆. Low voltage may normally be present in some of the leads, but not in all.

The *RS–T* junctions are often displaced upward, but rarely more than 2 mm.; they are seldom displaced below the isoelectric level, and then only a little below. The *RS–T* segments are usually short in duration and may be indistinguishable from the *T* wave.

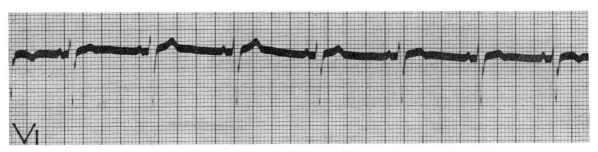

Fig. 36. Variations in the *T* waves associated with respiration in precordial Lead V₁.

wave has the greatest amplitude of the *Q*, *R* and *S* waves, but the duration of *S* may be greater than that of *R* (Fig. 34, *C*). The *Q* waves are never prominent. The *T* waves are nearly always upright, but rarely they are diphasic and, very rarely, inverted. Lead V₆ may resemble Leads 1, 2 or aV_F.

GENERAL REMARKS. The six precordial lead positions usually fall on both sides of the transitional zone which separates the negative and positive portions of the cardiac electrical field. Thus the chief *QRS* deflection is downwardly directed on the right side, upwardly directed on the left, and transitional in character at some point in between. Sometimes, particularly in children, a transitional *QRS* complex is seen in V₁ and it is necessary to obtain a curve from position V₃R or V₄R in order to obtain a *QRS* complex with the chief deflection downward. It is important to appreciate that the transitional zone may tend to be directed rather vertically or horizontally. In the former instance it is passed quite quickly, as shown in Figure 34, *B*; observe the small increase in *R* in V₁ through V₃ and the sudden change to a tall *R* in V₄. In contrast to this, when the transitional zone is rather horizontal, there is a gradual change in *QRS* as shown in Figure 34, *C*. *QRS* may be low in voltage at the transitional zone,

The transitional zone for the *T* wave may lie to the right of the V₁ position, in which case *T* in that lead is upright. Ordinarily a transitional *T* wave is found to the right of the transitional *QRS* complex. Either the *QRS* or the *T* wave (Fig. 36) may change with respiration in leads from over the transitional zone.

It is necessary for the electrocardiographer to become familiar with the form of the curves from positions around the entire thorax. These are illustrated in Figure 37. The individual variation is great except in regard to the general features. The amplitude of the waves falls off rapidly as the electrode is moved away from the heart. Curves obtained from the right and left shoulder region tend to resemble respectively aV_R and aV_L. Note that *rsr'* or *rsr's'* complexes may be obtained just above and to the left of the V₁ position.

Esophageal Leads

Multiple esophageal electrocardiograms are shown in Figure 38. A good "landmark" is the spiked *P* wave in Lead EV_a, indicating that the electrode is near the atrium. Above this level the *P* waves gradually become inverted, and below this level they become upright. At or near the level of EV_a the *QRS* complex has a transitional form *QR*, while above this level

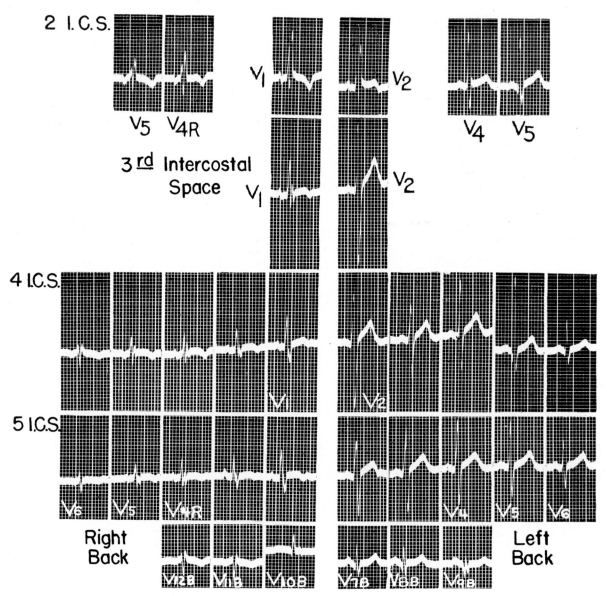

Fig. 37. Multiple chest leads obtained from a young healthy person. See text.

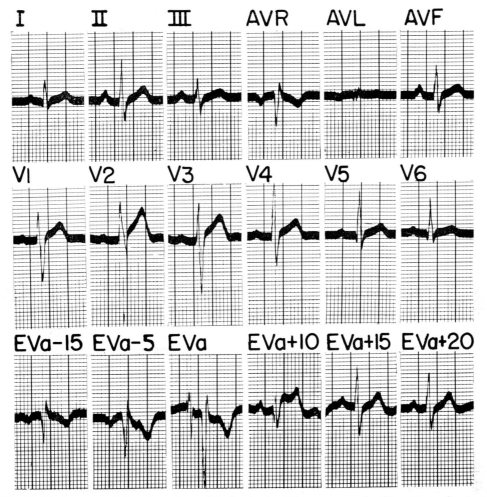

Fig. 38. Limb, precordial and esophageal leads obtained from a young healthy person. See text.

the chief QRS deflection is down (QR, sometimes QS) and below this level the chief deflection is upright. The T waves are usually inverted at the EV_a level and above, but become upright at lower levels. Although considerable individual variation is present, the general characteristics are the same: namely, that in multiple esophageal leads the deflections above the transitional zone for P, QRS and T are inverted, and below it they are upright.

CHAPTER 6

Limb Leads

Augmented Unipolar Limb Leads

A typical augmented unipolar limb lead electrocardiogram is shown in Figure 39. Strictly

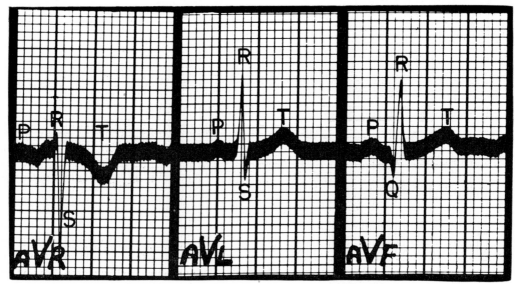

Fig. 39. Normal augmented unipolar limb leads.

speaking, these are bipolar leads, but inasmuch as the potential variations at the central connection are zero, they are commonly referred to as unipolar leads, which has the advantage of distinguishing them from the classical or bipolar limb lead electrocardiogram. Both the unipolar and the bipolar limb leads provide the same kind of information with respect to the electrical field of the heart. They differ in that they do not bear the same proportionality to the electrical force of the heart, and in the direction of the lead axes. The relationships between the bipolar and unipolar limb leads, and in turn their relationships to the electrical field of the heart, were discussed in detail in Chapter 4.

It is necessary at this point to make clear our position with regard to the use of bipolar and augmented unipolar limb leads. In many respects they have common advantages, and one is merely a substitute for the other. However,

each has its own advantages and serves to complement the other. Both should be taken routinely, but if this is not feasible, then preference should be given the bipolar limb leads because of our greater familiarity with them and because the unipolar leads as conventionally taken are more difficult to interpret. We have adhered to the custom of obtaining aV_R with waves inverted and of considering separately the findings in the bipolar and augmented unipolar limb leads. The reader should refer to Chapter 4 (p. 35) for a full discussion of the relationships between the so-called bipolar and augmented unipolar limb leads.

The general characteristics of the augmented unipolar limb leads are shown in Figures 40 and 41. The chief components in aV_R are downwardly directed; in aV_L they are transitional; and in aV_F they are usually upright. Normally the QRS complex is 0.1 second or less in duration and varies greatly in form and amplitude in the three leads. There may be low voltage of QRS in any one lead (Fig. 40, A), but the voltage should be greater than 4 mm. in at least one lead. The *RS–T* junction may begin as much as 1 mm. above or 0.5 mm. below the baseline normally. The *T* wave may vary a great deal in amplitude, but is usually in the same direction as the chief initial ventricular deflection.

RIGHT ARM LEAD. The chief components in this lead are nearly always downwardly directed, because the axis of this lead usually lies in the

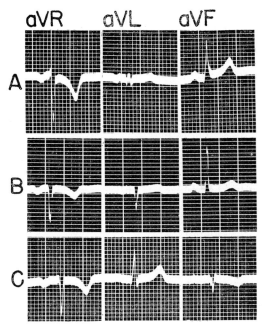

Fig. 40. Normal variations in augmented unipolar limb leads obtained from young healthy persons.

negative half of the cardiac electrical field. The waves are as a rule of considerable amplitude, because the lead axis corresponds fairly closely to the mean pathways taken by the depolarization and repolarization processes. The *P* wave is always inverted. The *QRS* complex usually consists of a small *R* and prominent *S* wave, but may consist of *QS* (Fig. 40 *B*), *rSr'* (Fig. 40, *C*) or *QR* (Fig. 41, *B*). The *RS–T* junction is frequently displaced slightly downward and rarely slightly upward. The *T* waves are always inverted.

LEFT ARM LEAD. The axis of this lead usually lies near the transition between the negative and positive halves of the electrical field; hence the waves may be upright, inverted or biphasic. The *P* waves are inverted in Figure 40, *A*, nearly isoelectric in Figure 41, *A*, and upright in Figure 41, *C*. The *QRS* complex may be nearly isoelectric (Fig. 40, *A*) or consist of *QS, RS,*

rS or *qR* (Figs. 40, 41). *Q* waves are frequently seen when the voltage is low. When the voltage of *R* is greater than 5 mm., a *Q* wave may also be present (Fig. 41, *C*) but it is normally less than one quarter the amplitude of *R* and less than 0.04 second in duration. *R* waves may be tall, especially if the heart lies horizontally, but abnormally high voltage is associated with left

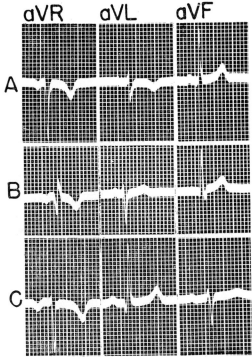

Fig. 41. Normal variations in augmented unipolar limb leads obtained from young healthy persons.

ventricular hypertrophy. The *T* waves are low or inverted when associated with a *QS* (Fig. 40, *B*), *rS* (Fig. 41, *A*) or *rSr'* pattern. *T* may be upright or inverted when associated with an *RS* pattern, but should be upright when the chief initial ventricular deflection is a tall *R* wave.

LEFT LEG LEAD. *P* is usually upright, but may be diphasic or even inverted. As in the other leads, the ventricular components vary a great deal, depending on the position of the heart, being highest when the heart is vertical. The chief *QRS* deflection may be upwardly or downwardly directed, or the pattern may be intermediate between the two extremes (Figs. 40, 41). The *T* waves tend to be in the same direction as the chief *QRS* deflection. Occasionally there is low voltage of all waves, in which case the *T* wave may be upwardly or downwardly (Fig. 40,

C) directed. This lead is sometimes helpful in the evaluation of *Q* waves which appear in the classical Lead 2 or Leads 2 and 3. *Q* waves may be present normally in aV$_F$ (Fig. 42), but are

electrocardiogram by a shallow depression of the *P–R* segment (Fig. 45), but is frequently "lost" in the *QRS* complex. It is unimportant except as it may alter the level of the *P–R*

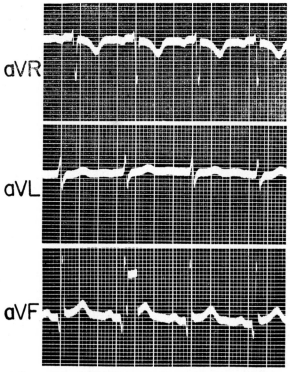

Fig 42. Prominent *Q* waves in AV$_{\overline{F}}$. Electrocardiogram obtained from a young healthy person.

nearly always less than 0.04 second in duration and less than half the amplitude of *R* if this wave is 5 mm. or more.

Bipolar Limb Leads

Although this section is devoted to a discussion of the variations encountered in the bipolar limb leads (Fig. 43), most of the illustrations include the augmented unipolar limb leads and the six precordial leads as well. Henceforth in this text these twelve leads will constitute the "standard" illustration.

P WAVE. The *P* wave is normally upright in Leads 1 and 2, but may be upright, inverted or diphasic in Lead 3. Some of the normal variations are shown in Figure 44. Tall *P* waves tend to be peaked, whereas low *P* waves tend to be rounded or slightly notched as in Lead 1 (Fig. 43). When *P* waves are diphasic, the first phase is upright (Fig. 44, *B*). The tallest *P* wave in any lead is rarely over 2.5 mm. in amplitude. The duration of *P* varies considerably, but is rarely greater than 0.12 second.

ATRIAL *T* WAVE. This is represented in the

interval or influence the contour of the early portion of the ventricular complex.

P–R INTERVAL. This is the interval between the onset of the *P* wave and the onset of the *QRS* complex (Figure 43). It can be measured with accuracy within 0.01 second unless the onset of *P* or *QRS* is poorly defined. It should be measured in the lead showing the most prominent *P* wave. If the initial portion of *QRS* is isoelectric or poorly defined, the total *P–QRS* duration should be measured; then in another lead in which *QRS* is well shown, its duration should be measured and this value subtracted from the total duration of *P–QRS*.

The average duration of the *P–R* interval in the first decade of life is 0.12 second; in the second, 0.14 second; and in the third, 0.16 second. However, in older children and adults the range is from 0.1 to over 0.2 second (Fig. 46). An exceptionally long *P–R* interval is shown in Figure 45. This record was obtained from an apparently healthy young person. It is possible that slight scarring in the atrioventricular junctional tissue may result from some

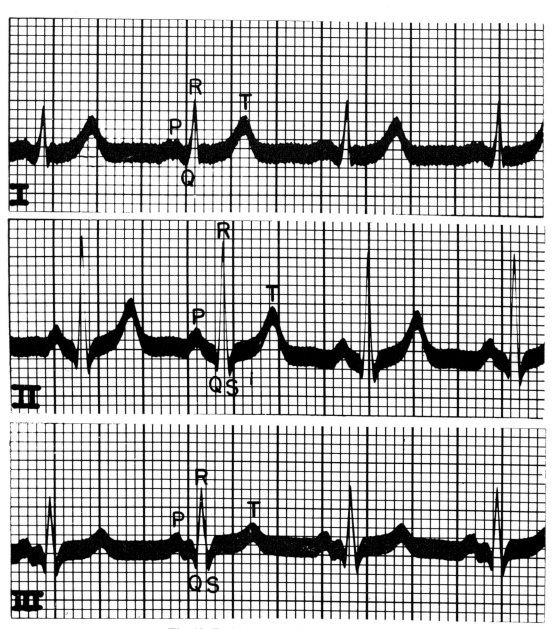

Fig. 43. Typical normal bipolar limb leads.

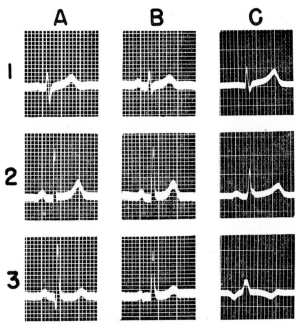

Fig. 44. Normal variations of the *P* waves in electrocardiograms obtained from young healthy persons.

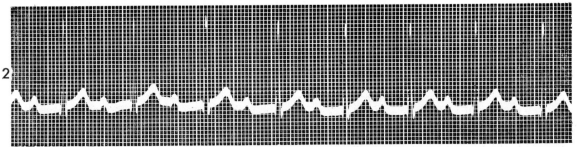

Fig. 45. Atrial *T* waves following *P* waves in an electrocardiogram obtained from an apparently healthy young person with unusually prolonged *P–R* intervals.

childhood infection in an otherwise perfectly normal person to account for otherwise unexplained prolongation of *P–R*, to, say, 0.22 second. The *P–R* interval varies inversely with heart rate; the difference is approximately 0.01 second for a change in rate of 20 beats a minute.

QRS COMPLEX. It is important to use exact terminology in referring to the several components of the *QRS* complex, and these have been carefully defined by the Committee of the American Heart Association for the Standardization of Electrocardiographic Nomenclature* as follows:

In order to indicate how the *QRS* complex should be subdivided for the purpose of assigning symbols to the deflections which it displays, we may describe a *QRS* complex which has three components in the following terms: The first deflection begins at the onset of the *QRS* interval when the trace first leaves the reference level. From this point the trace rises or falls to a turning

* J.A.M.A., *121:* 1347, 1943.

point where the direction of its motion is reversed. It may pass through a second or third turning point before crossing to the opposite side of the reference level.† At this crossing the first deflection ends and the second begins. The second deflection, necessarily opposite in direction to the first, must display one turning point and may display many; it does not end until the trace crosses the reference level for the second time. The third deflection begins at the second crossing and ends at the *RS–T* junction. No part of the *QRS* complex which does not display at least one turning point should be considered a separate deflection. If the *RS–T* junction is displaced and this junction and the last turning point lie on opposite sides of the reference level, that portion of the trace which lies between the last crossing and the *RS–T* junction should be considered part of the deflection to which the last turning point belongs.

† When the trace is descending it crosses the reference level at the instant when its lower margin reaches a position below that which it occupied at the beginning of the *QRS* interval. When the trace is ascending it crosses the reference level at the instant when its upper margin reaches a position above that which it occupied at the beginning of the *QRS* interval.

The earliest QRS deflection which lies above the reference level should be labeled R. Any downward deflection which precedes R, so defined, should be labeled Q. The first of any downward deflections which may follow R should be labeled S. The first of any upward deflections which may follow S should be labeled R', and the first of any downward deflections which may follow R' should be labeled S'. If it is necessary to label still later deflections of the QRS group, the symbols R'', S'' and so on should be used in accordance with the same principles. When R is absent, so that the QRS complex consists of a single downward deflection, this deflection should be labeled QS. In statistical studies QS, Q and S deflections should be considered separately.

A deflection is "notched" when it displays more than one turning point on the same side of the reference level. A deflection is "slurred" when it displays a distinct and local "thickening" on either limb or at its apex, owing to a sudden and pronounced change in the slope of the curve, or, in other words, in the rate at which the trace is rising or falling.

When the form of the QRS complex varies from moment to moment because of the effect of the respiratory movements on the position of the heart or for some similar reason, the classification of this complex should be determined by the variety of complex which is most abundant, or, if no type is numerically predominant, by the outline of the complexes which are of intermediate form. Very small QRS complexes (largest deflection less than 5 mm.) which display more than three components or multiple slurring and notching should be classed as "small and bizarre" or "vibratory."

The duration of the QRS complex should be carefully measured in the lead showing the longest interval. The average duration in young healthy persons is about 0.08 second, being slightly longer in the male than in the female. The range is from 0.06 to 0.11 or possibly 0.12

second. The upper end of the normal range merges almost imperceptibly into the right bundle branch block pattern. An example of a short QRS interval is shown in Figure 47 and of long QRS intervals in Figure 48; the electrocardiograms in both instances were obtained from healthy young persons.

The electrical axis of QRS was discussed in detail in Chapter 4 (p. 35). Here it is sufficient to say that moderate degrees of left and right axis deviation or shift may be seen in the records obtained from healthy persons. Left axis deviation is present when the net value for QRS is a plus value in Lead 1 and a minus value in Lead 3, and the R wave is taller in Lead 1 than in Lead 2. The electrocardiogram in Figure 49, obtained from a healthy young person, shows a moderate degree of left axis deviation. Right axis deviation is said to be present when the net value for QRS is a minus value in Lead 1 and a plus value in Lead 3, and the R wave is taller in Lead 3 than in Lead 2. A moderate degree of right axis deviation is shown in Figure 50; this record was obtained from a healthy young person with a "vertical" heart.

The electrocardiogram in Figure 51 shows slurring and notching of QRS. Such slurring and notching is to be regarded as normal if the voltage of QRS is low or if it occurs near the baseline. Exceptionally, as in this case, there may be thickening or slurring of the chief QRS deflection well above or below the baseline.

The electrocardiogram in Figure 52 was ob-

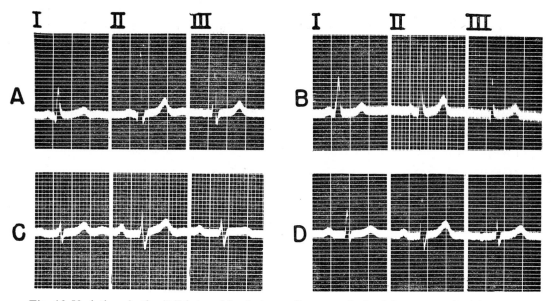

Fig. 46. Variations in the *P-R* interval in electrocardiograms obtained from young healthy persons.

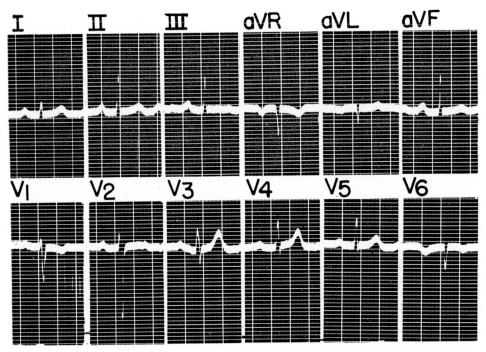

Fig. 47. Short *QRS* duration in electrocardiogram obtained from a young healthy person.

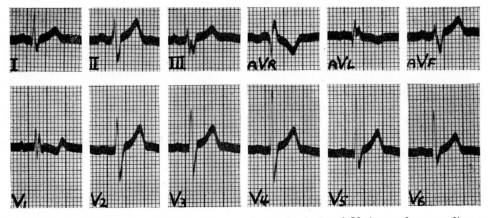

Fig. 48. Unusually long *QRS* duration together with an *rr'* complex in Lead V₁ in an electrocardiogram obtained from a young healthy person.

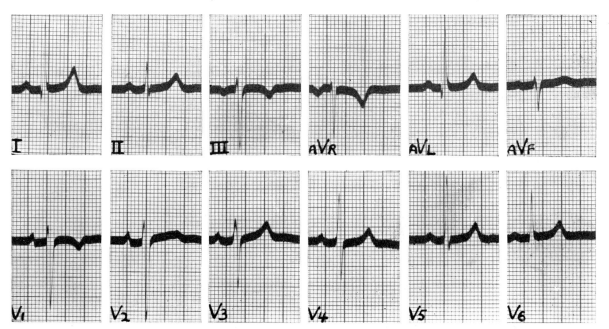

Fig. 49. Left axis deviation of both *QRS* and *T* waves in an electrocardiogram obtained from a young healthy person.

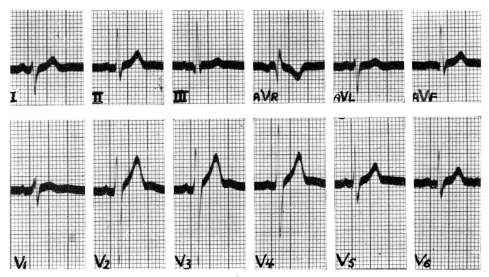

Fig. 50. Right axis deviation in an electrocardiogram obtained from a young healthy person.

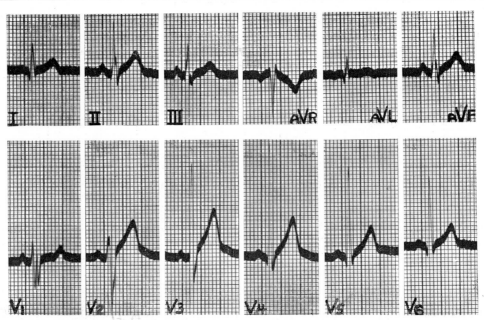

Fig. 51. Slurring and notching of *QRS* in an electrocardiogram obtained from a young healthy person.

tained from a healthy young person and shows remarkably low voltage in both the limb and precordial leads. Low voltage in the limb leads (all *Q*, *R* and *S* waves under 5 mm.) is uncommon but not rare.

Q WAVE. The electrocardiogram in Figure 53 shows rather prominent *Q* waves in Leads 1 and 2. These represent about the upper limit of the normal range with respect to the duration of *Q*, which is 0.04 second in Lead 2. The amplitude of *Q* is usually small in relation to *R*, which is 0.04 second in Lead 2. The amplitude of *Q* is usually small in relation to *R*, but it may be normally one third the amplitude of *R* in Lead 1 and one fourth the amplitude of *R* in Lead 2.

The record in Figure 54 shows prominent *Q* waves in Leads 2 and 3. In Lead 3 the *Q* wave is 0.04 second in duration, which is the upper normal limit. Note also that there is a prominent

Q in Lead aV$_F$. It is the rule to observe a small *Q* wave in Lead 3, but in exceptional instances it may, normally, form the chief component of *QRS*. It may be difficult to determine whether or not *Q* waves in Lead 3 have pathologic significance. *Q* waves are less likely to have pathologic significance (1) if they are absent in Leads aV$_F$ and 2 (Fig. 55), (2) if there are no associated abnormalities of *RS–T* and *T*, and (3) if they are seen only in association with shift in heart position.

R WAVE. The *R* waves vary greatly in amplitude, as shown by a comparison of Figures 52 and 53. In subjects with hearts which tend to lie horizontally, the *R* waves are tallest in Lead 1 (Fig. 49); if the heart tends to hang vertically, the *R* waves are usually tallest in Lead 3 (Fig. 50).

S WAVE. Prominent *S* waves may normally

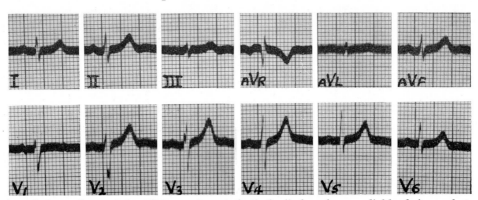

Fig. 52. Moderately low voltage of the *QRS* complexes in both the limb and precordial leads in an electrocardiogram obtained from a young healthy person.

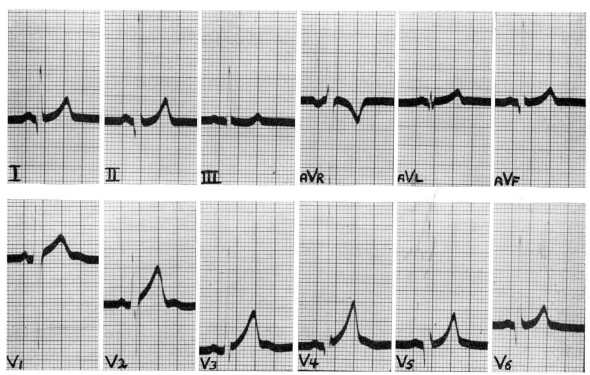

Fig. 53. Prominent *Q* waves in Leads 1 and 2 and in precordial Leads V₅ and V₆ in an electrocardiogram obtained from a young healthy person.

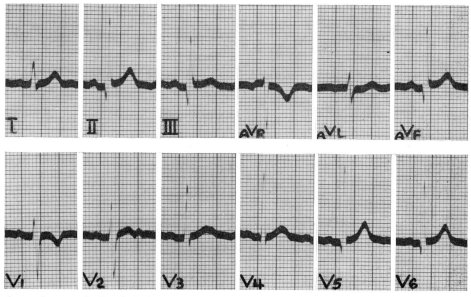

Fig. 54. Prominent *Q* waves in Leads 2, 3, V₅, V₆ and aVF in an electrocardiogram obtained from a young healthy person.

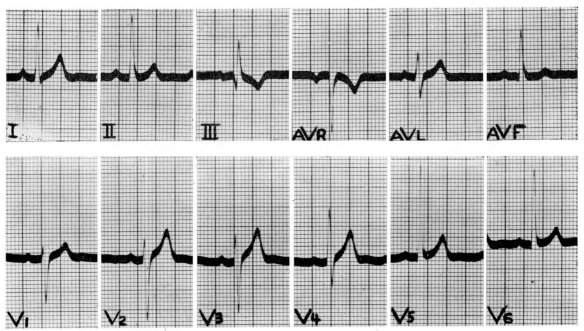

Fig. 55. Prominent *Q* waves in Lead 3, but not in aVF, in an electrocardiogram obtained from a young healthy person.

be seen in one or all of the limb leads. A typical example of prominent *S* waves in Leads 1 and 2 is shown in Figure 56. This is a characteristic pattern seen in records obtained from subjects with hearts which tend to hang vertically. The electrocardiogram in Figure 57 was obtained from a young healthy person and shows prominent *S* waves in Leads 2 and 3. In persons with horizontally placed hearts and a tendency toward left axis deviation prominent S waves are seen in Lead 3 (Fig. 49) or in Leads 2 and 3.

RS–T JUNCTION. Slight elevation of the *RS–T* junction is commonly observed as a variation of the normal. A typical example is shown in Figure 58. This elevation is rarely greater than 1.5 mm. and is usually seen in association with tall *T* waves. The *RS–T* junction is rarely displaced downward normally, and then never more than 1 mm. (Fig. 57).

RS–T SEGMENT. This segment is not always distinguishable from the *T* wave. It begins at the *RS–T* junction and lies at or near the baseline until it ends at the place where it is deflected to form the ascending limb of the *T* wave. It is usually described as flat, sloping, convex or concave. It may be displaced above the baseline

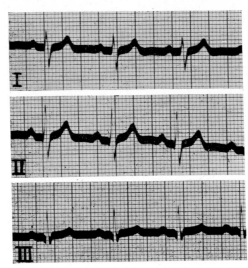

Fig. 56. Prominent *S* waves in Leads 1 and 2 in an electrocardiogram obtained from a young healthy person.

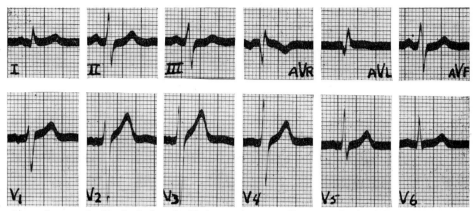

Fig. 57. Prominent *S* waves in Leads 2, 3 and aVF in an electrocardiogram obtained from a young healthy person.

as shown in Figure 59 and, more typically, Figure 54. Such upward displacement is rarely over 1 mm. Downward displacement of the *RS–T* segment is uncommonly seen in Leads 1 and 2, and then to only a slight degree (Fig. 60). In Lead 3, however, it is frequently seen displaced downward (Fig. 59).

T WAVE. The electrical axis of the *T* waves tends to lie in the same general direction as *QRS*; hence the amplitude and direction of *T* correspond to the amplitude and direction of the chief component of *QRS*. Accordingly, when the *R* wave in Lead 1 is of low amplitude, or if the *S* is more prominent than the *R* wave, *T* tends to be low in amplitude (Fig. 58), and if *R* is tall, *T* tends to be tall (Fig. 55). The *T* waves are normally upright in Leads 1 and 2, but may be upright, diphasic or inverted in Lead 3.

There are rare exceptions to this rule. In electrocardiograms obtained from tall thin persons with right axis deviation of *QRS*, *T* may be isoelectric or even slightly inverted in Lead 1. In stocky persons with horizontally placed hearts, and in some persons with vertically placed hearts, the *T* wave may be inverted in Lead 2 during certain phases of respiration (Figs. 65, 66). Still other exceptions are difficult to explain, as in the case illustrated in Figure 61. This record was obtained from a healthy young person, and the diphasic *T* waves in Lead 2 may be the result of anxiety, of overventilation or of other factors. Inversion of all complexes, *P*, *QRS* and *T* waves, in Lead 3 indicates the probability of a horizontal position of the heart, regardless of whether the heart is healthy or diseased.

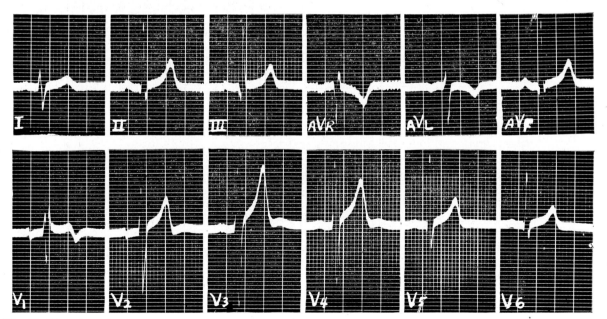

Fig. 58. Elevation of the *RS-T* segments in Leads 2, 3, aVF and V₃ in an electrocardiogram obtained from a young healthy person.

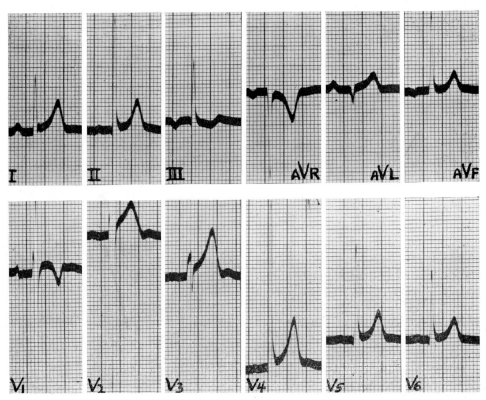

Fig. 59. Upward displacement of the *RS-T* segments in both limb and precordial leads in an electrocardiogram from a young healthy person.

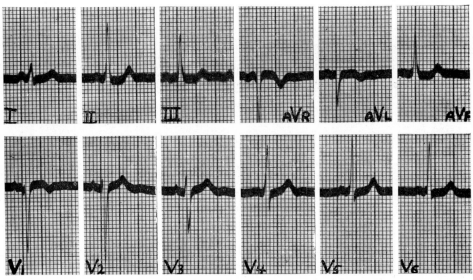

Fig. 60. Slight downward displacement of the *RS-T* segments in Leads 2, 3 and aVf in an electrocardiogram from a young healthy person.

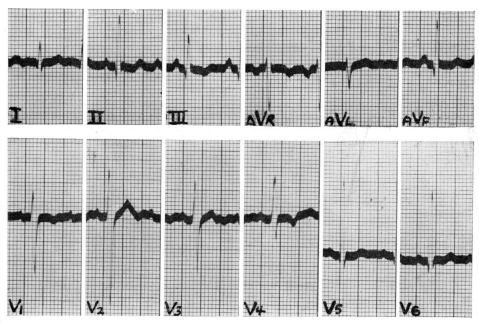

Fig. 61. Diphasic *T* waves in Lead 2 and low or inverted *T* waves in Lead 3 and precordial leads V₄ through V₆ in an electrocardiogram obtained from a young healthy person.

Q–T DURATION (OFTEN LOOSELY CALLED THE "*Q–T* INTERVAL"). The time interval from the beginning of the initial ventricular deflection (*QRS*) to the end of *T* represents fairly accurately the duration of ventricular systole. The *Q–T* systolic duration varies normally with the heart rate; at average rates ranging from 50 to 100 it measures 0.4 to 0.3 second (the faster the rate, the shorter the systole), while at rates of 30 to 50 it may be prolonged, even to 0.5 second or more, and at rapid rates of 120 to 150 it may

be reduced to 0.25 second or less. Certain factors, such as the lack of calcium, the effect of quinidine, cardiac enlargement, and heart block, prolong systole inordinately.

U WAVE. Sometimes there is a low summit following the *T* wave which has been termed the "*U*" wave. It follows the *T* wave in direction, whether upright or inverted, but is almost invariably much smaller; rarely in precordial leads it may be quite prominent (up to 2 mm.). Its mechanism is obscure.

CHAPTER 7

Electrocardiographic Variations Due to Physiologic Factors

There are minor variations in the electrocardiogram related to sex and more important variations associated with age. It is probable that differences in heart size are largely responsible for differences in duration of the time intervals in normal persons. This is strongly supported by comparison of the time intervals in the electrocardiograms of normal adult elephants (Fig. 62) with those of a human infant (Fig. 63).

Adult males have slightly longer *P–R* intervals and *QRS* durations and slightly shorter cor-

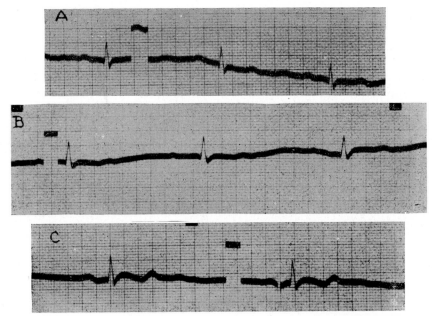

Fig. 62. The electrocardiograms of Lead 1 of three healthy elephants: Clara (*A*), Lizzie (*B*) and Juno (*C*). (Am. Hear J., *16*: 747, 1938. Courtesy of the C. V. Mosby Company.)

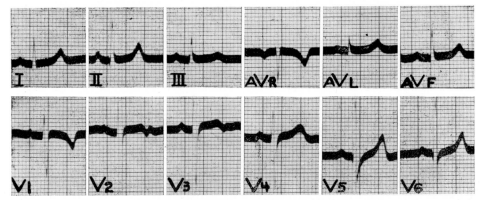

Fig. 63. Low or inverted *T* waves in precordial leads V_1 through V_3 in electrocardiograms obtained from a healthy female, age sixteen months.

rected QT durations than adult females. Large breasts in the latter may influence the voltage in the precordial leads.

In young infants the heart rate is rapid and there is slight right ventricular preponderance resulting in right axis deviation. In children with a large belly the heart may be pushed up to a semihorizontal position, so that, proceeding from right to left across the chest, the QRS transitional zone is not passed until position

taken from a healthy man of stocky build, thirty-two years of age, who was in the sitting position. They illustrate strikingly the effects of a change in the position of the heart, due to a respiratory change in the position of the diaphragm, on the electrical axis of both the QRS complexes and the T waves. Figure 66, A, is the control record taken during quiet respiration. The P waves, $P-R$ interval, QRS waves and T waves are all normal, although the T

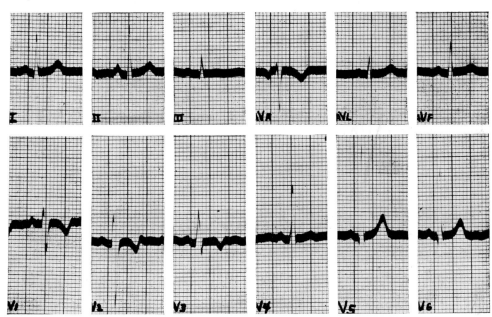

Fig. 64. Low or inverted T waves in precordial Leads V_1 through V_4 in electrocardiograms obtained from a female child eleven years of age.

V_4 or V_5 is reached (Fig. 63). The same is true for the T waves, as shown in Figure 64. In children the $P-R$ intervals and QRS durations are shorter than in adults, and there is often rather high voltage of the T waves or QRS complexes, or both.

Respiration may alter the electrocardiogram to an important degree in certain persons. The electrocardiograms in Figure 65 were obtained from a healthy man of stocky build while in the supine position. The control record was obtained during quiet respiration and the following two during inspiration and expiration respectively. The significant changes occurred during inspiration and are indicated by a shift of the electrical axis of QRS toward the right and lowering of the T waves in the limb leads. Considerable change is also seen in the precordial leads.

The electrocardiograms in Figure 66 were

waves are rather low in Lead 2 and inverted in Lead 3. There is normal, average axis deviation. The heart rate is 110. Figure 66, B, is a record taken in full inspiration with a much more vertical position of the heart, which is rotated to the right. Note the slower rate of 70, the tendency toward right axis deviation, which is now nearly 90 degrees (R is lower in Lead 1 and taller in Lead 3), and especially the inversion of the T waves in Lead 2, resembling "coronary T waves," with deeper T waves in Lead 3. Figure 66, C, taken in full expiration, shows a swing of the electrical axis up toward the left, as indicated by a taller R in Lead 1 and rr' in Lead 3. The T waves are not changed much from those of the control record.

The electrocardiograms in Figure 67 were taken from a healthy girl of twelve, who had recently recovered from a cold, and show the effects of a change in posture. Figure 67, A,

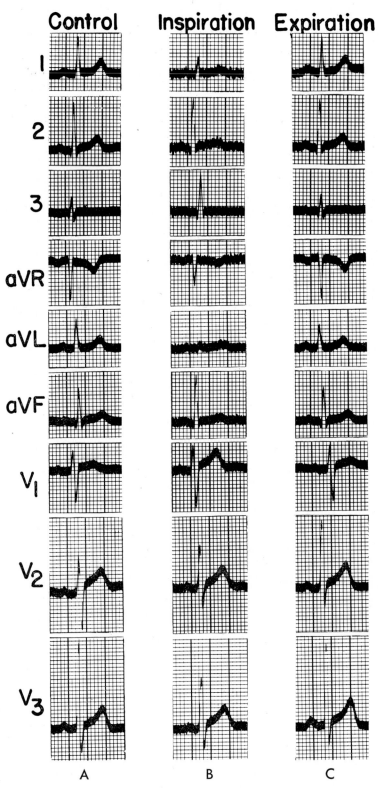

Fig. 65. Alterations in the electrocardiogram associated with changes in respiration: *A*, control; *B*, full inspiration; *C*, full expiration.

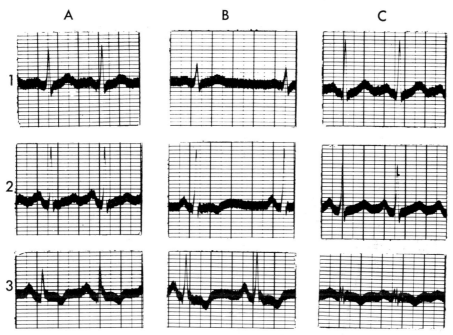

Fig. 66. Alterations in the electrocardiogram associated with changes in respiration: *A*, control; *B*, full inspiration; *C*, full expiration.

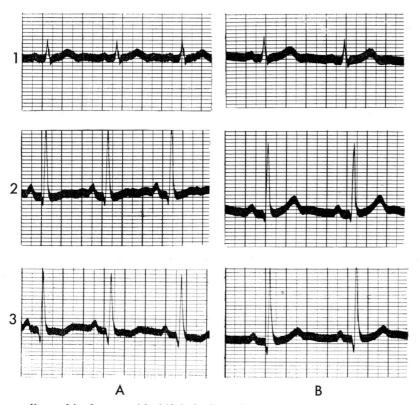

Fig. 67. Electrocardiographic changes with shift in body position in a healthy girl of twelve: *A*, seated; *B*, supine.

was taken in the sitting position and is normal throughout, with a rate of 90, although there is a low *T* wave in Lead 2. There is a tendency to right axis deviation, in accord with a vertical heart position. Figure 67, *B*, was taken with the subject recumbent and shows normal rhythm at a rate of 70; the *T* waves are now normally high, without much change in axis of the *QRS* waves. Changes in the anatomic position of the heart in any one of two, or indeed in all three planes, readily explain these differences. It must

slightly inverted in Lead 3. Two factors are probably involved in this change: one is an actual shift in the axis of the *T* waves, due to a change in heart position (which may be rotation on its longitudinal axis—the *QRS* axis changes little); the other, at times apparently more significant, is a direct sympathetic nerve action (or rather, change in the degree of action) with change in heart rate. Both factors may operate simultaneously. Further study of the mechanism of this phenomenon is needed.

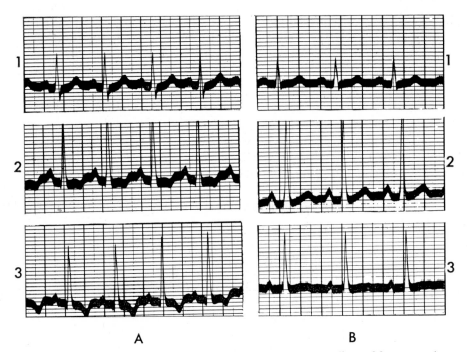

A   B

Fig. 68. Electrocardiographic changes with changes in body position in a schoolboy of fourteen: *A*, seated; *B*, supine.

be noted that the position of the heart when the *QRS* is written may be different from that in full systole when the heart is fully lifted at the peak of the *T*. A change from the recumbent to the upright position, if associated with orthostatic hypotension, also may result in *T* wave inversion; in such a case myocardial ischemia may be to blame.

The electrocardiograms in Figure 68 were obtained from a schoolboy fourteen years of age. These records also present an excellent illustration of a normal physiologic phenomenon. The inversion of the *T* waves in Leads 2 and 3 is a not uncommon normal variation found in certain persons with vertically placed hearts when they are sitting or standing. The assumption of the supine position raises the *T* waves, usually to an average normal status, upright in Lead 2, and upright, flat or only

Overventilation, with reduction of carbon dioxide tension in the alveoli, leads to alkalosis and characteristic electrocardiographic changes. These are illustrated in Figure 69 and consist of slight lowering of the *RS–T* segments and flattening or lowering of the *T* waves in the standard leads.

The electrocardiograms in Figure 70 were obtained from a healthy young man twenty-three years of age. The control record was obtained while he rested quietly on a bed. Then, while Lead 2 was being recorded, a pistol was fired near the subject. The four strips of Lead 2 in Figure 70, *B*, form a continuous record. The wide hatch marks near the end of strip 1 indicate the somatic tremor induced by the startle. This is followed by an increase in heart rate which gives way to bradycardia at the end of strip 3. Note the progressive lowering of the

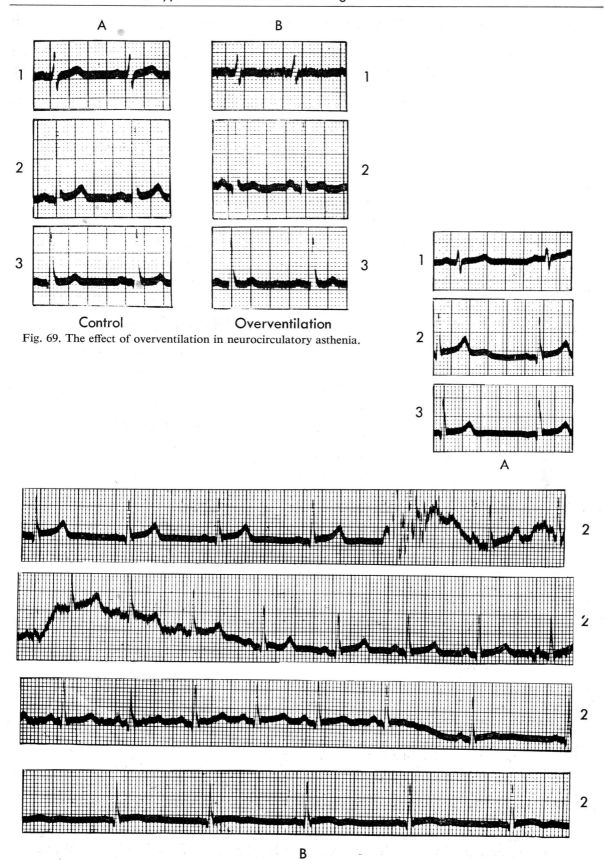

Fig. 69. The effect of overventilation in neurocirculatory asthenia.

Fig. 70. The startle reaction: *A*, control; *B*, continuous recording of Lead 2 before and after pistol shot.

T waves. In some instances the *T* waves may become inverted in reaction to startle.

Another effect produced by the same stimulus is shown in Figure 71. Comparison of the records obtained before and immediately after the startle shows that the *QRS* interval has widened considerably, temporarily producing right bundle branch block.

with which they appear argues against their being due to such mechanisms as overventilation, hormonal influence or other metabolic changes which require more time for their exhibition.

When a healthy person exercises strenuously, fairly characteristic changes occur in the electrocardiogram, in addition to the increase in heart

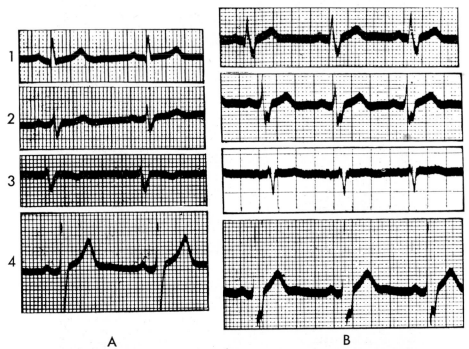

A   B

Fig. 71. Startle reaction producing bundle branch block: *A*, control; *B*, reaction. (Graybiel et al.: Analysis of the Electrocardiograms Obtained from One Thousand Young Healthy Aviators. Am. Heart J., *27:* 524, 1944.)

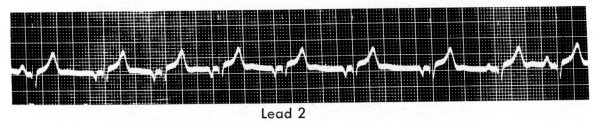

Lead 2

Fig. 72. Alterations in the *P* waves following a startle in a young healthy man.

Still another example is shown in Figure 72, wherein the *P* waves suddenly become inverted, and then gradually return to their original form. This shift of pacemaker is the commonest electrocardiographic alteration due to a startle, with the exception of changes in heart rate.

These examples of the electrocardiographic changes following startle indicate the sudden and rather remarkable effects on the sinoatrial node, intraventricular conduction, and the repolarization process in the ventricles brought about by a nervous stimulus. The suddenness

rate. During the exercise the *T* waves tend to become lower, owing possibly to alteration in sympathetic-parasympathetic balance with sympathetic predominance (Fig. 73). Immediately after exercise and during recovery further changes occur which are also illustrated in Figure 73. In the limb leads the *P* waves become taller after exercise and the electrical axis of *P* tends to shift slightly to the right. The *QRS* axis also tends to shift slightly to the right. There is slight lowering of the *RS–T* segments, and the amplitude of the *T* waves is slightly decreased.

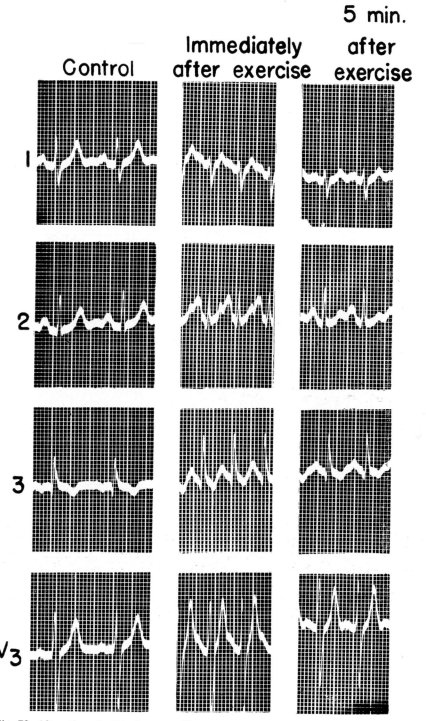

Fig. 73. Alterations in the electrocardiogram of a young healthy man after exercise.

The alterations are still present five minutes after exercise. Note the prominent *S* waves in Lead 1, the slight sagging of *RS-T* in Lead 2 and the rather low amplitude of the *T* waves in Leads 1 and 2.

Hyperpyrexia of moderate degree produces little change in the electrocardiogram save for an increase in rate. However, a severe degree of hyperpyrexia may cause considerable lowering of the *RS–T* segments and *T* waves.

The lowering of body temperature produces little electrocardiographic change. Marked lowering, however, such as may take place during hypothermia treatments or during excessive ex-

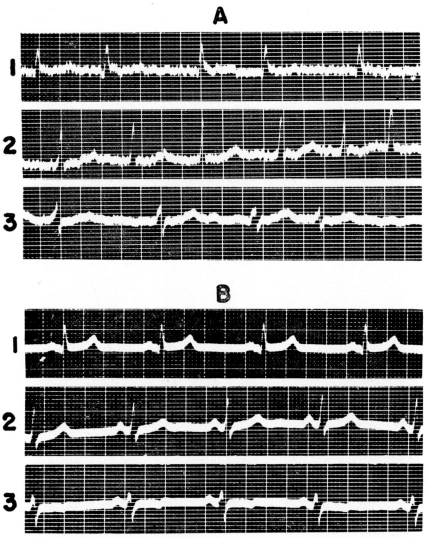

Fig. 74. *A*, Atrial fibrillation and other electrocardiographic alterations in a previously young healthy man suffering from exposure to cold. *B*, After recovery. (Graybiel, A., and Dawe, C. J.: Auricular Fibrillation following Hypothermia. Armed Forces Med. J., *1:* 418, 1950.)

posure in cold weather, may cause a slowing of the heart rate or the appearance of atrial fibrillation. The *RS–T* segments may become depressed and the *T* waves may become lower in amplitude. The electrocardiogram in Figure 74, *A*, was obtained from a previously healthy young man who nearly perished from cold as the result of accidental immersion in cold water. There are atrial fibrillation, slight sagging of the *RS–T* segments in Leads 1 and 2, and abnormally low *T* waves in Lead 1. These alterations were abolished after the patient's recovery from exposure (Fig. 74, *B*).

Exposure to reduced barometric pressure or reduction in the percentage of oxygen in the inspired air produces electrocardiographic changes even in young healthy subjects. The curves in Figure 75 were obtained before and after a healthy subject breathed 10 per cent oxygen for twenty minutes. Note the increase in heart rate and the lowering of the *T* waves in the limb leads and precordial leads V_4 and V_6.

The use of the "anoxia test" in the diagnosis of coronary insufficiency will be described in Chapter 21 (p. 265).

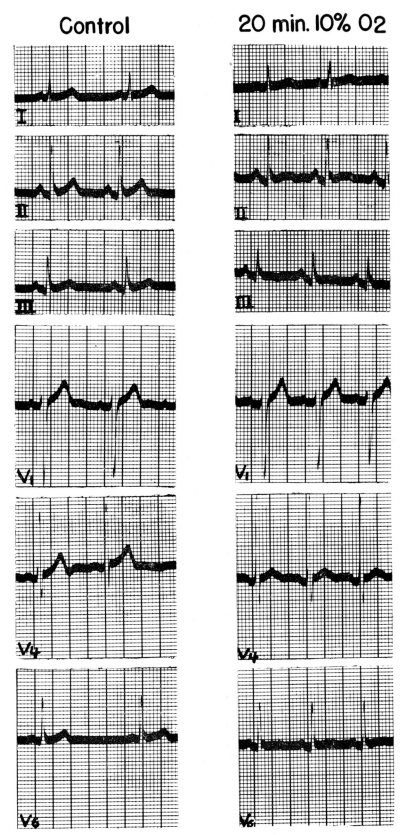

Fig. 75. E'ectrocardiographic alterations in a young healthy person exposed to 10 per cent oxygen for a period of twenty minutes.

CHAPTER 8

Artifacts and Technical Errors

There are many reasons why a particular curve does not bear interpretation. An error may have been made in obtaining or labeling the record, or the curve may be distorted from one of a number of causes. The difficulty may rest with the patient, with the operator, with the electrocardiograph and its connection to the patient, or with some other factor. The recognition and resolution of these simple but often neglected problems will come with experience, but a knowledge of their common causes is helpful.

Artifacts*

So far as artifacts inherent in the electrocardiograph are concerned, it is important to remember that an instrument utilizing the string galvanometer is quite different in mechanical operation from the more recently developed amplifier electrocardiographs. Each type has its own peculiarities, the details of which are well set forth in an article by Rappaport.†

Underdamped Oscillation

Figure 76, *A*, is a control strip of Lead 2, taken from a normal subject with an amplifier instrument. The curves are quite normal in form, and the standardization deflection is quite satisfactory, although it includes the *QRS* complex. One of the essential characteristics of an electrocardiograph is proper control of the motion of string or rotary coil in the galvanometer to prevent distortion of curves as a result of inertia of the moving string or coil. Motion will continue after the electrical stimulus has stopped, unless a "braking" effect is introduced. This is known technically as damping. Figure 76, *B* (same subject), shows the distortion produced by insufficient damping. In the stand-

ardization curve the upward deflection goes beyond the 10 mm. (1 millivolt) mark by 5 mm. (overshooting) and then returns to the 10 mm. mark. The second small deflection is due to the natural oscillation of the underdamped galvanometer. The third large deflection is the *QRS* complex, followed by a *T* wave. Shortly after the *T* wave the standardizing current was cut off and the downward deflection was produced. This also shows overshooting and natural underdamped oscillation. The curve in Figure 76, *C*, shows overshooting at each end. The distortion produced in the electrocardiogram in Figure 76, *B*, takes the form of high *R* waves, a "vibratory" *S* wave, and higher *T*'s.

Overshooting

Overshooting was an important artifact in the early days of electrocardiography, owing to polarization effects at the electrodes. The electrodes and paste used today do not produce these effects. In the modern string machine this artifact is seldom encountered, unless too heavy a string is used; and it is rare in the amplifier instrument, although a loose or weakened magnet may occasionally produce it. (See Figure 76, *C*.)

High Skin Resistance

High skin resistance does not produce overshooting in any electrocardiograph. In the string instrument, however, high skin resistance, especially when combined with lower magnetic field strength, may produce sluggish movement of the galvanometer resulting in deformity like that seen in Figure 76, *D*. Here the standardization curve shows slow deflection, and the *QRS* complexes are slurred. High skin resistance in amplifier types of electrocardiographs, especially when it varies in the three limbs, can cause distortion in unipolar electrocardiograms. This effect produces a deviation of the central terminal from "0" or approximately "0." In bipolar leads high skin resistance in the amplifier type

* We are indebted to Mr. Maurice B. Rappaport of the Sanborn Co., Cambridge, Massachusetts, for assistance in the preparation of this discussion.

† Rappaport, M. B., and Rappaport, I.: Electrocardiographic Considerations in Small Animal Investigations. Am. Heart J., *26:* 662, 1943.

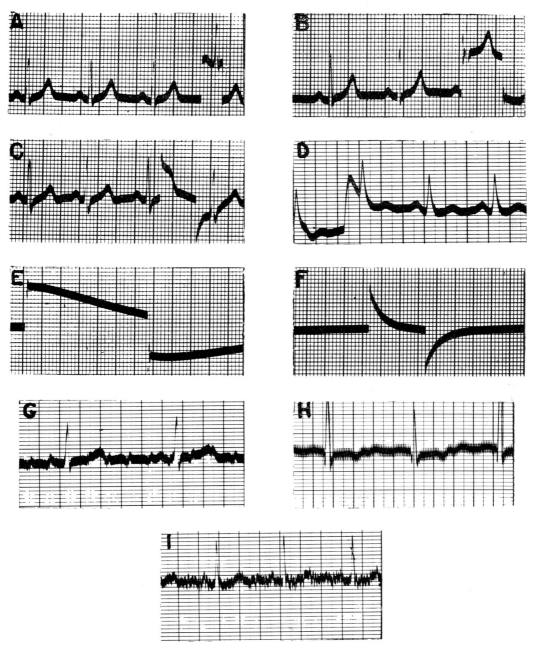

Fig. 76. *A*, Normal control (amplifier type electrocardiograph). *B*, Underdamped oscillation (amplifier type electrocardiograph). *C*, Overshooting (string galvanometer). *D*, Sluggish string (string galvanometer). *E*, Normal "decay" curve (amplifier type electrocardiograph). *F*, Rapid "decay" curve (amplifier type electrocardiograph). *G*, Muscle twitching (string galvanometer). *H*, Alternating current (string galvanometer). *I*, Somatic tremor (string galvanometer).

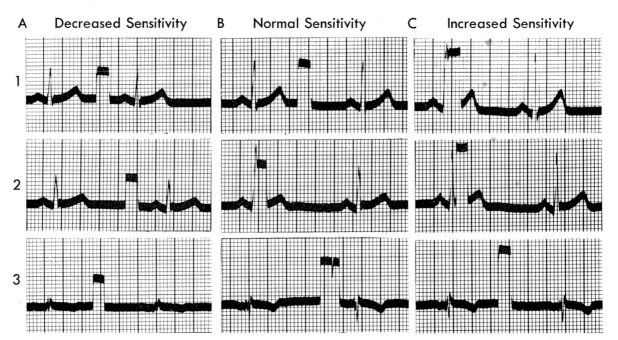

Fig. 77. Electrocardiograms illustrating the changes produced by both an abnormal decrease and an increase in sensitivity.

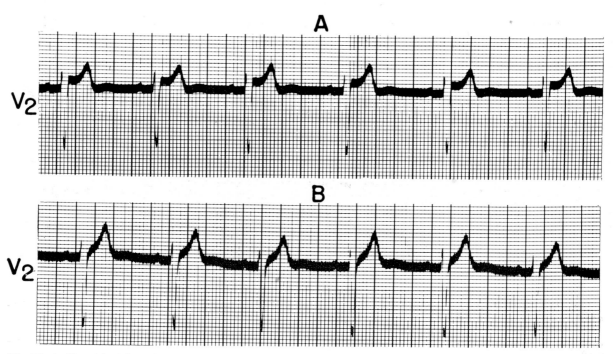

Fig. 78. Artifact (elevation of $RS\text{-}T$ segment) sometimes observed in obtaining precordial leads, particularly V_2 or V_3, caused by a poor contact between skin and electrode.

of electrocardiograph will not produce a distorted electrocardiogram, but may introduce alternating current interference.*

Decay of the Beam

Another kind of distortion is occasionally seen with the amplifier machine. It is a peculiarity of all such instruments that the beam does not remain deflected indefinitely when the 1 millivolt standardizing current is introduced, but gradually returns to the baseline. This phenomenon is known as decay of the beam, which ordinarily does not distort the complexes because the beam does not begin to decline appreciably for 0.12 second or more. The property of beam decay is utilized to provide automatic compensation for skin currents which would otherwise distort the electrocardiogram; different provision is made in the string instrument to eliminate this factor. Figure 76, E, shows a normal decay curve. Overshooting has been artificially produced at each end, but this does not affect the curve. The sudden drop in the middle of the curve occurs when the standardization button has been released, 1.26 seconds after the beginning of standardization. The curve then slowly rises toward the baseline. Slow decay of the beam is a condenser discharge effect. If condensers are faulty, the beam will fall rapidly, as shown in Figure 76, F, producing considerable distortion of the electrocardiogram. This is well shown in Figure 76, C (same subject as in Fig. 76, A, B). Here the S waves are deepened and the T waves lowered with slight late dip.

Other Artifacts

Figure 76, G, demonstrates one of the many artifacts which arise from outside the machine. Here regular, small deflections, at a rate of 300, simulating atrial flutter are seen. However, these were produced by rhythmic muscle twitching in a patient with Sydenham's chorea. The true P waves precede each QRS complex, but are somewhat obscured by the smaller deflections.

In Figure 76, H, 60-cycle alternating current from electric power lines has been picked up by the electrocardiograph. The fine oscillations of the baseline measure 60 per second exactly.

---

* Rappaport, M. B., and Williams, C., with ed· assistance of White, P. D.: An Analysis of the Relative Accuracies of the Wilson and Goldberger Methods for Registering Unipolar and Augmented Unipolar Electrocardiographic Leads. Am. Heart J., *37:* 892, 1949.

In Figure 76, I, the coarse, irregular vibrations obscuring the baseline are produced by somatic tremor, often seen in nervous persons.

Electrocardiograms are said to be properly standardized when the trace is deflected 1 cm. when 1 millivolt is introduced into the circuit. If the deflection is less than 1 cm. (Fig. 77, A), the sensitivity is too low and the resulting curve too small. If the deflection is greater than 1 cm., the sensitivity is too high and the resulting curve too large (Fig. 77, C).

A curious artifact is sometimes observed in obtaining precordial leads, particularly V_2 or V_3, in which the RS-T junction is abnormally elevated (Fig. 78, A). It may be due to a poor contact between electrode and skin, inasmuch as it is abolished when a better contact is made (Fig. 78, B).

Errors in Attaching Lead Wires

Incorrect application of the lead wires is far more likely to occur in the standard limb leads than in the unipolar precordial leads. A discussion of these errors may be approached from two standpoints: namely, the prediction of the electrocardiographic alterations when the error in applying the electrodes is known, and prediction of the error made in applying the electrodes by analysis of the alterations in the electrocardiogram.

With regard to the former, an illustration will serve to demonstrate the method to be followed in determining, for example, the changes to be expected when the left leg and left arm lead wires have been switched. First, draw a small triangle and indicate the correct lead connections and their polarity. Next, draw a larger triangle around the small one and indicate the error made in applying the lead wires and the *correct polarity* for that lead, as shown in Figure 79. In Figure 79, A, Lead 1 wires will record Lead 2, and the curve will be "upright" because the polarity is the same as that shown when the lead is obtained normally. Lead 2 wires will record Lead 1, which will be "upright" because the polarity is correct. Lead 3 wires will record Lead 3, but the curve will be upside down because the polarity is the reverse of the normal.

Ordinarily an error in applying the lead wires is first recognized when the electrocardiographer gets the record for interpretation, by which time it is too late to discover how the leads were applied. One basis for detection of the error is

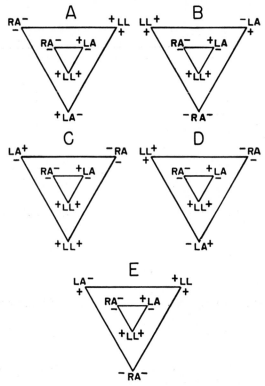

Fig. 79A. Sketch to be used in connection with the determination of errors resulting from misapplication of limb lead electrodes. See text.

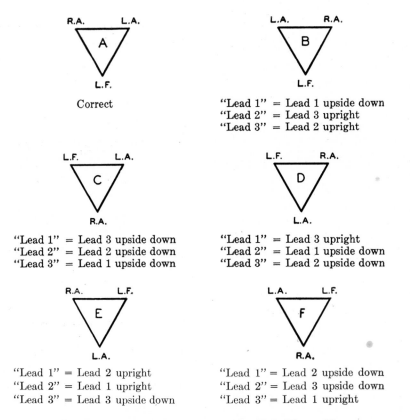

Fig. 79B. Key to artifacts (crossed leads) in Figure 80.

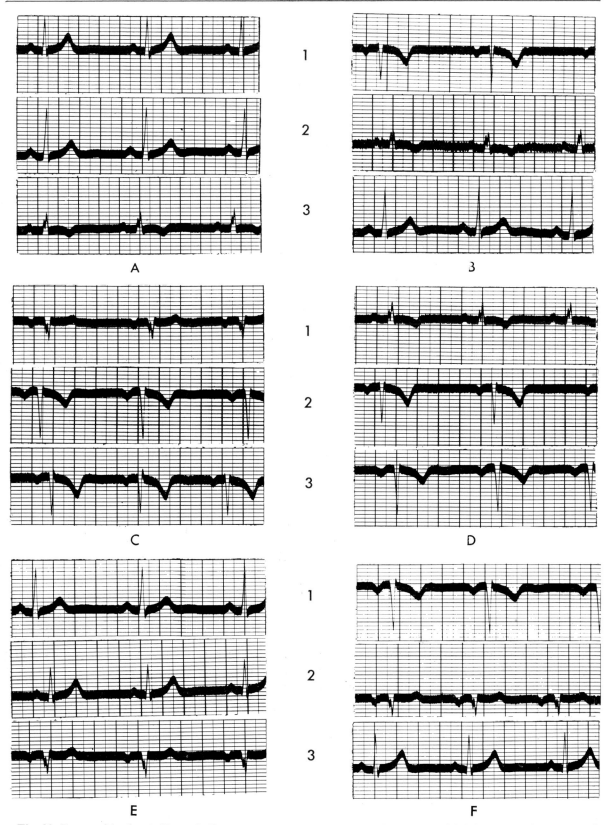

Fig. 80. Reversed leads. *A*, Normal; *B*, arm connections reversed; *C*, right arm and left leg connections reversed; *D*, clockwise rotation of all lead connections; *E*, left arm and left leg connections reversed; *F*, counterclockwise rotation of all lead connections.

Table 1. To Be Used in Connection with Determining the Errors Resulting from Misapplication of Limb Lead Electrodes. (See Text.)

	Arm connections reversed	Left arm and left leg connections* reversed	Right arm and left leg connections reversed	Clockwise rotation all lead connections	Counter-clockwise rotation all lead connections
Polarity strip 1	(↓)	↑	(↓)	↑	(↓)
Polarity strip 2	↑	↑	(↓)	(↓)	(↓)
Polarity strip 3	↑	(↓)	(↓)	(↓)	↑

* Most easily overlooked because Lead 3 is often normally inverted.

(↓) Strip or "lead" "upsidedown".

↑   Strip or "lead" "upright".

to note which lead or leads have been recorded upside down. Five possibilities account for all errors in application of the electrodes, as shown in Table 1.

If only the curve in strip 1 is upside down, the arm connections were reversed and strip 1 has become Lead 1 upside down, strip 2 has become Lead 3, and strip 3 has become Lead 2 (Fig. 80, *B*). If only the curve in strip 3 is upside down, the left arm and left leg connections were reversed and strip 1 has become Lead 2, strip 2 has become Lead 1, and strip 3 has become Lead 3 upside down (Fig. 80, *E*). If the curves in all three strips are upside down, the right arm and left leg connections were reversed and strip 1 has become Lead 3 upside down, strip 2 has become Lead 2 upside down, and strip 3 has become Lead 1 upside down (Fig. 80, *C*). If the curves in strips 2 and 3 are upside down, all the connections have been rotated clockwise and strip 1 has become Lead 3, strip 2 has become Lead 1 upside down, and strip 3 has become Lead 2 upside down (Fig. 80, *D*). If the curves in strips 1 and 2 are upside down, all the connections have been rotated counterclockwise and strip 1 has become Lead 2 upside down, strip 2 has become Lead 3 upside down and strip 3 has become Lead 1 (Fig. 80, *F*).

PART IV

Disorders of Rhythm and Conduction

CHAPTER 9

Disorders of Rhythm and Conduction

Electrocardiography was introduced in the clinic a generation ago largely to facilitate the interpretation of cardiac arrhythmia, tachycardia, and bradycardia. It has served this purpose admirably and still remains the best means of analyzing disorders of cardiac rhythm and conduction. With the passage of time, however, and with the great increase in our knowledge of electrocardiography and of its value in ascertaining the presence of myocardial disease, there has been a tendency to neglect intensive training in electrocardiographic interpretation of disorders of rhythm. We have, in fact, noted that on occasion physicians expert in the analysis of the electrocardiographic complexes in multiple leads and their significance in relation to heart position and disease may be puzzled by some obscure rhythm which should be quite easily interpreted. Thus this section of the book continues to be of routine importance.

With experience it is not infrequently possible to interpret at a glance an abnormality of rhythm, without detailed measurements of time intervals or of the individual complexes. For the beginner and in difficult cases, however, it is well to follow a definite procedure of identification of the atrial complexes with respect to rate and rhythm and their relationship to the ventricular complexes. The form, duration and amplitude, as well as the rate and rhythm, of the atrial and ventricular complexes are to be analyzed in doubtful cases.

Normal cardiac rhythm may be defined as the relatively regular sequence of cycles, usually between the rates of 50 and 100 a minute, although normal sinus tachycardia may occur at a rate as high as 120 or even higher, and normal sinus bradycardia may occur at a rate as low as 40. In normal cardiac rhythm the excitatory impulse arises in the sinoatrial node and proceeds normally through the heart to the ventricular musculature. As a variation of normal cardiac rhythm there is a condition which has been called sinus arrhythmia, in which, especially with respiration, there is a regular waxing and waning of heart rate (see Fig. 81). There is no need of therapy directed at these variations of normal rhythm per se, namely, sinus tachycardia (see Fig. 82), sinus bradycardia (see Fig. 83) or sinus arrhythmia. Important causes of excessive tachycardia, such as infectious disease or thyrotoxicosis, should naturally be identified and treated specifically. Sinus bradycardia is in itself usually an asset.

The cardiac arrhythmias are clinically significant for one or more of three reasons. They may (1) cause symptoms, (2) alter cardiac efficiency, and (3) reveal underlying heart disease or other disorder.

Symptoms may or may not be associated with reduced cardiac efficiency; for example, premature beats may be worrisome or annoying and yet have no significant effect on the circulation. Symptoms depend on (1) the nature of the arrhythmia (rate, regularity, and locus of impulse formation), (2) degree and type of underlying heart disease or other disorder, (3) sensitivity of the patient, and (4) complications such as embolism and thrombosis.

Cardiac efficiency may be increased, reduced, or remain unaltered by variations of rhythm. The result depends on the previous state of the circulation and on the nature of the arrhythmia. The sinus tachycardia associated with exercise usually increases cardiac efficiency and, under certain circumstances, the onset of complete atrioventricular block may be beneficial. Extremely fast ventricular rates or gross ventricular arrhythmias, however, reduce cardiac efficiency, and ventricular standstill for even a few seconds produces faintness or collapse.

Some of the cardiac arrhythmias neither cause symptoms nor alter cardiac efficiency, but are important simply because they are *signs of disease*. Bundle branch block and the first stage of atrioventricular heart block are examples.

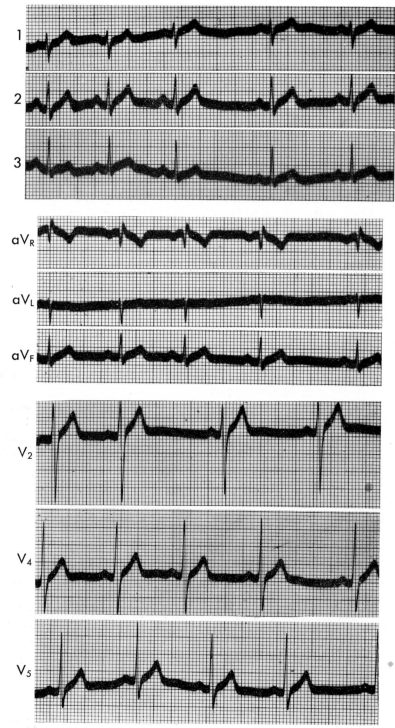

Fig. 81. Sinus arrhythmia.

Sinus arrhythmia in a young man of twenty-two with a normal heart.

INTERPRETATION. This record shows well-marked sinus arrhythmia with the heart rate varying from 80 at its maxi-
mum to 50 at its minimum. There is slight right axis deviation shown in the limb leads, which is well within normal
limits in a young person with a vertical heart position. The individual complexes and time intervals are normal in all
leads. Time intervals in this record and in those to follow are 0.20 and 0.04 second.

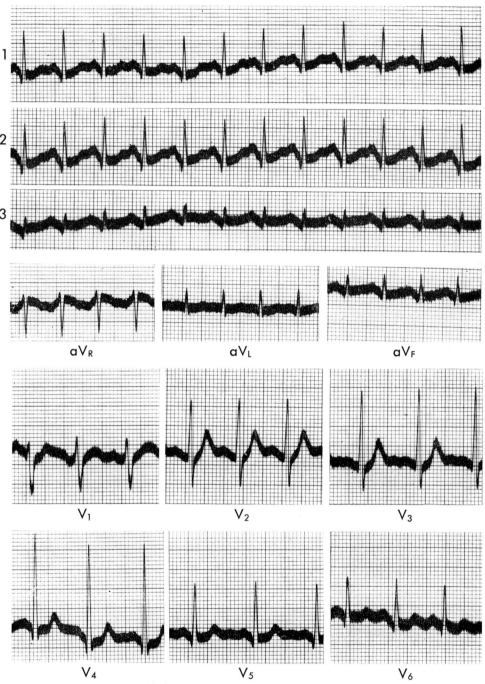

Fig. 82. Sinus (sinoatrial) tachycardia.

Sinus tachycardia in a woman of forty-seven with a normal heart.

INTERPRETATION. Normal rhythm at a rapid rate averaging 145. The *P–R* interval is rather short (0.12 second), consistent with this fast pulse. The *T* waves tend to be somewhat low in the limb leads and in V₆, also consistent with high sympathetic tone. It is of interest to know that at the end of the record, when the precordial leads over the left ventricle were taken, the heart rate had dropped to about 110, which is further confirmatory of variation in the rate of sinus rhythm as opposed to ectopic rhythm.

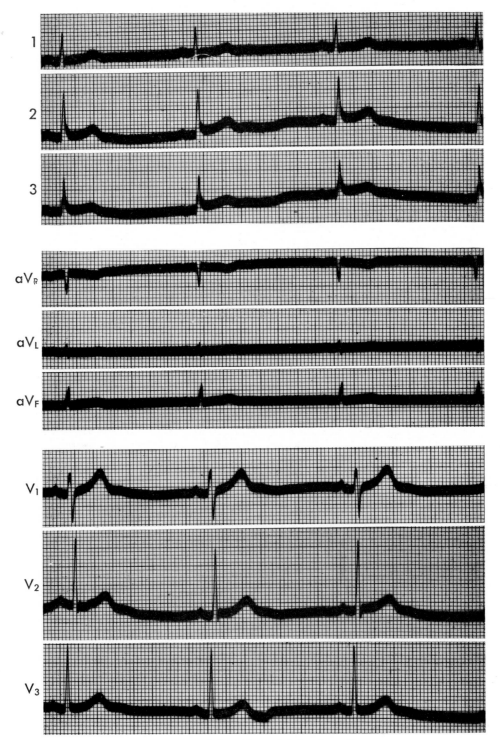

Fig. 83. Sinus (sinoatrial) bradycardia.

Sinus bradycardia in a fifty-seven year old barber with a diagnosis of prepyloric ulcer and a normal heart.

INTERPRETATION. Normal rhythm at a rate of 38 to 40. The *P–R* interval is normal (0.17 second). The *QRS* and *T* waves are normal throughout. There is slight elevation of the *S–T* segments in Leads 2 and 3, an occasional finding normally, especially with a slow heart rate. In the precordial leads there are rather prominent *U* waves that can be seen also, although less well, in the limb leads.

There may be some significance in the relationship of a high vagal tone shown by this patient and the presence of the peptic ulcer.

Sinus Arrhythmia

Sinus arrhythmia consists in a variation of rate of impulses coming from the sinus node, the normal pacemaker of the heart. The commonest type is that found normally in children, especially that associated with breathing. There is a quickening of rate at the beginning of inspiration and a slowing at the beginning of expiration. The atrioventricular conduction, or the *P–R* interval, and the ventricular complexes are completely normal, as are also the *P* waves themselves in all leads. On occasion, however, there may be gross sinus arrhythmia in which there is no relationship to respiration. In such cases the arrhythmia may closely resemble that of atrial fibrillation.

Sinus arrhythmia of slight to moderate degree is a common and entirely unimportant finding. It occurs most prominently in childhood, especially during convalescence from acute infections. When of high degree, it may be a toxic manifestation, as in digitalis or quinidine poisoning, or the result of coronary heart disease in some elderly persons, or it may be an otherwise unexplained vagotonic effect. Rarely it may reach a degree in which there are periods of cardiac standstill long enough to cause faintness or even syncope.

Sinoatrial Block

Sinoatrial block of the first degree consists in complete standstill of the whole heart for an interval approximating that of the time between two ordinary beats or of atrial standstill of that degree with ventricular escape (Figs. 84, 85; see also p. 134). On occasion, however, the standstill may be much longer, lasting for intervals equivalent to the time covering three, four, five or more beats. As in sinus arrhythmia, the *P*, *QRS* and *T* waves and the *P–R* interval are perfectly normal. The commonest type of sinoatrial block is that of the periodic omission of one sinoatrial stimulus with *P* waves not visible in any lead.

The *clinical significance* of sinoatrial block is generally nil. It is a somewhat exaggerated type of sinus arrhythmia. It may, however, be produced by disease or by toxic effect, for example, from digitalis action, and sometimes by carotid sinus pressure through a vagotonic action. In rare cases prolonged standstill of the sinus node results in Adams-Stokes attacks with syncope and convulsions.

The *treatment* of serious sinoatrial block includes omission of any causative toxic agent and a trial of atropine in large dosage parenterally, 0.6 mg. (1/100 grain) or more, or tincture of belladonna by mouth, 1 cc. or 15 minims p.r.n. Rarely in a case of carotid sinus syndrome, carotid sinus denervation should be considered.

Wandering Pacemaker

The term "wandering pacemaker" should be reserved for those rare cases in which the pacemaker varies in its position in the sinoatrial node from its usual site at the head of the node (with clearly upright *P* waves in Leads 1 and 2) to a midposition in the body of the node a centimeter or more below the head (evidenced by lower *P* waves) to a location at the tail of the node a full 2 cm. or more from the head of the node (with flat or even diphasic *P* waves). The lower the position of the pacemaker in the node, the slower its rate as a rule, so that such changes of position in the node tend to be accompanied by varying rates, constituting one type of sinus arrhythmia (see Fig. 86). In some cases the sinus node may cease to function altogether for a varying length of time, the atrioventricular node then assuming the role of pacemaker of the entire heart with slower rate and inverted *P* waves.

The *clinical significance* of a wandering pacemaker is but slight. It is rare and as a rule unimportant, being only of academic interest in most cases. Vagotonia from any cause may induce it, and digitalis is a more common toxic factor than any other specific cause.

The *treatment* would include measures already presented for the therapy of sinoatrial block.

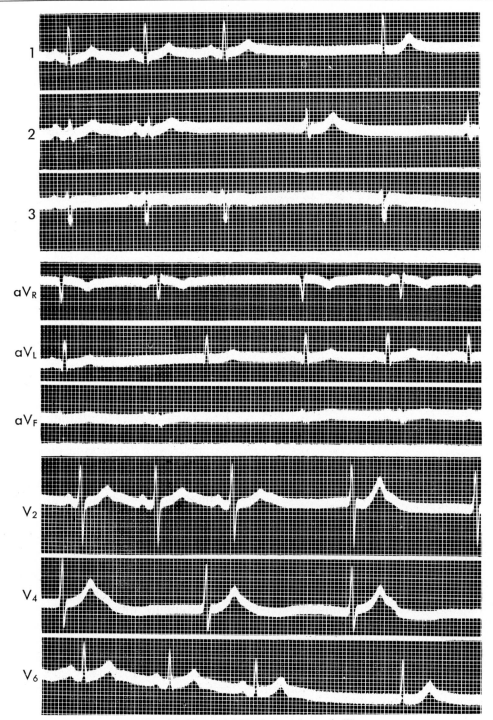

Fig. 84. Sinoatrial block (atrial standstill).

Sinoatrial block in a chef aged fifty-four who had been in and out of atrial fibrillation during the past month. This tracing was taken ten days after cholecystectomy, after which he had received digitalis and quinidine in an attempt to stabilize his heart rhythm.

INTERPRETATION. Marked sinus arrhythmia to the point of actual atrial standstill producing intervals of sinoatrial block. It will be noted that in Lead 1 no *P* wave is clearly seen after the first three. There may be one buried in either *QRS* or *T* wave, but it is possible that the atria are standing still throughout the balance of the strip of Lead 1. The same may be true of Lead 2 after the first two normal *P* waves. The fact that the third *T* is a little higher may not mean that a *P* wave is superimposed on the *T* wave: with a slower heart rate and increased vagus tone the *T* waves are higher normally. In lead V₄ no *P* waves can be distinctly identified; possibly they are superimposed on the descent of the first and third *T* waves.

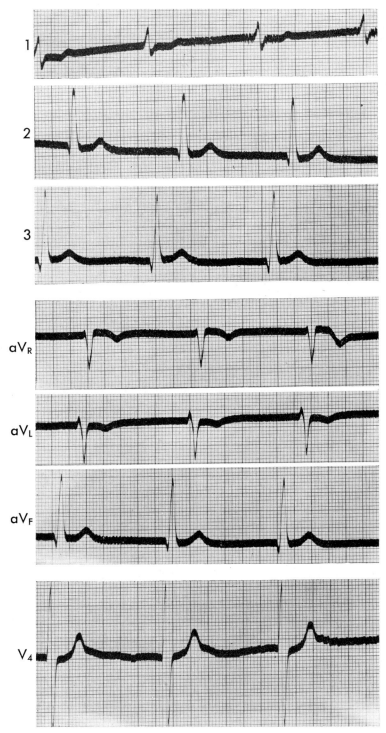

Fig. 85. Atrial standstill.

Atrial standstill in a fifty-five year old insurance collector with hypertensive, coronary heart disease. The tracing shown here was taken on the day of his death in uremia with pulmonary edema.

INTERPRETATION. Regular, probably idioventricular rhythm at a slow rate of 45 to 50, with no evidence of atrial action in any lead. Although it is possible that there are P waves buried in QRS or T waves, it is more likely that the atria are completely paralyzed throughout the time of this record. Two other less likely possibilities are that there is atrioventricular nodal rhythm with inverted P waves buried in the QRS complexes, or that atrial fibrillation with hardly discernible atrial activity is present with complete atrioventricular block. The occasional, slight rapid oscillations of the baseline are doubtless due to tremor (Lead 1) or extraneous current (Lead aVF).

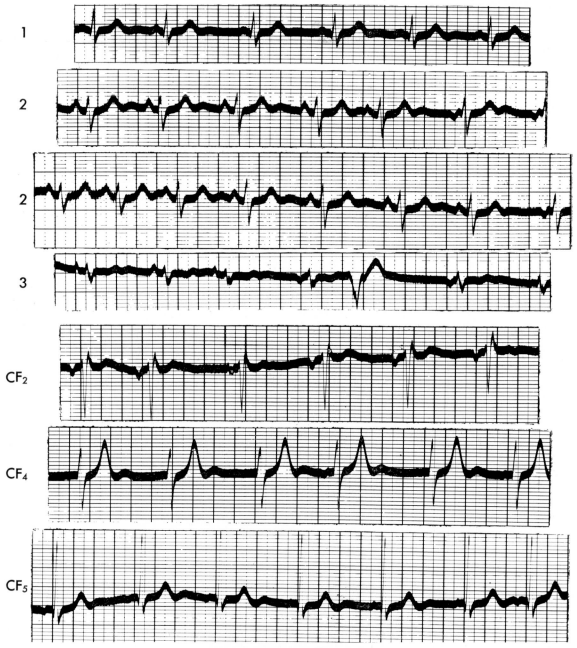

Fig. 86. Wandering pacemaker.

Wandering pacemaker in a woman of fifty-two, with slight cardiac enlargement and possible coronary heart disease. She had had palpitation and choking sensations for a period of twenty years, present almost constantly at this time and related to moving about. For the past year she had experienced "shortness of breath" on carrying bundles or climbing hills, a sensation which disappeared with rest. Although she had been able to play badminton without difficulty during the past year, it was considered possible that she had mild angina pectoris on unusual exertion. She had not been taking digitalis.

INTERPRETATION. Arrhythmia due in part to premature beats (one atrial in Lead 2 and one ventricular in Lead 3) and in part to sinus arrhythmia (best shown in Lead 2) and to shift of the pacemaker either to a low position in the sinus node or to the atrioventricular node (best shown in the last beats of Leads 2 and 3). The *P–R* interval remains fairly constant at 0.12 to 0.15 second when the *P* waves are upright, but with the inverted *P* waves the *P–R* interval is a little shorter. The heart rate averages about 85, varying from 105 to 70. The *QRS* and *T* waves are normal throughout.

This rare disorder of rhythm is of academic interest only. It has been encountered both in persons with heart disease and in those without.

ATRIAL ARRHYTHMIAS

Atrial Premature Beat

An atrial premature beat is shown by the premature occurrence of a *P* wave, almost invariably of abnorma shape and frequently diphasic or even inverted in Leads 1 and 2 (see Fig. 87). It is not followed by a "compensatory pause," as is the usual ventricular premature beat; that is, the time interval between the preceding beat and the following beat is shorter than the sum of systoles and diastoles of two normal beats. This is due to the interruption of the normal building up of the impulse in the sinus node. A technique of spacing the beats of a mechanical graphic record (arteriogram or cardiogram) permits one to distinguish between atrial and ventricular premature beats in most cases, but the electrocardiogram enables one to identify these beats at a glance and thus is easier and more accurate (see Figs. 88, 89).

If premature beats are represented by *P* waves of normal shape, they are called *sinoatrial;* such beats do not differ in significance from the usual type, so far as we know (see Fig. 90). The ventricular response (*QRS* and *T* waves) to an atrial premature beat is as a rule normal; but on occasion, especially in patients with defective conduction, either atrioventricular or bundle branch, there may be either no ventricular response at all or one showing bundle branch block (see Fig. 288, p. 357).

The *clinical significance* of an atrial premature beat is relatively slight, although somewhat greater than that of a ventricular premature beat. If it occurs commonly—that is, every few beats or at least many times a day—it may be troublesome and cause palpitation, but it can occur off and on for many years without doing any harm. It is somewhat more common in persons subject to atrial paroxysmal tachycardia or to atrial fibrillation or flutter than in those not so subject.

Omission of an exciting factor such as tobacco, coffee, indigestion or fatigue often helps when this arrhythmia is disturbing, and, if necessary, the administration of quinidine sulfate, 0.2 gm. (3 grains) orally p.r.n., triple bromides, 0.5 to 1 gm. (7½ to 15 grains), or both.

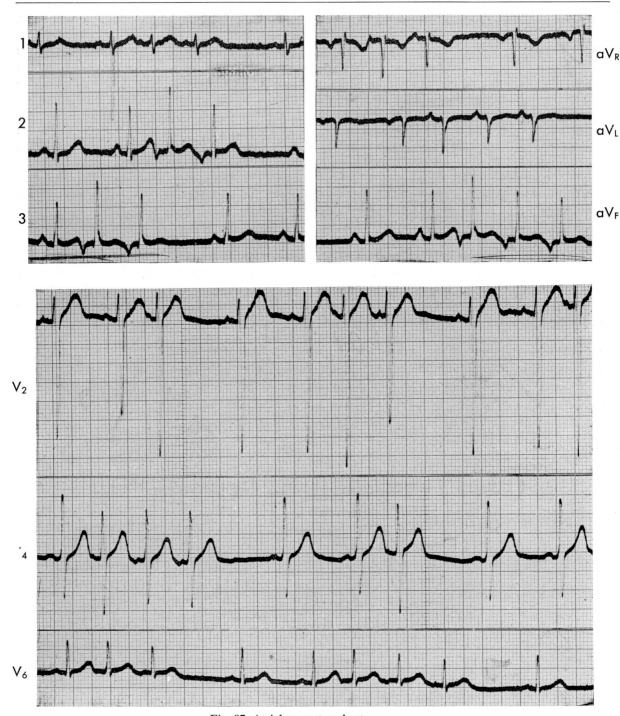

Fig. 87. Atrial premature beats.

Atrial premature beats with inverted *P's* in a boy of eighteen with a normal heart. This patient had been subject to episodes of ectopic atrial tachycardia since the age of thirteen. He was taking quinidine, 3 grains twice daily, at the time of the electrocardiogram shown here. He was not aware of the irregular heart rhythm manifested thereon, which was due to single or multiple premature beats and was dispelled by exercise.

INTERPRETATION. Frequent atrial premature beats in runs of two to four. The heart rate during normal rhythm, of which there are relatively few beats, is approximately 65. During the runs of atrial premature beats the rate has increased to about 140. The *P* waves of the atrial premature beats are clearly abnormal, being inverted in Leads 2, 3 and aV_F and upright in aV_R and aV_L. The *P* waves are less well marked in the precordial leads; that is the usual finding. The ventricular complexes are not remarkable.

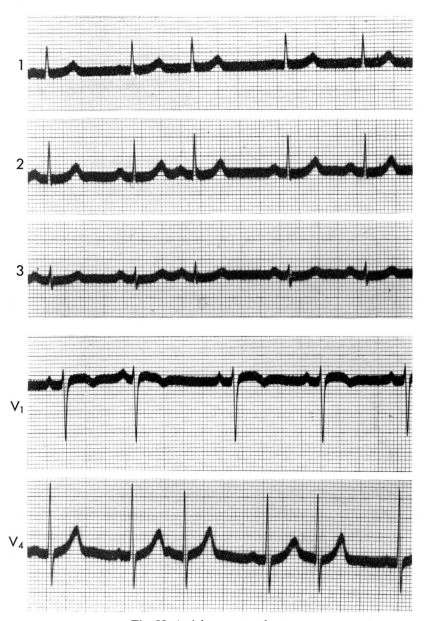

Fig. 88. Atrial premature beats.

Atrial premature beats in a sixty-nine year old man with coronary heart disease and benign prostatic hypertrophy.

INTERPRETATION. Occasional atrial premature beats interrupting otherwise normal rhythm at a rate of 70. The abnormal *P* waves differ only slightly in shape from the usual *P* waves. For example, in Leads 1 and V$_4$ the premature *P* wave is isoelectric instead of being slightly upright; in Leads 2, 3 and V$_1$ it is a little broader and more notched than the usual *P* wave. The *QRS* and *T* waves are normal throughout.

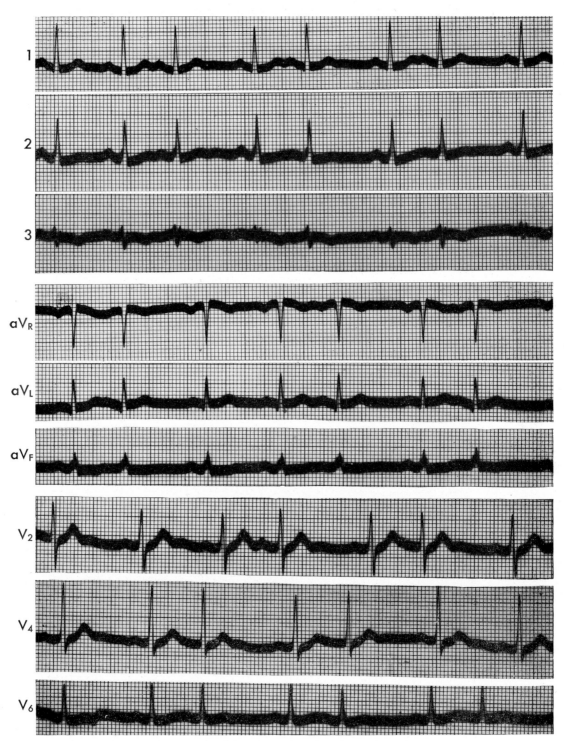

Fig. 89. Atrial premature beats.

Atrial premature beats in a man of forty-nine complaining of irregularity of heart rhythm.

INTERPRETATION. Frequently bigeminal rhythm due to atrial premature beats occurring as a rule every other beat at a heart rate of 85. The premature *P* waves are slightly different in shape from the normal.

These two examples (Figs. 88, 89) show the more common type of premature *P* waves in contrast to the inverted *P* waves (Fig. 87) which were at one time considered classical.

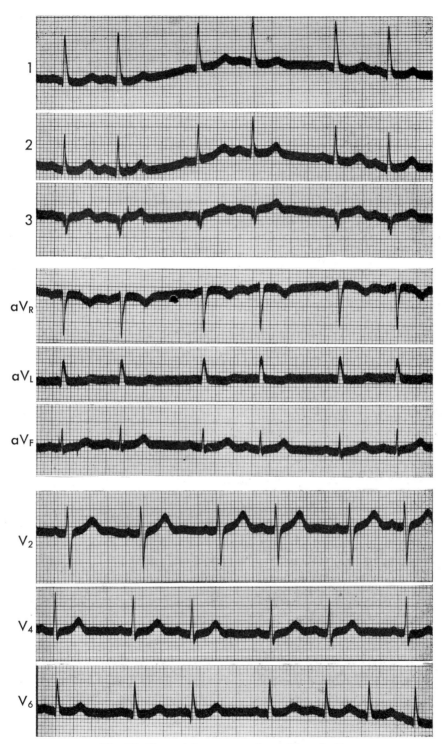

Fig. 90. Sinoatrial premature beats (bigeminal).

Sinoatrial premature beats producing bigeminy in a woman of seventy-nine with carcinoma of the cecum. (She was discharged home improved after right colectomy.)

INTERPRETATION. Frequent bigeminy due to atrial premature beats every other beat, at a heart rate of 80. The fact that the premature P waves have the same shape as the normal indicates that the starting point is in, or close to, the sinoatrial node. In the precordial leads there is some variation in the rhythm: in V_2 and V_4 there are only two premature beats; in V_6 there are four, the last three sequential.

Atrial Paroxysmal Tachycardia

This disorder of rhythm is indicated by the rapid regular occurrence of abnormal *P* waves in the electrocardiogram (inverted, diphasic or upright, depending on the lead) at rates ranging from 100 up to 200 or somewhat more, but usually at a lesser range of 140 to 180. The onset and offset are abrupt as a rule. The ventricular complexes are generally of normal configuration and the atrioventricular conduction time also normal, but variations occur, as, for example, bundle branch block and various grades of atrioventricular block, transiently or constantly. After an attack of atrial paroxysmal tachycardia the *T* waves may be reversed for a few hours or days, apparently a "fatigue" phenomenon (this is also true of ventricular paroxysmal tachycardia). The term "nomotopic" has been applied to a paroxysm which shows *P* waves of normal shape apparently arising in or near the sinoatrial node. See Figures 91 to 96 for examples of atrial paroxysmal tachycardia.

The *clinical significance* of atrial paroxysmal tachycardia is as a rule not great. It has chiefly a nuisance value, but it may in the presence of actual heart disease precipitate or aggravate coronary or myocardial insufficiency. A status anginosus persisting throughout the duration of the paroxysm may occur in the face of serious coronary heart disease and be mistaken for acute myocardial infarction, or long-continuing pulmonary edema may be found when the left ventricular myocardium is weak. The paroxysms themselves vary from brief, infrequent, quite unimportant attacks to prolonged, weekly or daily attacks that are incapacitating.

The *treatment* will vary according to the amount of trouble occasioned. Reassurance is usually the most important therapy, along with the measures mentioned, especially the use of quinidine sulfate, for the treatment of disturbing atrial premature beats when necessary.

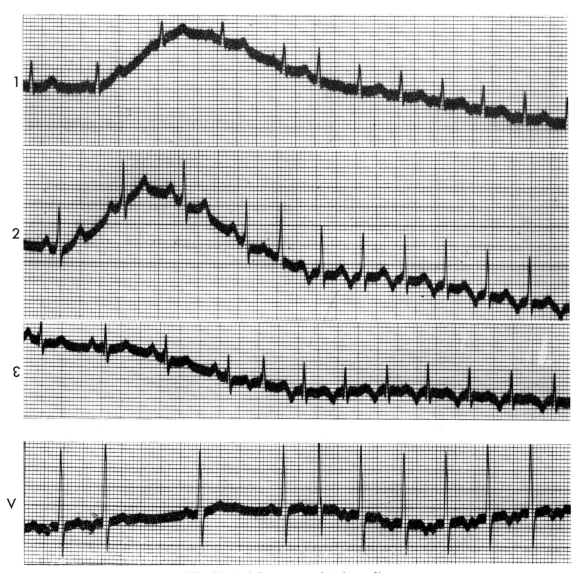

Fig. 91. Atrial paroxysmal tachycardia.

Atrial paroxysmal tachycardia (with inverted *P's*) in an eight year old boy with an appendiceal abscess upon whom surgery was contemplated. The patient was digitalized prior to operation, and an appendicectomy was successfully performed despite an episode of tachycardia during the procedure. Atrial premature beats and further bouts of tachycardia were observed subsequently by electrocardiogram.

INTERPRETATION. In each of the four leads presented there appears the onset of a paroxysm of atrial tachycardia, initiated by *P* waves which are deeply inverted in Leads 2 and 3 in contrast to the normal *P* waves. In Lead V$_4$ there is also seen the termination of a paroxysm. The heart rate during the normal rhythm averages 90; during the paroxysms the rate is about 140. The *QRS* and *T* waves are essentially normal throughout, except for lowering and apparent late inversion of the latter during the paroxysm in Lead V$_4$.

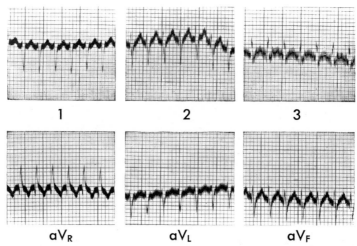

Fig. 92. Atrial paroxysmal tachycardia.

Atrial paroxysmal tachycardia at a rapid rate in a twelve day old male infant without evidence of heart disease prior to the onset of this attack (February 24, 1949). The infant responded to cedilanid with a drop in heart rate from 350 to 150 and improvement in heart sounds and in color. There were no murmurs. By March 1 it was no longer necessary to keep him in an oxygen tent; his pulse rate was regular at 110 to 140. An x-ray film of the chest on February 25 showed the heart to be definitely enlarged, with a cardiothoracic ratio of 6.7:9.4 cm., but upon re-examination by roentgenogram five days later the heart size was normal as was also its configuration. The infant was continued on digitoxin until his discharge home on March 4.

INTERPRETATION. Extreme atrial tachycardia at a rate of 350, with otherwise normal complexes in all six limb leads. There is well-marked right axis deviation, normally found during the first week or two after birth. This record is characteristic of the instances of extreme tachycardia in infants, on occasion responsible for serious cardiac enlargement and failure, as described by John Hubbard in 1941 (Am. J. Dis. Child., *61:* 687, 1941).

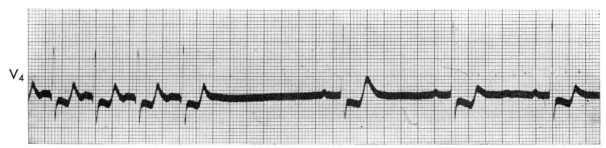

Fig. 93. Atrial paroxysmal tachycardia, showing end of paroxysm.

Atrial paroxysmal tachycardia with end of paroxysm in a man of sixty-nine with coronary heart disease and angina pectoris which followed probable myocardial infarction two years before. The heart was enlarged. A_2 was greater than P_2, and there were no murmurs. The lungs were clear. The liver was not palpable. The patient was receiving digitoxin at the time of the electrocardiogram shown here.

Although he was considered a moderately poor operative risk, it was believed that he could tolerate radical surgery for carcinoma of the prostate. A perineal operation was carried out on March 30, 1949, and he was discharged home, his condition unchanged, on April 5, on digitoxin therapy.

INTERPRETATION. The termination of a paroxysm of atrial tachycardia at a rate of 125 is shown. The ectopic *P* waves are difficult to identify, but are probably represented by the slight depressions of the baseline following the *T* waves. After an interval of nearly two seconds, sinus rhythm returns at a slow rate of 45 to 50. The *S–T* segments are deeply depressed throughout. The *T* wave in the first normal beat after the long pause following the termination of the paroxysm is unusually high, a common finding after prolonged cardiac standstill.

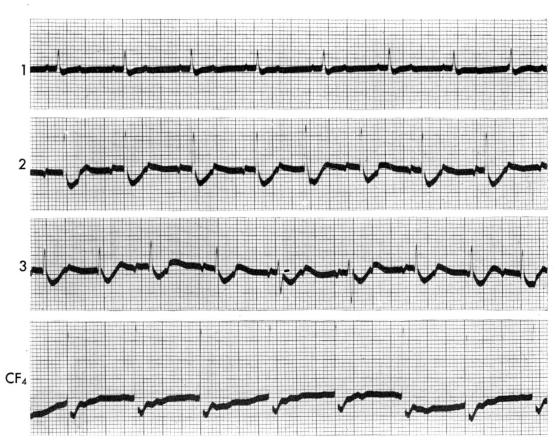

Fig. 94. Atrial paroxysmal tachycardia, with 2:1 block.

Sudden arrhythmia in a woman of sixty-two during the course of hospitalization for malnutrition and avitaminosis. This electrocardiogram, showing an atrial paroxysmal tachycardia with 2:1 atrioventricular block, was taken on September 4, 1949. The heart was not remarkable save for occasional extrasystoles until this day, when, one half hour after the administration of a final digitalizing dose of cedilanid, a grossly irregular rhythm was noted. She was maintained thereafter on digalen without further cardiac abnormality until her death on September 20. Postmortem examination confirmed the diagnosis of sprue.

INTERPRETATION. Atrial paroxysmal tachycardia with atrioventricular block, mostly 2:1, but occasionally 3:2. The atrial rate is 170, the ventricular rate 85 during 2:1 block and 114 during 3:2 block. The P waves are plainly ectopic, being inverted in Leads 2 and 3. The S–T segments are deeply depressed in Leads 2 and 3, and the T waves are flat throughout. This abnormality of the S–T segments and T waves is confirmatory of serious myocardial depression.

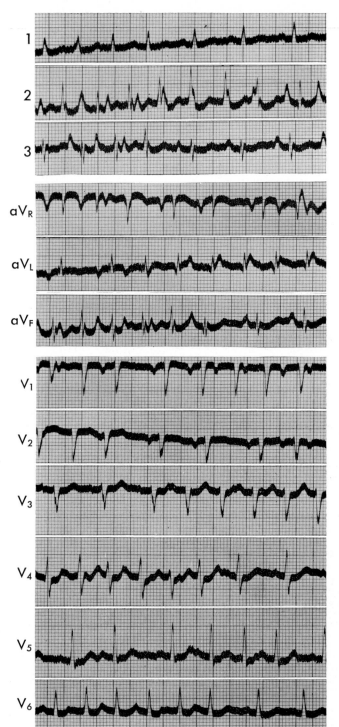

Fig. 95. Atrial paroxysmal tachycardia.

Atrial paroxysmal tachycardia, a variation, in a fifty-one year old carpenter with the diagnoses of alcoholism, gastritis and malnutrition. The patient was apparently unaware of the cardiac irregularity manifested in this tracing, taken on the day following hospital admission.

INTERPRETATION. Unusual type of tachycardia and arrhythmia associated with a fast atrial rate averaging about 160. There are a few normal beats, as indicated particularly in the last three beats of Lead 1, at a rate of 95 to 100. There is some ventricular arrhythmia during the paroxysm of atrial tachycardia, due apparently to atrioventricular block, the P–R interval varying from 0.16 to 0.28 second. On occasion the abnormal P waves are blocked altogether, which is true of the third from the last P wave in Lead 2: this P wave falls just prior to the R. The next ventricular response is delayed and at a normal time interval after the P wave which succeeds the blocked P. This variation of conduction time produces at times a bizarre superimposition of P waves on R waves. The T waves are not remarkable. The ectopic P waves are abnormally high and sharp in Leads 2 and 3.

(Legend continued from facing page, Figure 96)

C (January 31, 1951), Extreme tachycardia apparently of atrial origin in this same patient, with wide ventricular complexes closely resembling those in Lead 2 of the records shown in *A* and *B*. The heart rate on the average exceeds 300 during the first part of the paroxysm, but there is some arrhythmia, which may be that of atrial fibrillation. During the early part of the paroxysm shown here the rate is about 330 per minute. Also during this paroxysm there is at times apparently an alternation of amplitude of the *QRS* and *T* waves, although it is difficult to identify the *T* waves because of the extreme tachycardia. Arrhythmia of the ventricular responses is evident, particularly during the latter half of the tracing, when there is a slower heart rate averaging about 200.

This patient, a characteristic case of the Wolff-Parkinson-White syndrome (see Fig. 141), had had infrequent paroxysms of atrial tachycardia for a number of years. The final and fatal paroxysm occurred nine days after the death of her husband, which had resulted from acute fulminating myocardial infarction. Death occurred within an hour of the onset of this paroxysm. Postmortem examination of the heart showed no pathologic change. The heart weight was 310 gm.

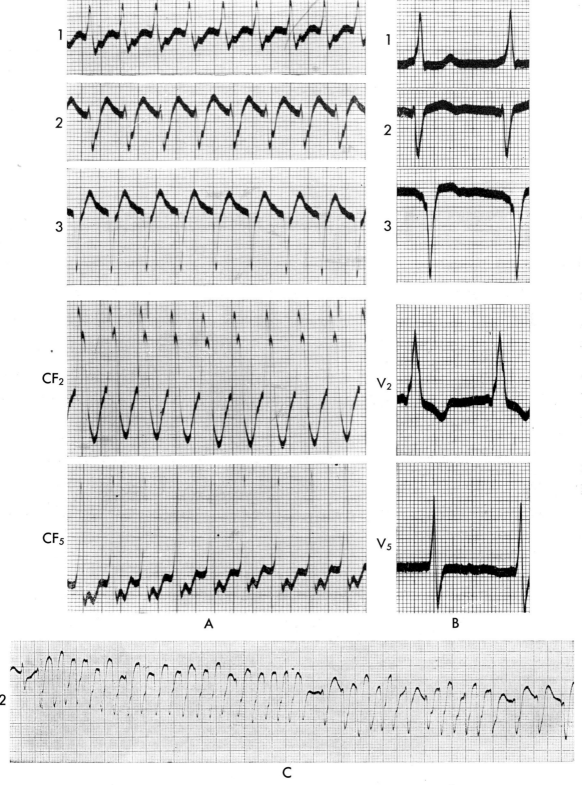

Fig. 96. Atrial paroxysmal tachycardia in Wolff-Parkinson-White syndrome.

A, Atrial paroxysmal tachycardia in a case of Wolff-Parkinson-White syndrome with otherwise normal heart in a woman aged forty-three. *B*, Tracing taken two years later showing normal rhythm in the Wolff-Parkinson-White syndrome. *C*, Tracing taken three years later, about fifteen to twenty minutes before sudden death during tachycardia.

INTERPRETATION. *A* (July 21, 1948), Atrial paroxysmal tachycardia at a heart rate of 160 with ectopic *P* waves falling on the *S–T* segments, and wide *QRS* waves characteristic of the Wolff-Parkinson-White syndrome.

B (July 3, 1950), Normal rhythm at a rate of 65, short *P–R* interval of about 0.08 second, and wide *QRS* waves with typical slurred upstrokes in Lead 1. *(Legend continued on opposite page)*

Atrial Flutter

Atrial flutter is shown electrocardiographically by an excessively rapid regular sequence of *P* waves of abnormal shape, consisting in Lead 2, as a rule, of constant oscillations of the baseline of diphasic nature without intervening level intervals, making it difficult or impossible in that lead, at least, to determine the time of onset or offset of the impulses, although in leads over the atria clear-cut individual complexes can be identified. The atrial rate varies from 200 to 360 (averaging 300) and is accompanied generally by 2 to 1 atrioventricular block, thus giving a ventricular rate of 100 to 180 (averaging 150). Rarely there is a 1 to 1 rhythm, with extreme tachycardia, and sometimes, especially after digitalis therapy, there are higher grades of block, particularly 4 to 1, which produce a regular pulse rhythm at a normal rate, that is, 60 to 80 per minute. The grade of block may be irregular, and this disorder of rhythm may then resemble that of atrial fibrillation except in the electrocardiogram, which permits quick identification. Once in a while the ventricular complexes may change, as a result of fatigue, particularly to those of bundle branch block during the more rapid heart rates. Ventricular premature beats or paroxysmal tachycardia, constant bundle branch block, or even complete heart block, may coincidentally complicate atrial flutter. See Figures 97, 98, 99 for examples of atrial flutter.

The *clinical significance* of atrial flutter is about midway between that of atrial paroxysmal tachycardia and that of atrial fibrillation. It may occur in the presence of heart disease, or it may disturb an otherwise normal heart. The more serious the heart disease and the faster the ventricular rate in atrial flutter, the more likely are important symptoms and signs, in particular congestive heart failure and coronary insufficiency, to supervene. Atrial flutter is as a rule paroxysmal, but the paroxysms are generally longer in duration than are those of atrial tachycardia, sometimes lasting for weeks, months or even years, and they tend to be more resistant to therapy with quinidine, digitalis, or other drugs. Indeed, they are not infrequently more difficult to abolish or to modify than is atrial fibrillation itself. The mechanism, at one time attributed to a circus movement about the sinoatrial node, has in recent years been ascribed to excitation from one focus ("ectopic"), as in paroxysmal tachycardia, but at a much more rapid rate.

The *prevention* of paroxysms of atrial flutter is best effected by omission or amelioration of exciting factors and by the use of quinidine sulfate orally.

The *treatment* of established atrial flutter is preferably by digitalization to increase the grade of atrioventricular block, to induce atrial fibrillation, or in some cases to help restore normal rhythm, with or without the aid of quinidine.

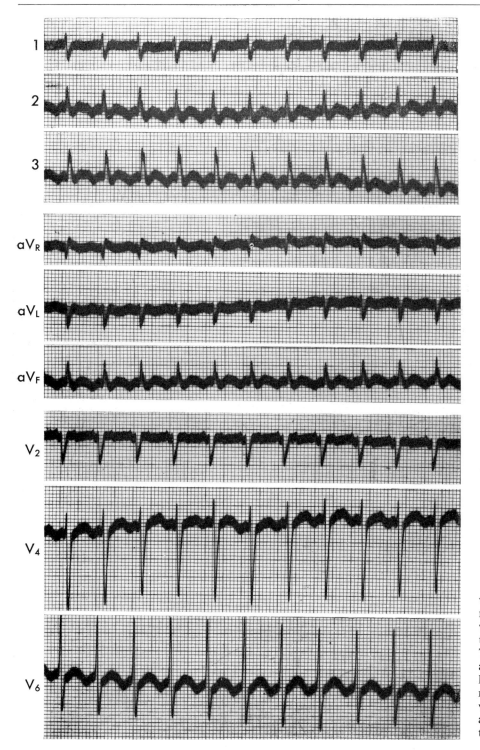

Fig. 97. Atrial flutter.

Atrial flutter with 2:1 ventricular response in a retired crane-operator with emphysema, bronchitis and acute heart failure. The patient improved on a course of cedilanid followed by digitalis leaf in maintenance dosage. He was not receiving digitalis at the time this record was taken.

INTERPRETATION. Atrial flutter with 2:1 block, atrial rate 290, ventricular rate 145; slight right axis deviation shown in the limb leads with prominent S waves in V_4 and R waves in V_6. The T waves are low throughout, essentially flat in Lead 1, but slightly upright in Leads 2, 3, V_4, and V_6. The flutter waves are best seen in Leads 2 and 3 with R waves superimposed on the middle of every other P wave.

This record is characteristic, so far as rhythm is concerned, of the electrocardiographic finding in atrial flutter as usually first discovered in any case. There is almost invariably 2:1 atrioventricular block, and these rates of close to 300 for the atria and 150 for the ventricles are the rule. Digitalis, the therapy of choice, results in improvement by increasing the grade of block. The right axis deviation here may have been due to heart position rather than to any intrinsic heart disease.

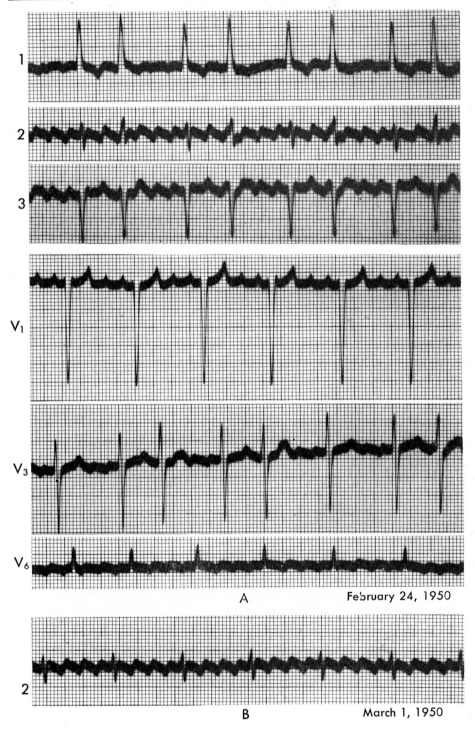

Fig. 98. Atrial flutter.

Atrial flutter in a sixty-seven year old salesman with carcinoma of the lung. On February 7, 1950, an electrocardiogram showed normal rhythm with a long *P–R* interval of 0.24 second. Pneumonectomy was performed on February 17, and the patient was given quinidine prophylactically thereafter. On February 22 an electrocardiogram demonstrated probable atrial flutter with 2:1 block at an average ventricular rate of 150. At this time digitoxin was started. The tracing shown in *A* was taken on February 24; the block varies, is generally 4:1, sometimes alternating with 2:1. *B*, taken on March 1, shows a constant 4:1 block. The patient was discharged on March 8, with atria still fluttering in 4:1 block, on digitalis therapy. It seemed unwise at this time to attempt reversion to normal rhythm with large doses of quinidine.

A   February 24, 1950

B   March 1, 1950

INTERPRETATION. *A*, Atrial flutter with varying grades of block, from 2:1 to 4:1; atrial rate 320, with ventricular rate varying from 160 to 80. There is left axis deviation shown by the limb leads, with inversion of the *T* waves in Lead 1, prominent *S* waves in Lead V₁, and flat *T* waves in V₆.

B, Atrial flutter with 4:1 block; atrial rate 320, ventricular rate 80.

These two records, *A* and *B*, are characteristic of the evolution of atrial flutter, in the course of treatment, from the 2:1 block shown in Figure 97 to a satisfactory heart rate, with or without later return to normal rhythm or change to atrial fibrillation. Digitalis is responsible for this favorable evolution.

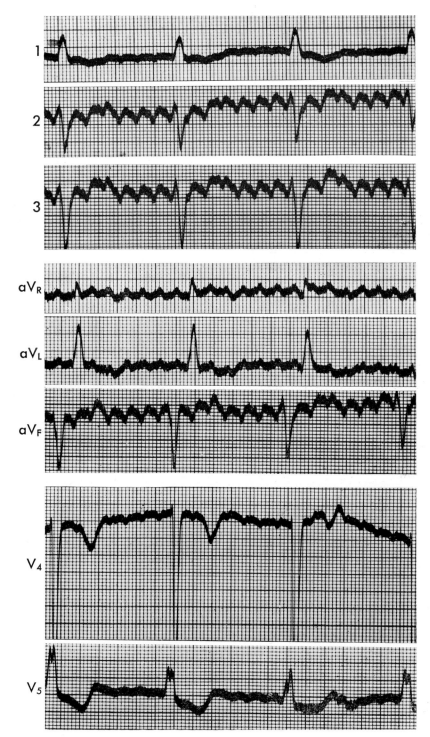

Fig. 99. Atrial flutter, with atrioventricular and left bundle branch block.

Atrial flutter with 7:1 atrioventricular block and left bundle branch block in a man of seventy-eight with infectious hepatitis, congestive failure on a basis of hypertensive, coronary heart disease, and benign prostatic hypertrophy. He was maintained on a dosage of 0.1 mg. of digitoxin daily.

INTERPRETATION. Atrial flutter with high grade atrioventricular block, probably partial, at 7:1, although complete dissociation is a possibility. The atrial rate is 300, the ventricular rate 44. There is also left bundle branch block, as indicated by the wide upright R waves in Lead 1 and wide notched R waves in Lead V₅. The T waves are slightly inverted in Lead 1, low in the other leads except for deep inversion in Lead V₄ and moderate inversion in Lead V₅.

This record is characteristic of the effect of age, with coronary obstruction producing both atrioventricular block and bundle branch block. The small dose of digitalis is not alone adequate to explain the high grade of atrioventricular block.

Atrial Fibrillation

Closely related to atrial flutter in mechanism, but much more common and much more often chronic, is fibrillation of the atria. In the electrocardiogram it is shown by two characteristics: (1) rapid and generally uncoordinated atrial complexes, of varying size and shape in most leads except those directly over the atria (right sternal precordial and esophageal leads), where regular, uniform waves may be shown at rates varying as a rule between 300 and 500 per minute; and (2) grossly irregular and rapid ventricular rates, but with normal ventricular complexes as a rule. The ventricular rate may be reduced by digitalis or disease to increase the grade of atrioventricular block, and the atrial rate may also be changed by drugs, e.g., quinidine to lower and regularize its rate and to transform the arrhythmia to that of atrial flutter. See Figures 100, 101, 102, 103, 104, 105 for examples of atrial fibrillation.

The *clinical significance* of atrial fibrillation has long been recognized. Although it may occur as a short paroxysm lasting a few minutes or a few hours in an otherwise normal heart irritated by temporary nervous or toxic factors, it is much more often of long duration and usually permanent in a person with heart disease or atrial strain, especially mitral stenosis. However, with proper control of the ventricular rate by digitalis, atrial fibrillation may persist for many years without doing any harm, although on occasion arterial embolism may complicate this arrhythmia because of the tendency for stasis to develop and for thrombi to form in the fibrillating left atrium.

Atrial Flutter-Fibrillation

This term has been applied to an arrhythmia which is midway between flutter and fibrillation, less regular in both atrial and ventricular rhythms than flutter, and behaving clinically more like fibrillation. It has also been called "coarse atrial fibrillation" and "impure atrial flutter." The distinction is not of much importance. See Figures 106 and 107.

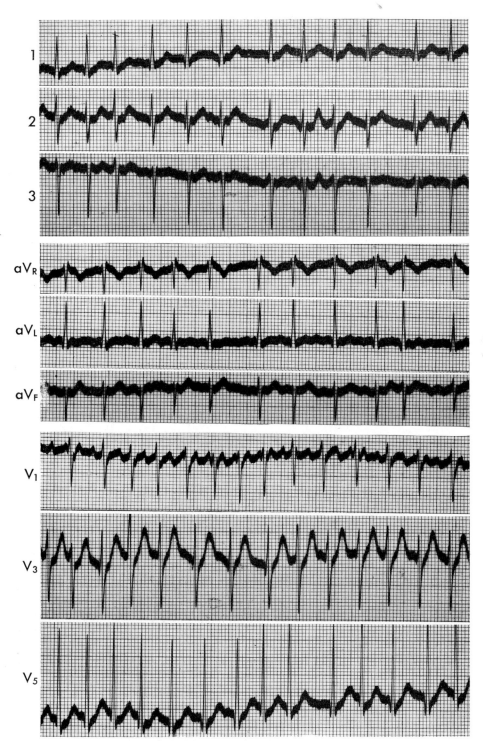

Fig. 100. Paroxysmal atrial fibrillation.

Uncontrolled atrial fibrillation in a woman of seventy-four with a toxic nodular goiter and a basal metabolic rate of plus 16 (pulse of 96; weight 54.2 kilograms) on this occasion. The tracing shown here was taken at 10:45 A.M. Two hours later, after five to ten minutes of lying recumbent, her pulse was checked and the rhythm was observed to be regular at 90. Normal rhythm, with the *P–R* interval prolonged to 0.22 second, in an electrocardiogram on the following day confirmed this impression of paroxysmal atrial fibrillation.

INTERPRETATION. Paroxysmal atrial fibrillation of coarse type with atrial complexes best seen as usual in precordial lead V₁. The atrial rate is 400, and the ventricular rate rapid and irregular, averaging 190. There is slight left axis deviation with high *R* waves in Lead V₅. The *T* waves are low in the limb leads.

This record is characteristic of paroxysmal atrial fibrillation of coarse type, such as is commonly encountered in the early stages of this arrhythmia. It can be found in thyrotoxicosis or in many other conditions. Thyrotoxicosis was apparently the causative factor here.

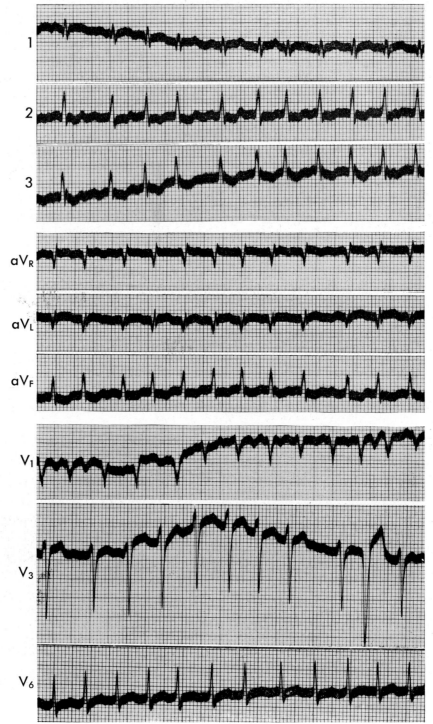

Fig. 101. Atrial fibrillation.

Atrial fibrillation with rapid ventricular rate in a man of sixty-five with diagnoses of coronary heart disease and a dissecting aneurysm of the abdominal and thoracic aortas. He was digitalized with subsequent restoration of rhythm to normal, but died five days after admission from rupture of the aneurysm into the left pleural cavity.

INTERPRETATION. Atrial fibrillation with uncontrolled ventricular rate of 160 to 170. There is absolute arrhythmia, although on a few occasions the intervals between beats are nearly equal. Otherwise there is no abnormality, except for unusually low T waves, which can be, in part at least, ascribed to the fast heart rate and effect of sympathetic stimulation. Oscillation of the baseline due to the atrial fibrillation is best seen in Lead V₁ (over the right atrium).

This is a characteristic record of atrial fibrillation before treatment in the presence of serious heart disease. However, such a record can be found also without actual organic cardiovascular disease.

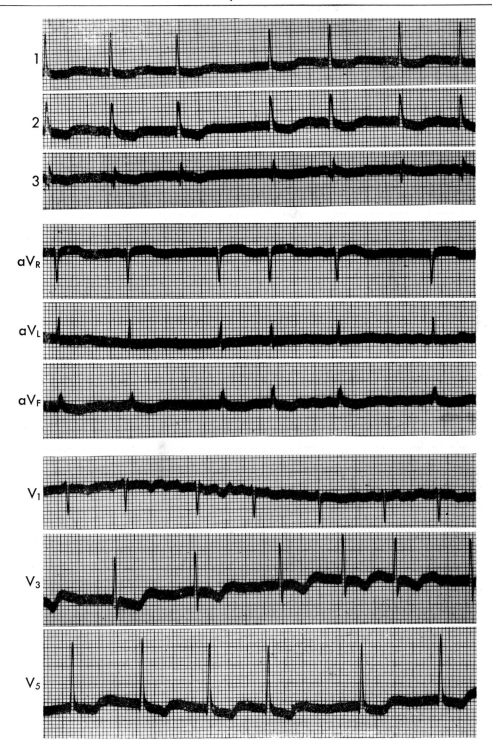

Fig. 102. Chronic atrial fibrillation.

Atrial fibrillation, chronic, with little atrial action in a seventy-five year old carpenter with coronary heart disease receiving daily digitalis.

INTERPRETATION. Atrial fibrillation with little evidence of atrial action except in Lead V_1, where oscillations at a rate of 300-odd can be seen, particularly after the second and third ventricular complexes. The ventricular rate is well controlled at an average of 75 to 80. The $S-T$ segments are depressed in Leads 1, 2, aVF, V_3 and V_5, and the T waves are much flattened in these leads, doubtless owing in the main to the effect of digitalis.

This record is characteristic of atrial fibrillation of long duration with the ventricular rate well controlled by digitalis action.

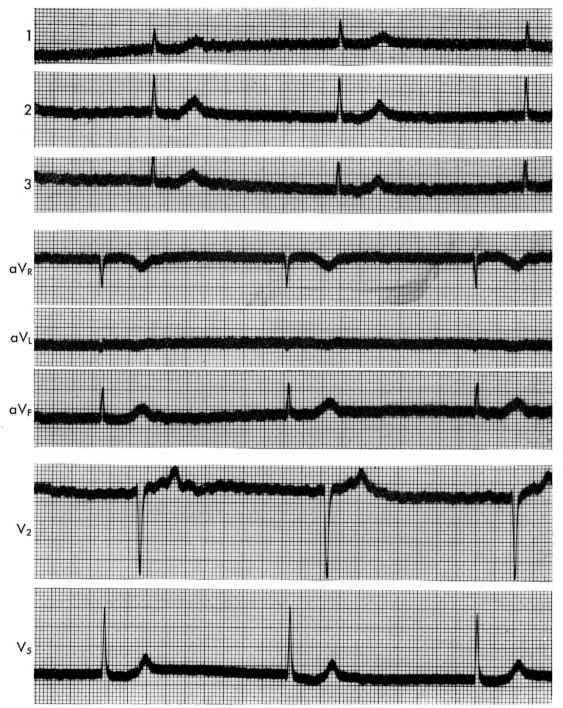

Fig. 103. Atrial fibrillation with complete block.

Atrial fibrillation with complete heart block in a sixty-four year old carpenter with chronic cystitis. The patient had had no symptoms of myocardial or coronary insufficiency, or of dizziness, syncope or paralysis, and no past history of rheumatic fever or diphtheria. There was a Grade 1 apical systolic murmur. The arrhythmia was thought most likely to be on the basis of coronary heart disease, and in preparation for cystoscopy epinephrine in oil (1:500) was suggested as a precaution against the occurrence of an Adams-Stokes attack. Digitalis was considered unnecessary, and quinidine contraindicated.

INTERPRETATION. Atrial fibrillation with complete atrioventricular block. The atrial action is poorly seen except in Lead V_2, where an atrial rate of 400 is evident. The ventricular rate is very slow at about 32, characteristic of idioventricular rhythm. The T waves are well marked, and the Q–T interval is considerably prolonged (0.56 second), as should be expected at this heart rate.

This record showing complete atrioventricular block complicating atrial fibrillation, although uncommon, is now and then encountered in old age, doubtless in large part due to coronary heart disease.

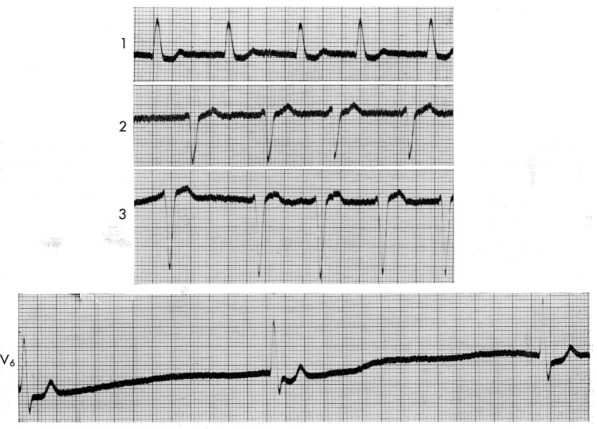

Fig. 104. Atrial fibrillation with slowing of ventricular rate by vomiting.

Atrial fibrillation in a man of seventy-nine years, following an intracapsular cataract extraction of the left eye. He was getting digitalis postoperatively, and for the past ten years had been taking this drug (with an increase from one pill to two daily during the week prior to admission). Two days after the operation he complained of distress in his left chest. While the electrocardiogram shown here was being taken, the patient vomited, and the subsequent slowing of his heart rate is recorded thereon. The chest pain persisted until the following day. Further diagnoses included coronary heart disease with atrial fibrillation, chronic pulmonary emphysema and fibrosis, and bronchiectasis.

INTERPRETATION. Atrial fibrillation with somewhat less irregular heart rhythm than when the ventricular rate is faster. The rate averages 80. There are wide QRS waves indicative probably of left bundle branch block. The T waves in Lead 1 are low but upright. Lead V_6 shows a marked slowing of the ventricles to a rate of about 24 from an excess of vagal action at the time of the vomiting. This slow rate is not completely regular.

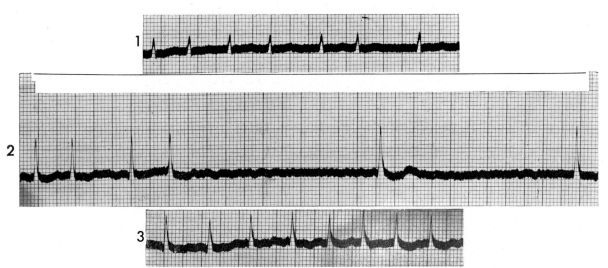

Fig. 105. Atrial fibrillation with slowing of ventricular rate by carotid sinus pressure (as indicated by white strip at top ot Lead 2).

Atrial fibrillation, preoperatively, in a seventy-five year old man with adenocarcinoma of the epiglottis. He had had no cardiac symptoms and no medication. There was no evidence of congestive failure. Upon left carotid sinus pressure the rate slowed, as demonstrated in this figure. Digitalization was instituted, and a laryngoscopy with biopsy was performed successfully under local anesthesia on the following day.

INTERPRETATION. Atrial fibrillation with rather rapid heart rate averaging about 120. During the taking of Lead 2 there was marked slowing of the ventricular rate by carotid sinus pressure to about 25. The T waves are low in all three leads.

COMMENT. Figures 104 and 105 show the pronounced vagal effect of different factors on the ventricular rate despite the presence of atrial fibrillation. In Figure 104 the vagotonic factor was associated with vomiting, and in Figure 105 with carotid sinus pressure (as signaled by white strip at top of Lead 2).

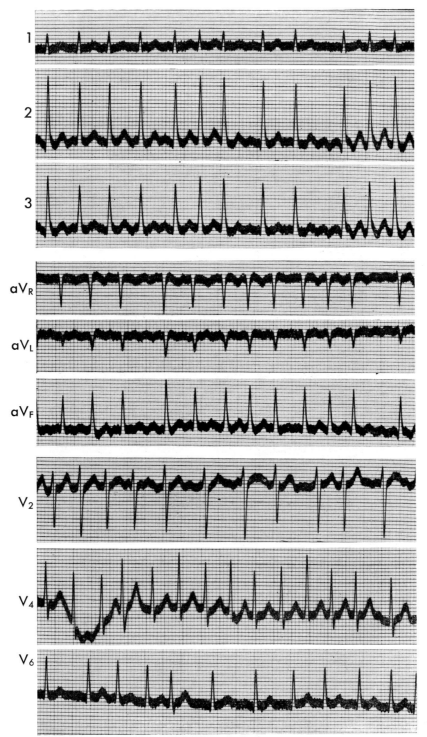

Fig. 106. Atrial flutter-fibrillation.

Atrial flutter-fibrillation in a retired porter of seventy-eight years with coronary heart disease and benign prostatic hypertrophy, for which a transurethral resection was later performed. Prior to this operation the heart rhythm was controlled by digitalis therapy. A follow-up electrocardiogram seven months later showed a return to normal rhythm.

INTERPRETATION. Rapid atrial arrhythmia of flutter-fibrillation type, with atrial rate shown by coarse complexes throughout, averaging about 400. The ventricular rate is regular and fast at a rate averaging 170. There is a tendency toward slight right axis deviation, probably due to a vertical heart position. The T waves are normal throughout.

This record is characteristic of early instances of coarse atrial fibrillation before therapy has been started, in which the rhythm closely resembles that of flutter. This condition has been labeled flutter-fibrillation.

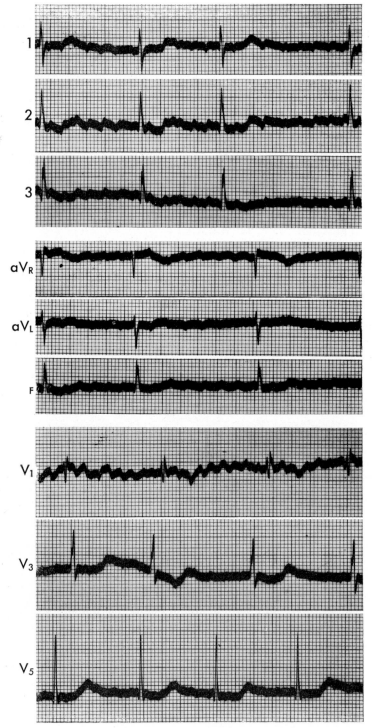

Fig. 107. Atrial flutter-fibrillation.

Atrial flutter-fibrillation in a woman of forty-two with the diagnosis of cirrhosis of the liver ascribed to chronic congestion and with cardiac enlargement and failure of undetermined cause. Electrocardiograms in the past had demonstrated atrial flutter with partial atrioventricular block. She had been taking "one digitalis leaf pill daily."

INTERPRETATION. Atrial fibrillation of coarse type, sometimes called flutter-fibrillation, with high grade atrioventricular block. The atrial rate, best counted in Lead V_1, is about 440. The ventricular rate is slow for this rhythm and averages 55 to 60. The S–T segments are depressed in Leads 1, 2, aVF, V_3 and V_5, suggesting a digitalis effect.

This instance of atrial fibrillation, of coarse type and probably relatively recent, illustrates the vigorous action of digitalis in inducing a high grade partial block and the establishment of a more satisfactory mechanism.

Ventricular Arrhythmias per Se

Ventricular Premature Beat (Extrasystole)

A ventricular premature beat is shown in the electrocardiogram by the early appearance of an abnormal *QRS* wave, followed as a rule by a full compensatory pause. The ventricular pause is called compensatory when the two ventricular intervals, pre-extrasystolic and post-extrasystolic, when added together, are equal to the sum of two normal beats. This is a natural result of the persistence of the dominant rhythm of the atria temporarily interrupted by the ventricular premature beat. One can distinguish by arteriogram between atrial and ventricular premature beats by applying by means of calipers the method of spacing to determine the presence or absence of a compensatory pause, but the distinction is much more quickly and accurately made by electrocardiogram.

On rare occasions when the heart rate is slow, a ventricular premature beat is *interpolated* between two normal beats with slight delay in the appearance of the post-extrasystolic beat, owing to prolongation of the *P–R* interval which is best ascribed to transient fatigue (see Fig. 112). Sometimes the premature beat occurs every second or third beat, producing a bigeminy or trigeminy, and infrequently there are two or three ventricular premature beats in a row. See Figures 108, 109, 110, 111 for examples of ventricular premature beats.

Ventricular premature beats are generally of no importance whatsoever and sooner or later occur in nearly all persons as they grow older. They may be likened to the appearance of gray hairs. Often they are not felt by the persons showing them, but in sensitive, nervous persons they may be annoying and should be treated by more than simple reassurance, which is, however, of prior importance. When they are induced by effort, especially in a person subject to coronary insufficiency, or when they are excessively numerous and arise from different sites, they should be regarded with more respect and the victim studied and treated with greater care, as in the case of atrial premature beats.

Ventricular Paroxysmal Tachycardia

More important, but much less common, than atrial paroxysmal tachycardia is ventricular paroxysmal tachycardia. Electrocardiograms show a rapid succession of abnormal *QRS* waves, usually of the same shape and fairly, though often not completely, regular. The rate ranges as a rule from 120 to 200. The onset and offset are sudden, and it may be possible to identify normal *P* waves appearing at a considerably slower but regular rate. See Figures 113, 114, 115 for examples of ventricular paroxysmal tachycardia.

The *clinical significance* of ventricular paroxysmal tachycardia is generally serious. There are exceptions, however, in which, in the absence of heart disease, some irritating factor initiates ventricular instead of the more usual atrial paroxysmal tachycardia. Severe coronary heart disease, as in acute myocardial infarction, is one of the most common causes of this arrhythmia. Digitalis intoxication is another cause. In any case, the condition is to be regarded as important, demanding as a rule emergency treatment by quinidine sulfate or procaine amide (pronestyl).

The distinction between ventricular paroxysmal tachycardia and atrial paroxysmal tachycardia (or flutter with 2 to 1 atrioventricular block) is often difficult clinically. An electrocardiogram is the only satisfactory differential test in the majority of instances, and even then there are rare cases of atrial paroxysmal tachycardia with bundle branch block that may simulate ventricular paroxysmal tachycardia, except at the onset of the paroxysm or after it has stopped (when the bundle branch block may be present with the normal rhythm also). It is true that sometimes there is a little arrhythmia in cases of ventricular paroxysmal tachycardia that can be detected clinically, or a different intensity of the heart sounds, increased when an independent atrial contraction coincides with a ventricular contraction, but these findings are not always clear cut. However, for what they are worth, possible differences are listed in Table 2 (p. 126).

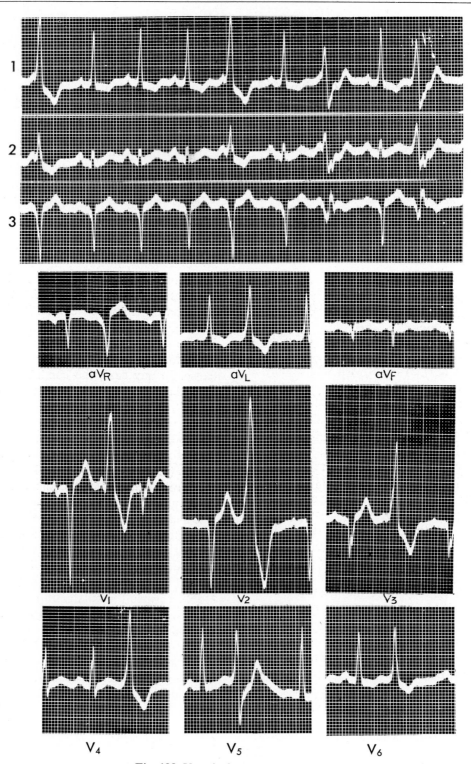

Fig. 108. Ventricular premature beats.

Ventricular premature beats in a man aged sixty-nine with hypertensive, coronary heart disease and a history of anterior and posterior myocardial infarcts twelve years before. He had had no cardiac symptoms thereafter until two years before his present hospitalization, when angina pectoris developed, occurring on exertion and relieved by nitroglycerin. During the past six months he had suffered from dyspnea, which had become increasingly severe. This record was taken before treatment was started. Digitoxin and diuretics caused a weight reduction of $4\frac{1}{2}$ pounds in two days. He was made comfortable on a regimen of daily digitoxin, ammonium chloride, and no added salt to his diet.

(Legend continued on facing page)

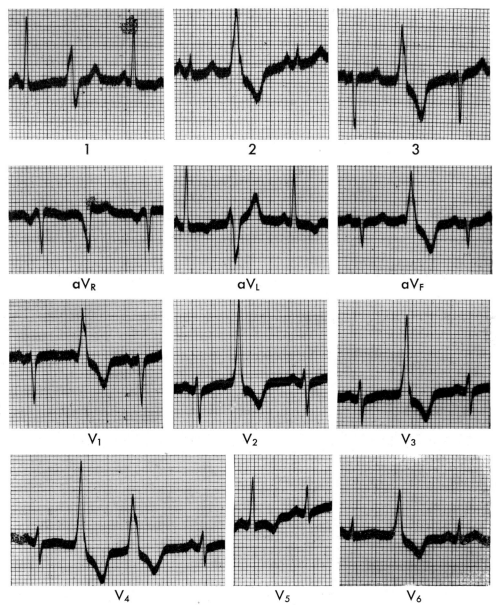

1   2   3
aV_R   aV_L   aV_F
V₁   V₂   V₃
V₄   V₅   V₆

Fig. 109. Ventricular premature beats.

Ventricular premature beats in a woman of sixty-eight who was admitted to the hospital for chronic simple glaucoma without definite cardiac complaints, save for some shortness of breath on stairs and on exertion, and irregularity of heart rhythm. For years she had been accustomed to sleep on two pillows at night, and for years she had been grossly overweight. At this time she weighed 225 pounds. Her blood pressure was 150 mm. of mercury systolic and 90 mm. diastolic. This electrocardiogram was taken four days after an iridencleisis had been performed on the right eye.

INTERPRETATION. This patient showed many premature beats at a rather fast heart rate of slightly over 100, which is somewhat unusual. The premature beats are always of one type and vary little in the degree of prematurity. On occasion, particularly in Leads aV$_F$ and V$_1$, it is possible to see the P wave on which the abnormal QRS wave is superimposed. Otherwise the P waves fall with the ectopic QRS waves. In Lead V$_4$ there are two ventricular premature beats in a row. In addition to the premature beats, there is left axis deviation with low T waves in Lead 1 and in the precordial leads.

(*Legend continued from opposite page, Figure 108*)

INTERPRETATION. This record shows many ventricular premature beats occurring at varying time intervals after the previous normal beat. They are of two different shapes: for example, in Lead 1 there are two, the first and the fifth QRS waves, that are only slightly premature falling near the top of the normal P waves, while the last two premature beats in that lead have wide S waves and occur much more prematurely, especially the last beat of all. There is a compensatory pause after each premature beat. In addition to these frequent ventricular premature beats, there is left axis deviation in the limb leads, with inverted T waves in Lead 1, QS waves in aV$_F$, and absent R waves in precordial leads V$_1$ to V$_3$ inclusive, in accord with the clinical story of myocardial infarction in the past. Thus this is a very irritable heart and probably should be treated with quinidine sulfate.

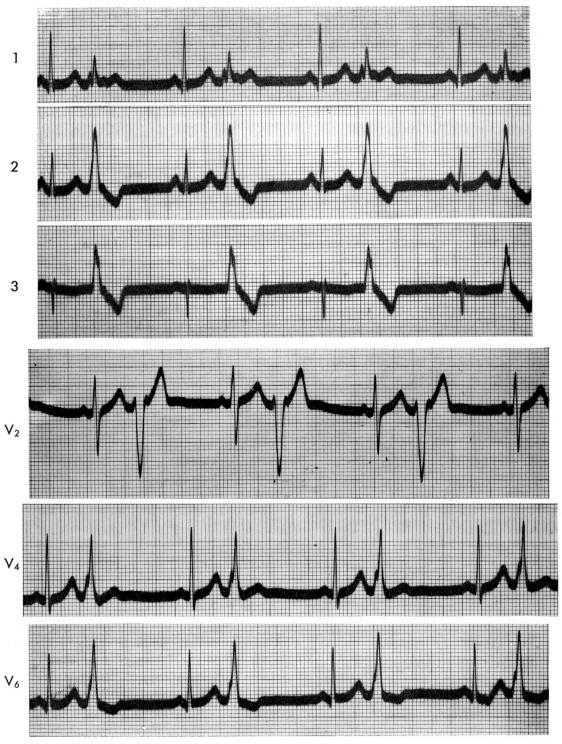

Fig. 110. Ventricular premature beats (bigeminal).

Ventricular premature beats with bigeminy in a woman aged forty-eight with an irritable normal heart. Six months later, after cutting down on her consumption of coffee, Coca-Cola, and cigarettes, there were no evidences of cardiac irregularity.

INTERPRETATION. Frequent ventricular premature beats producing a coupled or bigeminal rhythm at a heart rate of 85. The premature beats are all of one shape and degree of prematurity, and except for this arrhythmia the electrocardiogram is perfectly normal. It is quite likely that sources of irritation such as tobacco can explain this disturbance.

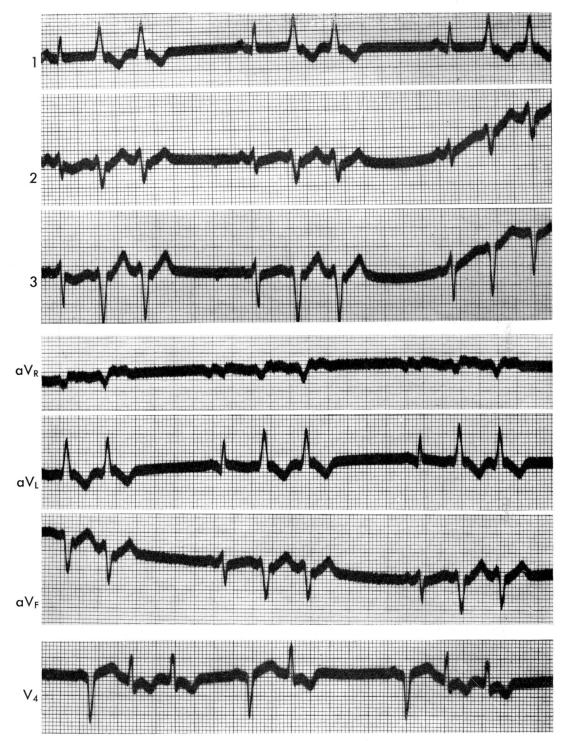

Fig. 111. Ventricular premature beats (trigeminal).

Ventricular premature beats with trigeminy following acute pulmonary edema in a sixty-five year old man with coronary heart disease and myocardial infarction. The patient was receiving digitalis.

INTERPRETATION. This is a more advanced disorder of rhythm than that shown in Figure 110. Here there is trigeminal rhythm at a heart rate of about 100. Trigeminy of this type is rare and probably important, indicating much irritability of the heart which may precede ventricular paroxysmal tachycardia. The common type of trigeminy due to premature beats every third beat is of no special importance. The atrial complexes on which the ectopic ventricular beats are superimposed are difficult to make out. In addition to this arrhythmia, there is flattening of the T waves in Lead 1, sagging of the S–T segments in Lead 2, which may be due to the effect of digitalis, and absence of the R waves in V4. Besides the presence of heart disease in this case, it is possible that digitalis intoxication may be a factor in the production of the arrhythmia.

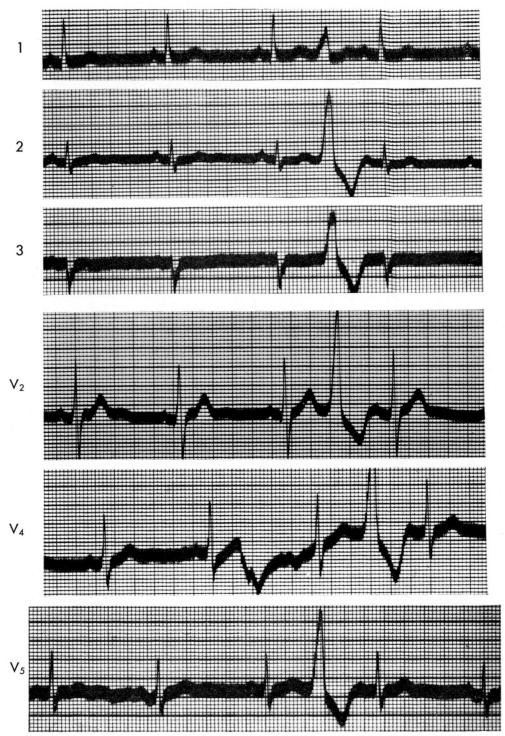

Fig. 112. Ventricular premature beats (interpolated).

Ventricular premature beats, interpolated, in a salesman aged sixty, occurring preoperatively a few days before subtotal gastrectomy for carcinoma of the stomach.

INTERPRETATION. This is a rather rare arrhythmia due to ventricular premature beats. Here they are interpolated between normal beats at a slow heart rate of about 55. In fact, it is this slow heart rate that allows the premature beats to be true "extra" systoles. The P–R intervals after the premature beats are slightly longer than the usual P–R intervals. This is probably the result of fatigue of the conduction tissue and is commonly found with interpolated ventricular premature beats even in the absence of heart disease.

Ventricular premature beats per se, whether interpolated or not, are in themselves no indication of heart disease, which seems to be true in this case.

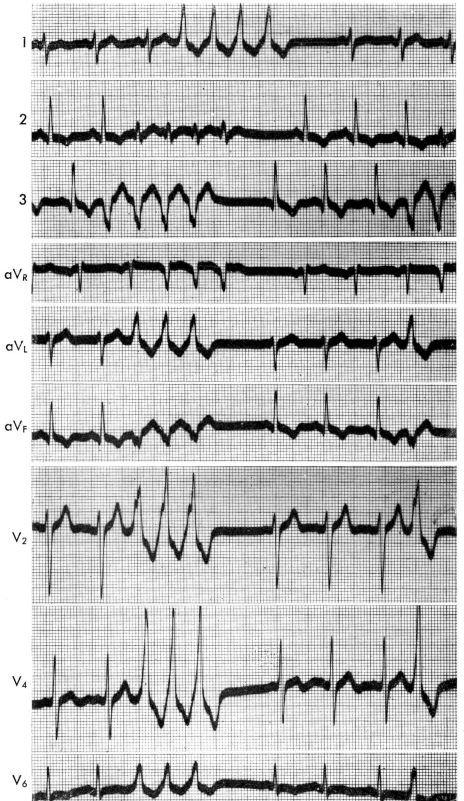

1

2

3

aV_R

aV_L

aV_F

V_2

V_4

V_6

Fig. 113. Ventricular paroxysmal tachycardia (in short runs).

Short runs of ventricular paroxysmal tachycardia in a forty-five year old ice-manufacturer with thyroid disease. A basal metabolic rate at this time was minus 25. On a previous admission for thyrotoxicosis four and a half months before, his basal metabolic rate had been plus 24 and his electrocardiogram had been considered borderline, showing a normal rhythm at a rate of 90 with slight slurring of the *QRS* waves and low *T*s in Lead 2, consistent with coronary heart disease. Treatment of his thyrotoxicosis had included thiouracil over the past few weeks. For this heart rhythm quinidine sulfate, 0.2 gm. orally four times a day, was prescribed.

INTERPRETATION. This record shows a slightly more advanced arrhythmia than is seen in Figures 110 and 111, which illustrate bigeminy and trigeminy. Here there are mostly three or four ventricular premature beats at a time, actually composing short paroxysms of ventricular tachycardia. The heart rate during normal rhythm is about 90. During the paroxysms of ventricular tachycardia the rate averages about 160.

In addition to the arrhythmia there is inversion of the *T* waves in Leads 2, 3, aV_F, and at times V_6. There are small *Q* waves in Leads 2, 3 and aV_F. Although clinically there was no clear story of coronary heart disease, such may be present to explain this high degree of cardiac irritability and the other abnormalities in the electrocardiogram.

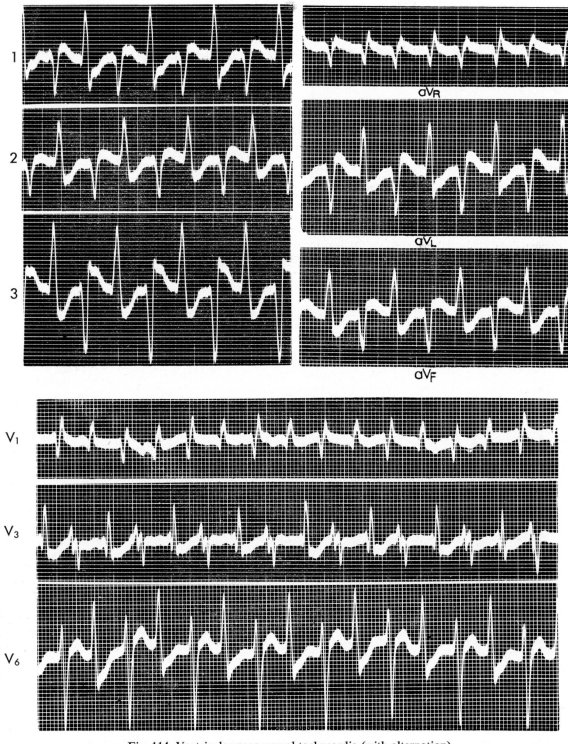

Fig. 114. Ventricular paroxysmal tachycardia (with alternation).

(*See facing page for legend.*)

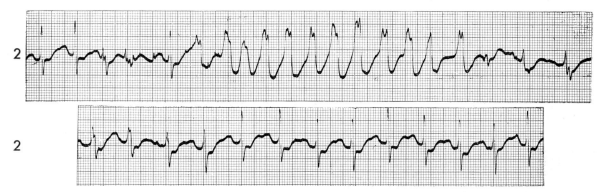

Fig. 115. Ventricular paroxysmal tachycardia.

Ventricular paroxysmal tachycardia occurring as a complication during mitral valve commissurotomy for relief of advanced mitral stenosis in a woman of thirty-five.

INTERPRETATION. The ventricular tachycardia consists of a series of eleven ectopic contractions in the first strip of this figure, varying slightly in rhythm. The rate averages 160. During the normal rhythm, which persisted and followed this paroxysm, the P waves are wide, which is typical of mitral stenosis, and the P–R interval is prolonged to about 0.22 second. The heart rate in the normal rhythm averages about 110.

In addition to the paroxysm of ventricular tachycardia, there are a few other premature beats and probably aberrant ventricular complexes.

(*Legend continued from opposite page, Figure 114*)

Ventricular paroxysmal tachycardia with alternation of direction of complexes in a fish-peddler aged sixty-two with malignant hypertension, uremia and congestive heart failure. This patient was hospitalized for one and one-half months after entry on September 13, 1949. Although his blood pressure dropped dramatically on protoveratrine therapy, this drug was discontinued because of toxic manifestations (nausea and vomiting). Oral veratrum viride also proved unsatisfactory. Digitoxin was started on October 2. A second course of protoveratrine beginning October 6 and continued through October 23 was unsuccessful. Digitoxin was stopped on October 19, on which day potassium acetate (20 per cent solution) was begun. By October 20 it was observed that he had slipped rather rapidly into cardio-renal failure, and by October 21 there was constant coupling of the pulse with an apical rate of 96; this was also present on October 23. On October 24 occasional extrasystoles were observed and digitalization was again instituted. The electrocardiogram shown here was taken on October 25. A subsequent electrocardiogram, obtained the following day, showed a slower rate with atrial flutter and block varying from 2:1 to 3:1. The patient was discharged to a nursing home on November 1 on a moderate low-salt diet, daily digitalis, bed rest, and phenobarbital.

INTERPRETATION. This electrocardiogram shows one of the most serious types of arrhythmia known, namely, alternating ventricular complexes in ventricular paroxysmal tachycardia. The heart rate averages 170. The alternation in direction of the ventricular complexes is best seen in the classical leads and in Leads aVF and V_6; in Leads aVR and V_1 there is relatively little difference. Digitalis intoxication, toxicity of the myocardium from other cause, and extensive coronary heart disease are the usual factors behind this extremely serious type of arrhythmia.

Table 2. Comparison of Findings in Ectopic Tachycardias

MECHANISM	DURATION	RHYTHM	AUSCULTATION	HEART DISEASE	CAROTID SINUS PRESSURE	PROGNOSIS
Atrial paroxysmal tachycardia	Variable, but usually minutes to hours	Regular as a rule	Symmetrical intensity of heart sounds	Usually none, but occasionally rheumatic	Sometimes stops attack at once	As a rule favorable as to life
Atrial flutter	Often days to weeks	Regular or regularly irregular	Symmetrical when regular	Usually present, especially rheumatic	May transiently slow pulse	Depends on heart disease present
Ventricular paroxysmal tachycardia	Variable, usually minutes to hours	Often slightly irregular	Variable intensity of heart sounds, often but slight	Almost always present, especially coronary heart disease (digitalis intoxication is also an important occasional cause)	No effect	Grave as a rule

Ventricular Fibrillation and Flutter

When the ectopic ventricular rate becomes very rapid and irregular, it approaches a hazardous state which may end in uncoordinated contraction of the ventricular muscle and death (see Figs. 117, 118). There tends to be a transitional state of so-called ventricular flutter (see Fig. 116). If surgical aid is at hand, as in the operating room, direct massage of the heart or/and electrical defibrillation may in rare cases restore normal rhythm and save life. When ventricular fibrillation threatens, as during the first ten or twelve days after acute myocardial infarction, or in patients subjected to cardiac or pericardial or even pulmonary surgery, rations of quinidine sulfate every few hours (e.g., 0.2 gm. [3 grains] at four to six hour intervals) may prevent this arrhythmia.

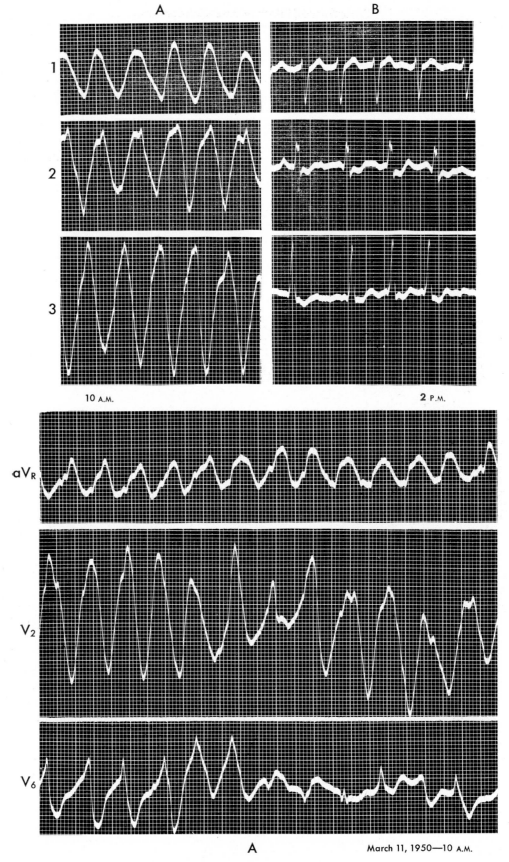

Fig. 116. Ventricular flutter.

(*See facing page for legend.*)

(Legend continued from opposite page, Figure 116)

Ventricular flutter in a woman of forty with a diagnosis of rheumatic heart disease, mitral stenosis and regurgitation, aortic regurgitation, congestive failure and paroxysmal arrhythmia. This arrhythmia occurred on March 11, 1950, almost one month after hospital admission following cerebral and splenic embolism. On March 8 she began to have increasing nausea and vomiting, although she had had no digitalis for the past four days. On March 10 she had a convulsive episode similar to several in the past and complained of dyspnea and severe pleuritic pain over the spleen.

The electrocardiogram shown in *A* was obtained at 10 A.M. on March 11 during one of these attacks of cyanosis, apnea and pulselessness (on this occasion immediately after a swallow of milk), beginning spontaneously and lasting for three minutes. Quinidine lactate was administered, and by 2 P.M. the rhythm had changed to the atrial fibrillation shown in *B*. She was still vomiting frequently and ran a downhill course until her death on March 13. (An electrocardiogram on that day showed probable atrial tachycardia with an atrial rate of 160, ventricular rate 80, and 2:1 atrioventricular block. The *Q–T* interval was 0.4 second.)

INTERPRETATION. During the paroxysm of rapid ventricular contractions shown in Leads 1, 2, 3, aVR, V_2 and V_6, the rate varied somewhat, but averaged 170. Best shown in Lead 1, there are constant wide excursions of the baseline without evidence of atrial action. This resembles somewhat the smaller oscillations of the baseline seen in atrial flutter, but here not interrupted by the sharp *QRS* waves which are invariably present in atrial flutter. The arrhythmia is most pronounced in Lead V_2, and there is a considerable change in the shape of the complexes in Leads V_2 and V_6. Evidently the effect of this disorder of rhythm on the cerebral circulation was severe, but perhaps on occasion during the periods of paroxysms there may have intervened actual ventricular fibrillation in addition to this ventricular flutter. This disturbance of rhythm, namely, ventricular flutter or fibrillation, is an occasional cause of so-called Adams-Stokes attacks.

The electrocardiogram shown in *B* is the more ordinary record of atrial fibrillation with a rather rapid ventricular rate averaging 120. There is, however, a high degree of right axis deviation in this record indicating a high degree of right ventricular enlargement secondary to mitral stenosis.

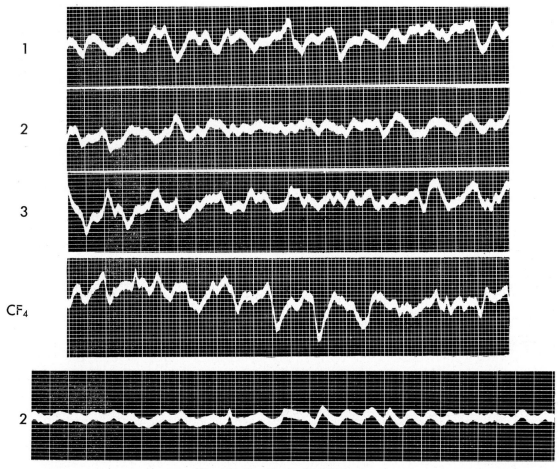

Fig. 117. Ventricular fibrillation.

Terminal ventricular fibrillation in a forty-one year old salesman who was hospitalized on September 28, 1948, for a question of myocardial infarction. His history included electrocardiographic and clinical evidence of myocardial infarction in March, 1947 (anterior), and again more recently, in September, 1948 (posterior). In the week before this admission he had had two to three daily attacks of substernal pain unrelated to effort and unrelieved by nitroglycerin, lasting about ten minutes. After entry he was comfortable on bed rest and quinidine, free from pain or symptoms of congestive failure. No dicoumarin was given. On the fourth hospital day he had been examined on evening ward rounds and found to be comfortable, without pain, with a perfectly regular pulse. Two minutes later he gasped, became cyanotic, and ceased to breathe. No heart sounds could be heard. Quinidine lactate and intracardiac epinephrine were administered without avail, and within five minutes of the onset of this acute attack (during which the electrocardiogram shown here was obtained) he expired.

INTERPRETATION. This record is typical of ventricular fibrillation, which very likely followed a brief period of ventricular tachycardia or flutter. The ventricular rate can be made out roughly in Lead 1 at close to 300 per minute, but there is probably a quite uncoordinated activity which has resulted in simultaneous contractions of various parts of the ventricular myocardium. In the last strip of Lead 2 the complexes are flattening out and are about to subside altogether.

This is a characteristic, and probably the commonest, cause of abrupt death in acute myocardial infarction or in angina decubitus such as this man had, doubtless due to a coronary thrombosis with or without infarction.

(*Legend continued from facing page, Figure 118*)

By the time the precordial leads were taken the condition had become obviously desperate, and there seems to be a coalescence of QRS waves and $S–T$ segments in V_2 and V_4. These extraordinarily wide complexes, which reach in V_4 a duration of 0.36 second, do not resemble the complexes of bundle branch block. The duration of systole, although hard to measure in these precordial leads, is obviously greatly prolonged. It can be made out in the next to the last beat or in the first and third beats of Lead V_2 to measure nearly 0.8 second in duration. At that time the heart rate had dropped to about 40, but picked up again to a rate of 65 in V_4. V_6 is a typical record of ventricular fibrillation and was obtained on this patient at the time of death.

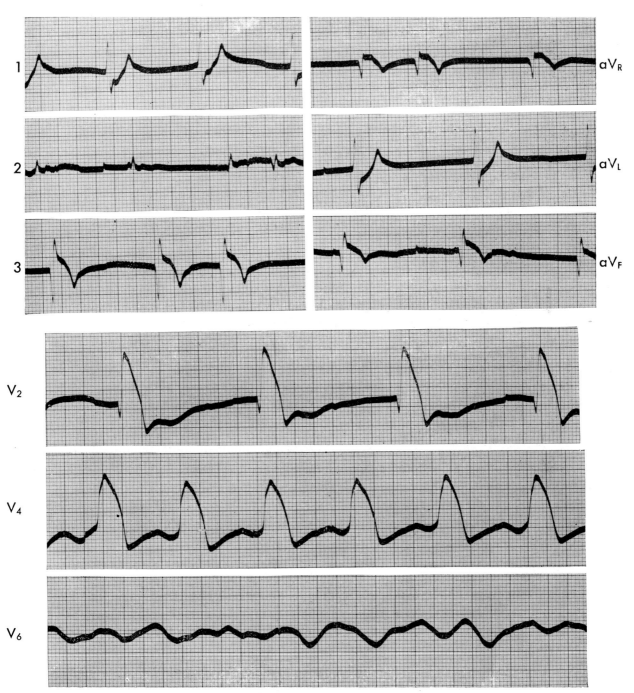

Fig. 118. Ventricular fibrillation.

Terminal ventricular fibrillation in a man of sixty-five. There had been no complaints suggestive of heart disease. On October 17, 1948, and again on October 25, laminectomy of L2 and L3 had been performed for relief of spinal cord compression caused by a malignant tumor of the vertebrae. The patient seemed to be doing well after the second procedure until about eight hours postoperatively, when he suddenly was seized with substernal pain and rapidly became unresponsive. Death followed within a few minutes. It was believed that he had sustained extensive pulmonary embolism, and this was confirmed by postmortem examination.

INTERPRETATION. This is an interesting record of a moribund patient showing infrequent small complexes that may represent futile atrial contractions and otherwise idioventricular rhythm (rate varying from 50 to 80, averaging about 60), with deep depression of the $S-T$ segments in Leads 1 and aVL, with high elevation of the $S-T$ segments in Leads 3, aVR and aVF, and prominent Q waves in Leads 3 and aVF, strongly suggestive of a fresh posterior myocardial infarct.

(Legend continued on opposite page)

ARRHYTHMIAS ASSOCIATED WITH ATRIOVENTRIC-
ULAR NODAL AND BUNDLE IRRITABILITY,
AUTOMATICITY, AND DEPRESSION

Atrioventricular Nodal Premature Beats and Paroxysmal Tachycardia

Rare types of premature beats and paroxysmal tachycardia arise in the atrioventricular node. They are shown electrocardiographically by the early appearance once or in rapid succession of normal QRS waves followed by reversed P waves (due to the retrograde transmission of the excitation wave from the atrioventricular junc-tional tissues, the sinus node remaining inac-tive). The timing of the premature beats is like that of ventricular premature beats, while that of atrioventricular nodal paroxysmal tachy-cardia resembles the timing of either atrial or ventricular paroxysmal tachycardia. See Figures 119 and 120 for examples of atrioventricular nodal premature beats and paroxysmal tachy-cardia.

The *clinical significance* of atrioventricular nodal premature beats and paroxysmal tachy-cardia is much like that of atrial arrhythmias. They are rare disturbances of rhythm and are relatively unimportant.

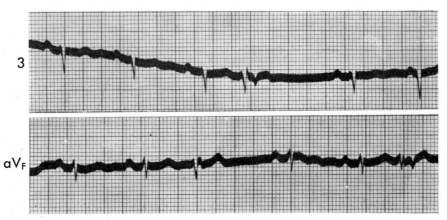

Fig. 119. Atrioventricular nodal premature beats.

Atrioventricular nodal premature beats in a woman of seventy with a diagnosis of acquired hemolytic anemia. In the course of her seventh hospital admission and three days after an exploratory laparotomy with dilatation and curettage, her pulse was discovered to be grossly irregular, owing to the premature beats demonstrated in this figure.

INTERPRETATION. Atrioventricular nodal premature beats, interrupting normal rhythm at a rate of 80. In Lead 3 the fourth QRS wave is premature and is followed by an inverted P wave, undoubtedly indicative of a retrograde atrial beat directly from the atrioventricular node. There is a compensatory pause. It is of interest that the last QRS wave of Lead 3 is slightly premature and, because it falls right at the end of the P wave, is not succeeded by a retrograde atrial contraction.

In Lead aVF there are two premature beats. The third QRS wave is only slightly premature and falls on top of the normal P wave. The last QRS in this lead is much more premature and so is succeeded by an inverted P wave. Thus actually we have strictly only two atrioventricular nodal premature beats in this record and two other premature beats which involve the atrioventricular nodal stimulus to the ventricle alone.

The atrioventricular nodal type of premature beat is of no clinical importance, but is of considerable academic interest; it is rather uncommon.

(Legend continued from facing page, Figure 120)

INTERPRETATION. Regular tachycardia at a rather slow rate of 115, with inverted P waves in Leads 2, 3, aVF, and V_5 immediately following slurred QRS waves of the shape usually found in other records of this patient. There is an $R–P$ interval of about 0.16 second. The P waves in most of the other leads are poorly shown, but can be made out faintly on the upstroke of the T waves in precordial lead V_4.

At first glance the inverted P waves in Leads 2, 3 and aVF simulate T waves, but actually the T waves are flat in these leads and are much longer in duration, as clearly shown in Leads V_2 and V_4. Thus the actual $Q–T$ time or dura-tion of systole, as measured best from Lead V_2, is 0.34 and not 0.22 second, as would be the case if we relied on Leads 2 and 3 only. The duration of systole expected at this heart rate is that found definitely in Lead V_2. It would be unlikely that the inverted P waves represent atrial paroxysmal tachycardia with long $P–R$ intervals of 0.4 second.

This type of paroxysmal tachycardia is rare in contrast to the frequency with which atrial paroxysmal tachycardia is seen, or indeed even in contrast to the frequency of occurrence of ventricular tachycardia. It is per se of little impor-tance and should be grouped, so far as clinical significance is concerned, with atrial paroxysmal tachycardia.

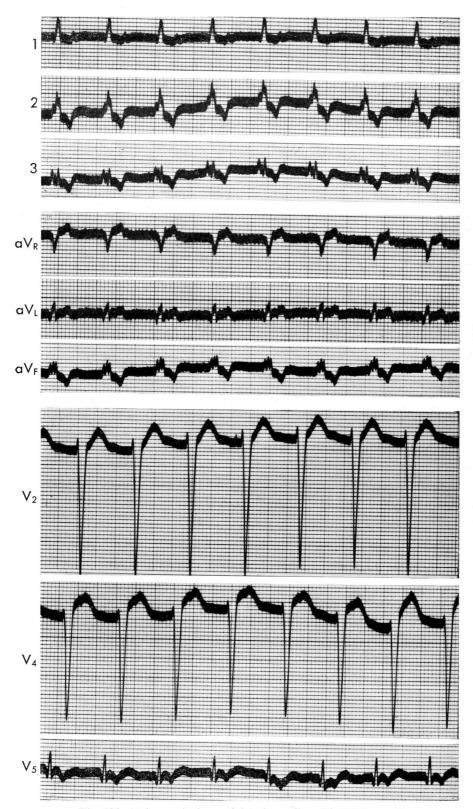

Fig. 120. Atrioventricular nodal tachycardia, with *R-P* interval.

Atrioventricular nodal tachycardia (with *R–P* interval) in a fifty-one year old man with coronary heart disease in congestive failure. The electrocardiogram taken on admission (July 8, 1948) showed a nodal tachycardia at a rate of 150. By the next day and after the administration of quinidine sulfate, the rate had dropped to 115, as shown in the electrocardiogram illustrated here. Quinidine was stopped at this point, but mercuhydrin and ammonium chloride were continued, with the loss of 6 pounds and resumption of normal rhythm by July 13. Purodigin, 0.2 mg. daily, was not started until July 14.

(*Legend continued on opposite page*)

Ventricular Escape, or Interference Dissociation

Escape of the ventricular pacemaker in the atrioventricular node is shown in the electrocardiogram by the appearance of a normal *QRS* complex independent of an atrial complex, generally when the sinoatrial nodal rate is temporarily slowed (e.g., into the fifties or forties) and the automatic ventricular pacemaker is unusually irritable. Rarely there may be ventricular escape at a normal sinus rate (60 to 80 per minute) and still more rarely at an accelerated rate (80 to 100 per minute). See Figures 121 and 122 for examples of ventricular escape.

Ventricular escape is of *no clinical importance*, although not infrequently it is an unnecessary cause for concern. It is, however, of considerable academic interest and is an excellent example of variations of physiologic function.

No *therapy* is needed unless digitalis intoxication is the cause; then the drug should be withdrawn until this disorder of rhythm clears.

Idioventricular Rhythm

This term is applied to any independent action of the atrioventricular node or bundle not controlled by or related to atrial action. Thus it is found in ventricular escape and in complete atrioventricular block and is considered under those headings here.

Atrioventricular Nodal Rhythm and Reciprocal Rhythm

Atrioventricular nodal rhythm is shown electrocardiographically by the regular sequence of normal ventricular complexes, of which the *QRS* waves are followed or immediately preceded by reversed *P* waves (inverted as a rule in limb leads 1 and 2). The *R–P* intervals average about 0.2 second, but may be longer or shorter according to the state of retrograde conduction from the atrioventricular nodal pacemaker to the atria (see Fig. 123).

In some cases of atrioventricular nodal rhythm the *R–P* interval may be so long that the ventricles, having escaped from their refractory state, respond to the atrial contraction, thus producing a reciprocal rhythm, as shown by an *R–P–R* sequence (see. Fig. 124). This is rare and of no clinical importance.

In some instances there is a *P–R* interval instead of an *R–P* one, when the conduction of the impulses back to the atria is faster than that forward to the ventricles, but such *P–R* interval is usually shorter than the average *P–R* interval with normal rhythm and measures 0.1 second or less (see Fig. 125). The atrioventricular nodal rate is as a rule slow, ranging from 35 to 50, in keeping with the lesser rate of automaticity of the idioventricular pacemaker.

There is but little *clinical significance* in the finding of atrioventricular nodal rhythm. Like ventricular escape, from which it differs only in that the ventricular pacemaker controls both atria and ventricles rather than ventricles alone, it is largely of academic interest, a physiologic variation as a rule, although it can cause the uninitiated observers to be unduly concerned. It may occur as the result of unusual inhibition or retardation of the sinoatrial pacemaker, which in turn can be "spontaneous" or secondary to some factor such as digitalis intoxication. It may be possible in atrioventricular nodal rhythm to block completely the retrograde conduction so that standstill of the atria may result.

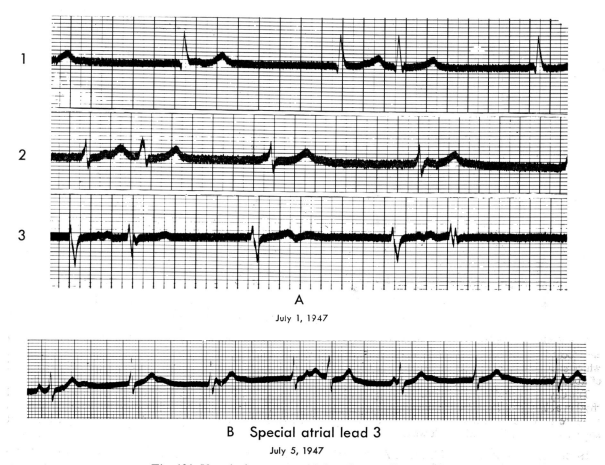

1

2

3

A

July 1, 1947

B Special atrial lead 3

July 5, 1947

Fig. 121. Ventricular escape with interference dissociation.

Ventricular escape with interference dissociation in a seventy-two year old man with optic atrophy from central nervous system syphilis and without significant cardiac symptoms. He was not receiving digitalis. On physical examination the pulse was slow at a rate of 54, with an occasional premature beat. His blood pressure was 165 mm. of mercury systolic and 70 mm. diastolic. The pupils reacted somewhat sluggishly to light. The neck veins were normal, and the lungs were clear. There were slight Grade 1 systolic murmurs in the aortic area and at the apex. The liver and spleen were not enlarged, and there was no edema. Dorsalis pedis pulses were feeble. There was enlargement of the heart by roentgenogram, most pronounced in the region of the left ventricle, and the aorta was tortuous. The cardiac enlargement was thought most likely to be on the basis of hypertension; there was no roentgenographic evidence of aneurysm or syphilitic heart disease. It was believed that the patient had mild hypertension with underlying coronary heart disease as a basis for the disturbance of rhythm.

INTERPRETATION. A (July 1, 1947), Infrequent P waves. In Lead 2 there is evidently a P wave which appears to be normal and precedes the second ventricular complex, which is rather widened, with a P–R interval of 0.24 second. The third ventricular complex in Lead 2 is superimposed apparently upon the top of a P wave. There may or may not be a P wave superimposed on the S–T segment of the fourth beat of Lead 2. In Leads 1 and 3 the only P waves that are evident occur with the three premature beats. The fundamental rhythm is that of the atrioventricular node (ventricular escape) at a rate of 40. The premature QRS waves occur consistently at about 0.55 second after the preceding ventricular complexes. The T waves are apparently normal. In Lead 3 at first glance there appears to be a small inverted P wave following the QRS of the second ventricular complex, but in comparing this complex with the last one of that lead it seems more likely that the M-shaped QRS wave can explain this appearance.

B (July 10, 1947), Here there is more evidence of atrial action, rather sharp P waves being noted just before the first ventricular complex, right after the fourth, just before the sixth, and directly after the eighth. There are a few other oscillations of the baseline which are probably artifacts, but which may be small atrial complexes. At two points there is probably a sequence of P and R complexes with conduction: on the first occasion with a P–R interval of 0.12 second in the case of the first beat, and later a P–R interval of 0.24 second in the case of the fifth beat. It is possible that intervening P waves are buried with the QRS waves, although such are not clearly evident. This special atrial lead was taken in order better to identify the atrial action.

These tracings are good examples of sinoatrial bradycardia or block and escape of the idioventricular pacemaker in the atrioventricular node.

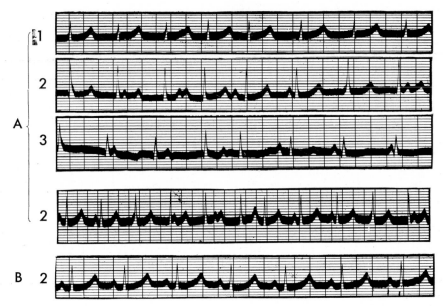

Fig. 122. Ventricular escape.

Ventricular escape in a nurse aged twenty-four who had had a tonsillectomy under ether four days before the first electrocardiogram (*A*) was taken. No drugs had been given. After operation she noticed slight but distinct palpitation which she had never experienced before. The heart rate was slightly irregular and higher than usual, 90 to 100 instead of about 70.

The day after the dissociation evidenced in the electrocardiogram was discovered, there was a resumption of normal rhythm at a rate of 78 to 83, as shown in the second electrocardiogram (*B*). However, either right or left carotid sinus pressure produced a temporary return of the arrhythmia. Aside from the electrocardiographic findings, the heart appeared normal. The patient felt well.

INTERPRETATION. *A* (March 10, 1916), Atrioventricular dissociation (interference dissociation) due to ventricular escape at a slightly higher rate (90) than that of the atria (80). There are a few sequences (the fourth and fifth beats in Lead 1, the fifth in Lead 2, the fifth in Lead 3, and the first and seventh beats in the second strip of Lead 2). Otherwise the record is normal.

B, The next day: normal rhythm at a rate of 80. The *P–R* interval is 0.16 second.

COMMENT. This is a perfect example of ventricular escape with temporary atrioventricular dissociation due to irritability of the atrioventricular nodal pacemaker, which controls the ventricles while the atria are still activated by the sinoatrial node. Return to normal sinus rhythm occurs when the *P* wave during the atrioventricular dissociation falls in such time sequence as to permit the impulse from the sinoatrial node to reach the ventricles before the atrioventricular nodal discharge. Ventricular escape is mainly of academic interest and does not as a rule indicate the presence of heart disease. This disorder has sometimes been inadequately referred to as "reciprocal rhythm."

(*Legend continued from facing page, Figure 123*)

with aortic regurgitation. Daily digitoxin had been started on February 24, the day after admission, and he was maintained thereon with the exception of three days (March 8, 9 and 10) when the heart rate had been around 56. The disturbances of rhythm demonstrated in these electrocardiograms were observed electrocardiographically on March 23 (*A*) and March 17 (*B*). The patient is now recovering from surgical exploration of the left kidney and unroofing of a cyst, which was successfully performed on March 23.

INTERPRETATION. *A* (March 23, 1951), Atrioventricular nodal rhythm of the usual type, with inverted *P* waves falling after the *QRS* complexes, best seen in Lead 2. The rate is 45, and the *R–P* interval is 0.28 second. There is also left axis deviation, with deep sagging of the *S–T* segments and flat *T* waves in Leads 1 and V₅ and low *T* waves in Lead 2.

B (March 17, 1951), An earlier Lead 2 of this same patient, with atrioventricular dissociation due to sinoatrial bradycardia of high degree and ventricular escape. The atrial rate is 38, and the ventricular rate is 40. There is one sequence of atrial and ventricular contractions with *P–R* interval of 0.3 second. This involves the first *P* wave and the second *QRS* wave.

COMMENT. Both disorders of rhythm shown in this case are equally rare, and when they do occur may be found in the same patient, as is illustrated here. The *R–P* interval is a little longer than usual, perhaps owing to some degree of atrioventricular block, confirmed by the length of the *P–R* interval in the one place in *B* where there is association between atria and ventricles. The effect of digitalis is suggested in these records.

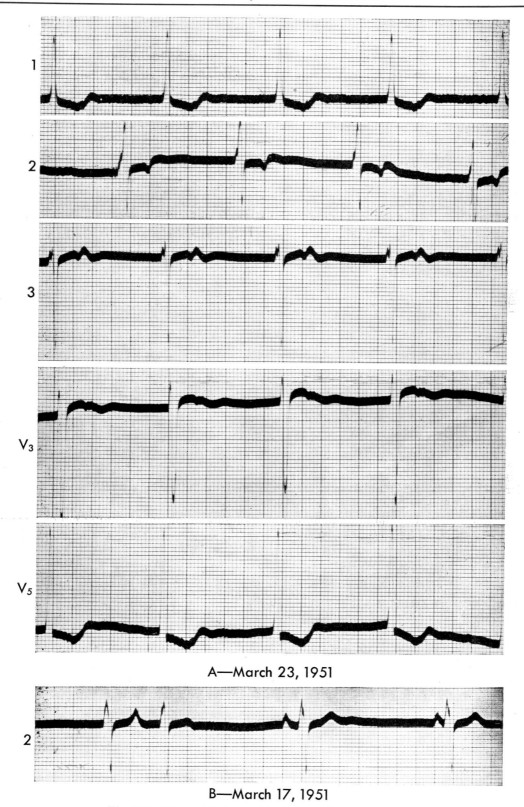

A—March 23, 1951

B—March 17, 1951

DR. WILLARD CARDWELL
GREENSBORO, N. C.

Fig. 123. Atrioventricular nodal rhythm, with *R-P* interval.

Atrioventricular nodal rhythm (with *R-P* interval) in a sixty-seven year old retired laborer on his tenth hospital admission, this time with the question of pulmonary embolism causing sudden collapse twenty minutes prior to entry. This episode was later believed more likely to be acute left ventricular failure on a probable basis of syphilitic aortitis

(*Legend continued on opposite page*)

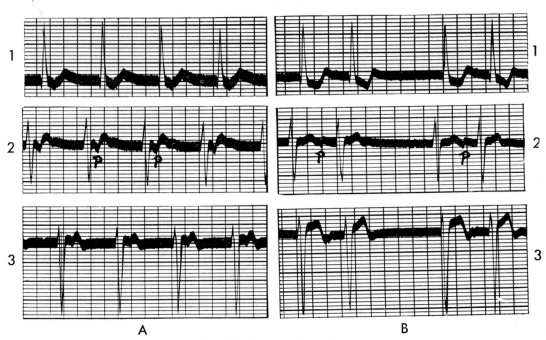

Fig. 124. Reciprocal rhythm.

Reciprocal rhythm in a man thirty-seven years of age who entered the hospital complaining of a knee injury. He had no cardiac symptoms or signs other than the disorder of rhythm.

INTERPRETATION. *A*, Atrioventricular nodal rhythm is present at a rate of 68. The excitation wave generated in the atrioventricular node reaches the ventricles first and the atria 0.18 second later, giving rise to the inverted *P* waves (the stimulus entering the atria from a direction the reverse of the usual when the rhythm is normal). Thus there is an *R–P* interval (of 0.18 second) in this case rather than a *P–R* interval. The *P* waves are poorly marked in Lead 1, but well seen in Leads 2 and 3. There is, incidentally, a high degree of left axis deviation (high R_1 and deep S_3), but with upright *T* waves in all three leads.

B, Record from the same case at a later date, showing a coupled rhythm (bigeminy) following digitalization. It will be noted that the inverted *P* waves of the atrioventricular nodal rhythm (best seen in Lead 2) are much delayed in their appearance, owing to the production of backward block, lengthening the *R–P* interval from 0.18 to 0.40 second. Such backward block results from the fact that the atrioventricular nodal junction between the atrium and the atrioventricular node is the most susceptible part of the atrioventricular conduction system. The ventricles are able to respond to the delayed atrial contractions with a *P–R* interval of about 0.22 second. Thus a curious rhythm results, consisting in a pair of ventricular contractions with one atrial contraction between them. No *P* wave follows the second *QRS* wave of each couple. This type of coupled rhythm has been called "reciprocal rhythm." The ventricular rate is 62, and the atrial rate 31; the latter rate is the fundamental rate of the atrioventricular nodal rhythm, depressed by digitalis effect (having previously been over twice that rate). The effect of the digitalis is further seen on the *S–T* segments of Lead 1 (sagging) and on the *T* waves of Lead 2 (lowered). The *QRS* and *P* waves are but little altered. Further digitalis abolished the *P* waves altogether, causing true atrial standstill.

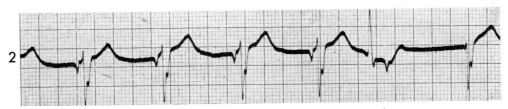

Fig. 125. Atrioventricular nodal rhythm, with *P–R* interval.

Atrioventricular nodal rhythm (with *P–R* interval) in a boy aged three and a half with atrioventricular heart block, probably on a congenital basis, and Adams-Stokes attacks on other occasions. The record shown here was taken forty-five minutes after an "excessive" dose of epinephrine (0.15 cc. of 1:200 adrenalin suspension).

INTERPRETATION. Regular heart rate, except for one premature beat with retrograde atrial conduction, at 70 per minute. Wide *QRS* waves indicative of intraventricular block and sharply inverted *P* waves with short *P–R* interval of 0.07 second. The last *QRS* complex in this strip is isolated without an evident *P* wave and doubtless represents response of the ventricle alone to the atrioventricular nodal stimulation, the impulse to the atria being completely blocked at that time, which would be consistent with the diagnosis of atrioventricular block made on other occasions.

The shape and direction of the P waves and the short *P–R* intervals establish this record as one showing atrioventricular nodal rhythm. In this instance the *P* wave precedes the *QRS* so that we have a *P–R* interval instead of the more usual sequence of the inverted *P* wave following the *R*, resulting in an *R–P* interval.

Atrioventricular Block

Depression or disease of the atrioventricular junctional tissues (node or/and bundle) may result in atrioventricular block, partial or complete. There are all grades from the slightest degree of block, shown by slight prolongation of the P–R interval, to, say, 0.22 second, up through the dropping of an occasional ventricular beat and higher grades of block, with ratios of atrial to ventricular complexes of 4 to 3, 3 to 2, 2 to 1, and 3 to 1, to complete dissociation with atrial rates of normal speed, e.g., 72 per minute, and idioventricular rates ranging from 50 to 25 and averaging 35. These various degrees of block may change from week to week or day to day, or even minute to minute, but sometimes they remain fixed for years, as in complete atrioventricular block. When there are occasional dropped beats only, there is often a curious ventricular and pulse arrhythmia due to the sequential lengthening of the P–R interval up to the time of the dropped beat, following which there is to be found the shortest P–R interval, resulting from the interval of rest. This mechanism produces occasional pauses (sometimes called "Wenckebach's periods") which are shorter than the sum of two normal beats. See Figures 126, 127, 128, 129, and 130 for examples of atrioventricular block.

Atrioventricular block is of considerable clinical significance. Although it can be transiently produced in lesser degree by vigorous vagal stimulation (e.g., carotid sinus pressure) or by digitalis intoxication in sensitive persons, it is as a rule the result of some disease process acting on the tissues themselves by inflammation or destruction. Acute rheumatic fever and anoxia secondary to coronary arterial blockage are the most frequent causative factors, but viruses and other more obscure or rarer conditions can also cause atrioventricular block. Not infrequently other disturbances of rhythm, in particular bundle branch block and atrial fibrillation, complicate atrioventricular block.

Adams-Stokes Attack

Prolonged standstill of the ventricles, usually in the course of serious high grade atrioventricular block, but on rare occasions dependent on high grade sinoatrial block (without ventricular escape), leads in the course of six to ten seconds to loss of consciousness and eventually to convulsions. This syndrome, described by Morgagni, Adams, and Stokes, may appear during the transitional period between partial and complete atrioventricular block and is shown electrocardiographically by prolonged absence of ventricular complexes with, as a rule, regular atrial rate at usual or somewhat increased speed (see Fig. 131). During the ventricular standstill the atrial T waves may be clearly evident following the P waves.

One other condition besides ventricular standstill may give rise to this syndrome: this is paroxysmal ventricular flutter or fibrillation followed by recovery. Although this is rare, it is important to recognize it, both because of its grave prognosis and because the therapy is different. Hence an essential feature of the examination of a patient with the Adams-Stokes syndrome is an electrocardiogram during an attack; this at once differentiates the various abnormalities of rhythm. (See Figure 132.)

The *therapy* of the usual Adams-Stokes attacks is best given in the form of epinephrine hydrochloride, 0.5 to 1 cc. of 1:1000 dilution subcutaneously as needed, with or without a trial of atropine parenterally also. When paroxysmal ventricular flutter or fibrillation, however, causes syncope, epinephrine is to be avoided and pronestyl or quinidine given instead.

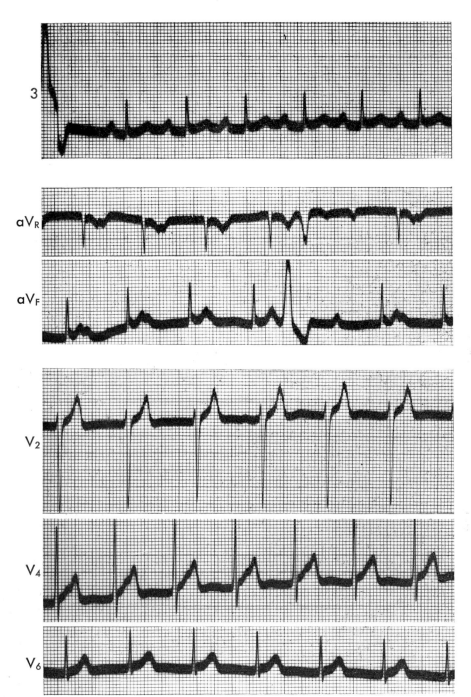

Fig. 126. Long P–R interval.

Long *P–R* interval in a young man of twenty-six with occasional premature beats and an otherwise normal heart. His past history included no serious illnesses. (An electrocardiogram taken one year later as a check on the partial heart block showed the *P–R* interval still varying from 0.22 to 0.50 second.)

INTERPRETATION. Partial atrioventricular block with occasional premature beats, after which the atrioventricular conduction may be either shortened or greatly lengthened or replaced by blocking of the atrial impulse and ventricular escape. The atrial rate and ventricular rate are generally equal at a rate of about 90. In Lead 3 the first *P–R* interval is relatively short, measuring 0.2 second. This is followed, however, by *P–R* intervals of 0.27 second, all apparently the same. In Lead aVR the *P–R* intervals are long at about 0.55 second, with the possibility that the ventricles are beating on their own (idioventricular rhythm due to ventricular escape), although atrioventricular block is more likely. There is one ventricular premature beat in Lead aVR and also one in aVF. In the precordial leads the *P* waves can be identified with difficulty, but can be seen on the upstroke of the *T* waves of V₄. In these leads the heart rate has slowed to about 80, but is regular.

There is apparently here a chronic state of defective atrioventricular conduction of variable degree. The cause of this defect is not clear from the history. The commonest explanation in young persons is serious infection in the past, usually either diphtheritic or rheumatic, or rarely virus. Congenital heart block is a remote possibility, but not likely. Except for the arrhythmia the record is normal.

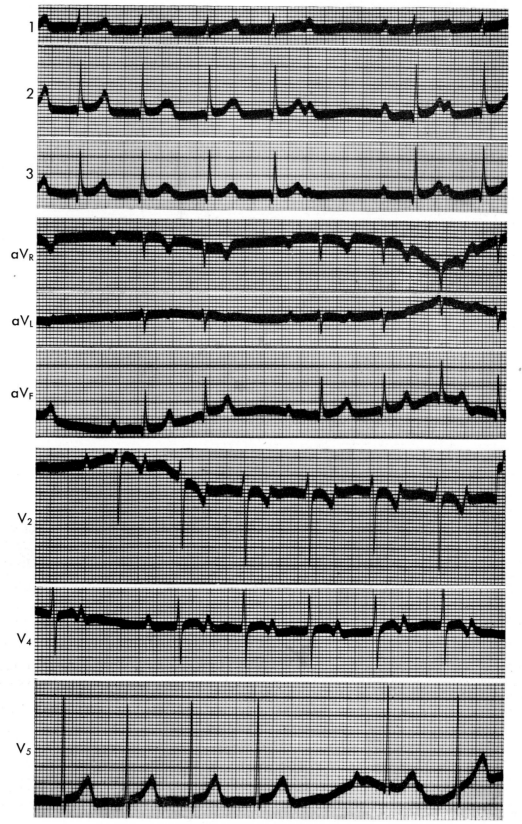

Fig. 127. Partial atrioventricular block with dropped beats.

(See facing page for legend.)

(Legend continued from opposite page, Figure 127)

Partial atrioventricular block with dropped beats (Wenckebach's periods) in a ten year old girl first seen in the clinic in May, 1948, complaining of frequent stomach aches. Upon examination the irregular heart rhythm demonstrated in Figure 127 was apparent. An x-ray film of the chest showed the heart to be normal in size and apparently normal in contour. The sedimentation rate was 5 mm., white blood cell count 7200 per cu. mm., hemoglobin 12.5 gm. per cent.

At the time of her examination on June 1 she looked well. Although somewhat nervous, she did not have true chorea. The most striking finding upon examination of the heart was a loud pulmonary second sound. Also audible were a Grade 1 soft systolic murmur at the apex and along the left sternal border and a Grade 1 short mid-diastolic rumble at the apex. On June 25 tonsillectomy and adenoidectomy were successfully performed.

There was some difference of opinion among the examiners as to whether this patient's cardiac signs were on a rheumatic or a congenital basis. The abnormal atrioventricular conduction first noted in the electrocardiogram shown here was of unknown duration and persisted in all subsequent tracings.

When last examined on March 1, 1951, she had been quite well. Her color was good. There were no nodules, no chorea, and no distention of the neck veins. The heart was not enlarged. P_2 was greater than A_2. Auscultation was described as follows: "in each sequence of beats a faint sound (? auricular sound) followed by a first sound of less than usual intensity and a loud second sound, then one or two similar beats, and finally a loud third sound—then pause and repeat." It was recommended that she lead a normal life and return in six months.

INTERPRETATION. Partial atrioventricular block with long *P–R* interval varying from 0.32 to 0.50 second. The atrial rate is 84, the ventricular rate somewhat slower, owing to the occurrence of occasional dropped beats. The *P–R* interval lengthens progressively up to the time of the dropped beats. The ventricular pause at the time of the dropped beat is approximately equal to the duration of two normal beats. Pauses like these have sometimes been called Wenckebach's periods.

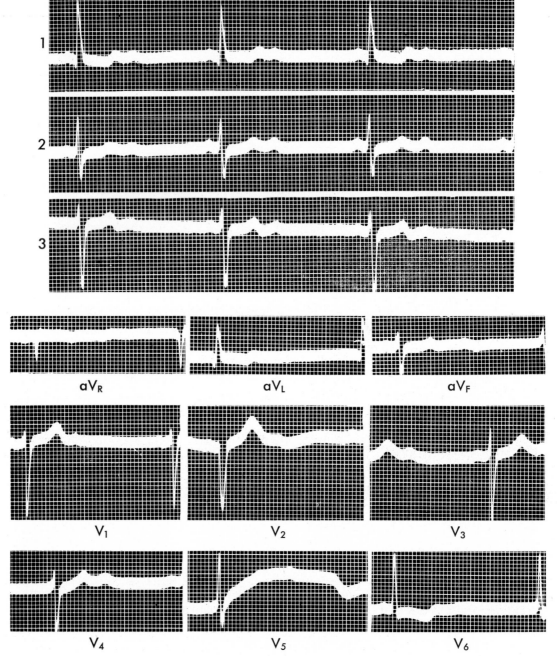

Fig. 128. Atrioventricular block (2:1).

Two-to-one atrioventricular block (with *P–P* intervals longer before the *QRS* waves) in a woman of seventy with a diagnosis of coronary heart disease and osteoarthritis. Her blood pressure was 220 mm. of mercury systolic and 90 mm. diastolic. An x-ray film of the chest showed the heart shadow to be enlarged in the region of the left ventricle, with a cardiothoracic ratio of 15:27 cm. and a tortuous aorta with calcification of the arch. Among other complaints was a "double beat" to her heart rhythm. On physical examination she had an apical systolic murmur and a moderately loud third sound regularly following the second sound in early diastole: it was considered probable that this represented an atrial sound in the presence of 2:1 block; this was confirmed by the electrocardiogram shown here. Inasmuch as her block was known to vary, the "double beat" episodes were explained on the basis of occasional 1:1 rhythm.

INTERPRETATION. Two-to-one atrioventricular block with atrial rate of 80, ventricular rate of 40. However, the atrial rate is not regular: it shows a bigeminy with blocked premature sinoatrial beats following the ventricular contractions, a common finding in atrioventricular block. There is left axis deviation, with slight depression of the *S–T* segments and low T waves in the limb leads and in the precordial leads over the left ventricle. In Lead V_6 the *T* waves are inverted.

This record is characteristic of the occasional grade of heart block in which every other atrial stimulus is blocked. As is doubtless true here, coronary atherosclerosis is the commonest cause of atrioventricular block.

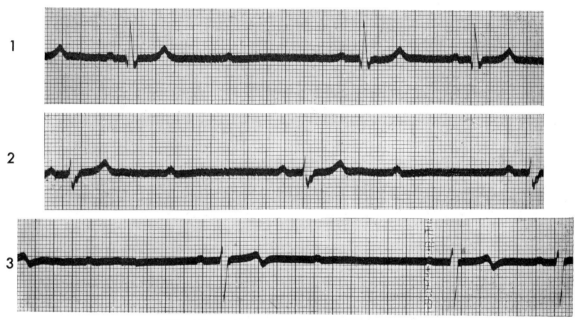

Fig. 129. Atrioventricular block (2:1 and 3:2).

High grade atrioventricular block in a seventy year old Dutchman with coronary heart disease and the onset of Adams-Stokes attacks several months before the tracing shown in this figure. The attacks had become so frequent and severe as to necessitate admission to the hospital. This electrocardiogram was obtained on November 16, 1943, and is transitional between his first tracing on September 16 of that year, which showed normal rhythm (with slight prolongation of the intraventricular conduction), and the establishment of complete atrioventricular block early in December.

This patient was having frequent Adams-Stokes attacks about the time this record was taken. On such occasions, of course, the grade of block would become much increased with ventricular standstill lasting several seconds. Adams-Stokes attacks are much more common during such a grade of atrioventricular block than early in the appearance of the block or after complete atrioventricular block has become established. There may be a great hazard from such attacks over a period of weeks or months. Epinephrine given parenterally at frequent intervals helped to prevent the Adams-Stokes attacks, and after a few weeks complete atrioventricular block developed and has continued since. With the disappearance of the Adams-Stokes attacks his health was restored, and so far as his heart is concerned he has remained well since. He is now under observation because of a pulmonary lesion.

INTERPRETATION. Sinus bradycardia at a rate of 50, with high grade partial atrioventricular block, varying from 3:2 to 2:1 ratio. The ventricular rate therefore varies between 25 and 33. When the ventricle responds, the *P–R* interval measures 0.22 to 0.26 second. There is also widening of the *QRS* waves with some degree of bundle branch block. The *T* waves are upright in Leads 1 and 2 and diphasic with late inversion in Lead 3.

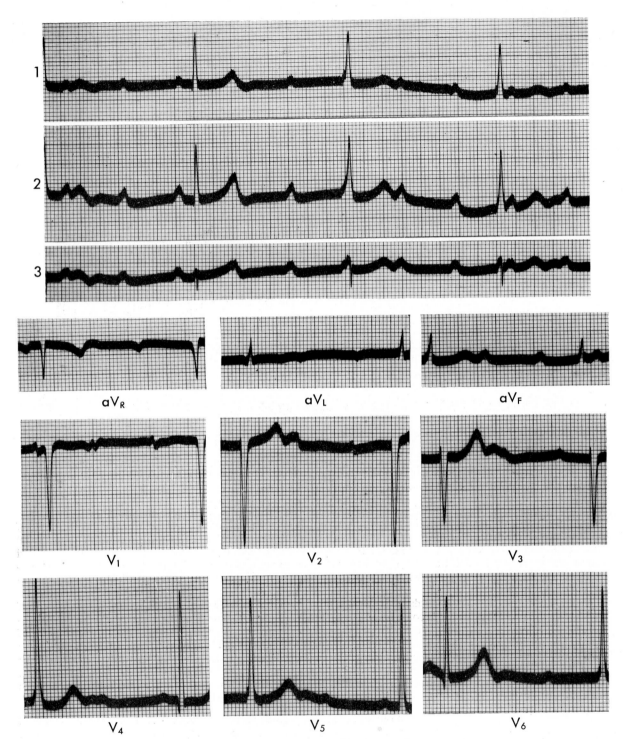

Fig. 130. Atrioventricular block, complete.

Complete atrioventricular block in a woman of sixty-eight with hypertensive, coronary heart disease. She had passed through a period of syncopal attacks, and an electrocardiogram taken two days before had demonstrated partial heart block (2:1). Ephedrine hydrochloride, 24 mg. every three hours, was prescribed. She had continued to do well on ephedrine when last seen one year later.

INTERPRETATION. Complete atrioventricular block with atrial rate of 100 and ventricular rate of 37, giving on occasion a false appearance of 3:1 ratio (see the first beats of Leads 1, 2 and 3). Otherwise the record is normal except for especially deep S waves in Lead V₂ and high R waves in Leads V₄, V₅ and V₆, indicative of enlargement of the left ventricle.

This record is characteristic of complete atrioventricular block in a person who has passed through a period of paroxysmal atrioventricular block with Adams-Stokes attacks. Coronary heart disease is, as in this case, the usual explanation.

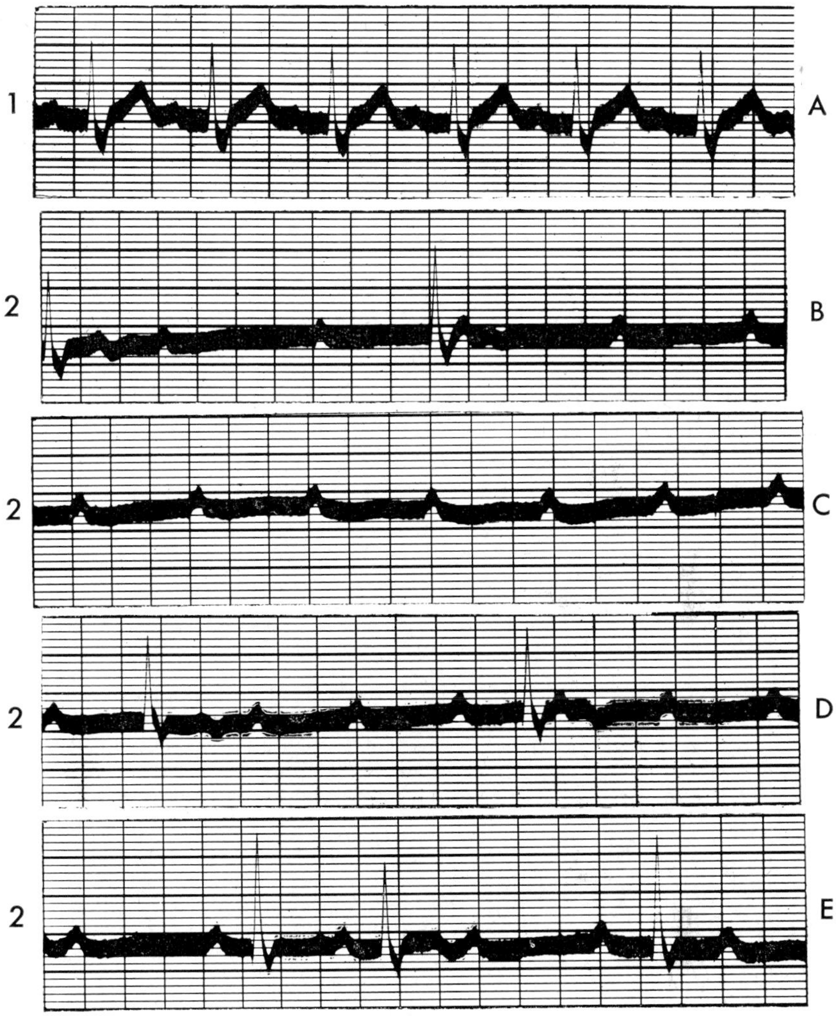

Fig. 131. Ventricular standstill in an Adams-Stokes attack.

Adams-Stokes attack with ventricular standstill in a forty-five year old salesman with no history of heart disease or of cardiac symptoms. In August, 1916, four months prior to hospital admission, he began to have chills, occurring about twice a week, lasting for from thirty minutes to one hour, and followed by severe sweats. For these he saw his local doctor, who later reported a positive blood serology. During the next two months he continued to feel weak and "dragged out," and on November 27 he first experienced "faint spells" which he described as "hot flashes," beginning in his stomach and going quickly to his head, lasting about thirty seconds, without associated pain or palpitation. These episodes would occur several times daily, and he believed that they would have caused him to fall had he not been holding on to something each time they occurred. There was no aura, no tremor, and no apparent loss of consciousness or ability to speak during the attacks.

On physical examination he appeared in no discomfort. The heart sounds were regular, slightly rapid, but of good quality. P_2 was greater than A_2, which was slightly accentuated. There was a soft systolic murmur in the pulmonary area. No thrill was felt. There was no edema and no clubbing of the extremities.

An x-ray film of the chest on November 29 revealed the right heart to be somewhat enlarged, with considerable prominence in the region of the great vessels and thickening of both lung roots.

During the patient's hospital admission he was seen during one of the attacks, in which there appeared to be a hot flash migrating to the head, then dyspnea, and for a few seconds inability to speak. Pallor succeeded by flushing was observed, with a sudden drop in heart rate to 26. He then appeared slightly cyanotic. The electrocardiogram shown here was taken on the third day after admission. Subsequently the patient experienced many attacks, but claimed on the fifth hospital day that he had had none for several hours and that he was "cured." He refused medicine (potassium iodide) and on December 5 was discharged against advice, with the diagnoses of heart block and syphilis. It was later reported that he died in April, 1917.

The etiologic factor behind the Adams-Stokes attacks in this case is not clear: usually coronary insufficiency or coronary thrombosis is the cause; rarely diphtheria, syphilis and rheumatic fever may be responsible. It is possible that syphilis was the cause in this case, but even though it may have been present, coronary atherosclerosis in this man aged forty-five is much more likely.

INTERPRETATION. *A*, Lead 1 shows a normal rhythm at a rate of 100, with slightly prolonged *P–R* interval measuring 0.22 second and wide *S* waves indicative of right bundle branch block.

B, Lead 2, showing complete atrioventricular dissociation, with atrial rate 75 to 80 and ventricular rate 30, with slightly inverted *T* waves.

C, Lead 2, showing ventricular standstill, with atrial rate 105.

D, Lead 2, showing high grade atrioventricular block, probably complete, atrial rate 120, ventricular rate 32, inverted *T* waves and bundle branch block as before.

E, Lead 2, showing partial atrioventricular block, varying in grade from 2:1 to 3:2, with atrial rate 90, ventricular rate about 52, the *T* waves still slightly inverted.

COMMENT. This series of electrocardiograms illustrates very well a common sequence of events before, during and after an Adams-Stokes attack. Starting with simple delayed conduction, there is an abrupt change to high grade heart block, with ventricular standstill and then recovery somewhat in the same sequence. Such electrocardiograms as this cover an interval as a rule of a very few minutes.

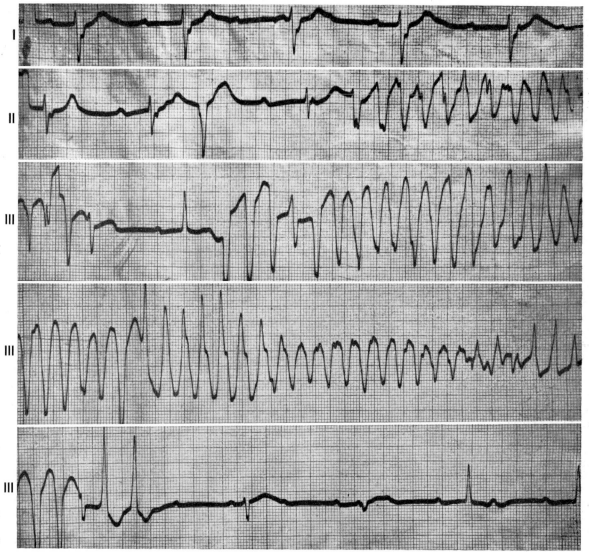

I

II

III

III

III

Fig. 132. Syncope in complete heart block.*

Syncope in complete heart block in a seventy-five year old housewife with hypertension and the present complaints of "dizziness," weakness, and nausea, which had persisted for one week. On physical examination the lungs were clear. The blood pressure was 210 mm. of mercury systolic and 80 mm. diastolic. The apical heart rate was 52, the radial pulse 37. Sounds were of fair quality, the first sound varying in intensity at the apex, where a soft blowing systolic murmur was audible with transmission to the base. P_2 was greater than A_2. There were numerous premature beats.

On the morning after admission, after complaining of dizzy spells, the patient became unconscious, and it was impossible to obtain her heart rate or pulse. There were slight convulsive movements, and during one period of syncope which lasted about twenty-five seconds complete heart block followed by rapid ventricular action was demonstrated electrocardiographically. She was given two doses of quinidine, 3 grains, and was to have received more, but on the second day her pulse rate was 16 and the quinidine was discontinued. On the third hospital day she had episodes of Cheyne-Stokes respiration with loss of consciousness, after which premature beats were again observed at the apex. The electrocardiogram shown in this figure was taken four days after entry and the day before she died. There was no autopsy.

INTERPRETATION. ? Complete atrioventricular block with bundle branch block and occasional ectopic beats interrupted by paroxysms of ventricular flutter sufficiently prolonged and disturbing to cause syncope, thus imitating Adams-Stokes attacks.

This is an unusual type of syncope, the more common being that of prolonged ventricular standstill. In this type, of course, epinephrine would be contraindicated.

* Courtesy of Dr. Stanley August.

Bundle Branch Block

One of the few disorders of the cardiac mechanism that can be identified by electrocardiogram only, and so is usually an unexpected finding, is that of bundle branch block. As a rule, the sinus rhythm is present at normal rate with normal atrioventricular conduction, so that the electrocardiogram appears to be normal except for the deformity of the QRS and T waves. The diagnostic criterion is that of an abnormally prolonged duration of the QRS wave to 0.12 second or more in the absence of an abnormally short $P–R$ interval of 0.1 second or less (Wolff-Parkinson-White syndrome) (see p. 159). There is a borderline often of uncertain interpretation between the time durations of 0.10 and 0.12 second, which may not even be cleared by the precordial leads, for it has been shown (p. 46) that the R wave may be normally M-shaped in Lead V_2 at 0.10 or even longer, at 0.11 second duration. There may be great variation in the duration of the QRS complexes above the time interval of 0.12 second, and figures close to 0.20 second have been recorded.

It has been shown by histologic study that involvement of the bundle branches is almost invariably bilateral, but, since one branch as a rule conducts better than the other, we distinguish electrocardiographically between left and right bundle branch block. Also there are varying degrees of such preponderance in conduction, so that one speaks of lesser and greater grades of bundle branch block. The situation is further confused by the possibility in rare instances of "arborization block," that is, of abnormality of areas of the terminal fibers. Electrocardiographically, however, it is probably wiser to limit one's diagnostic terminology to "bundle branch block, left or right, of lesser or greater degree," until more accurate data are obtained by correlation of detailed myocardial histologic findings in the entire atrioventricular conduction tract with the electrocardiogram.

The presence of bundle branch block, especially left bundle branch block, in the electrocardiogram can often obscure other abnormalities or at least add to the difficulties of their detection.

Left bundle branch block is apparently slightly more common than right. The classical bipolar limb leads show as a rule a wide R wave with inverted T wave in Lead 1, a wide S wave with upright T wave in Lead 3, and a more or less isoelectric Lead 2 (due to neutralization of Leads 1 and 3). On occasion, however, the T_1 waves may be upwardly directed along with the QRS_1 waves.

This disorder of rhythm is shown best in the unipolar precordial leads; in Leads V_5 and V_6 (and sometimes V_4) the broad R wave is deeply notched and M-shaped. In leads over the right ventricle there are wide, slurred S waves. The T waves in the precordial leads are oppositely directed from the chief initial ventricular complex if the bundle branch block is uncomplicated. (See Figures 133 and 134.) In rare instances in which the heart is unusually vertical in position the classical limb leads may be misleading, the effect of the heart position neutralizing the usual characteristic pattern of left bundle branch block in Leads 1 and 3, and necessitating a correct interpretation by survey of the precordial leads (see Fig. 135).

Right bundle branch block is, as one would expect, the complement of left bundle branch block. The classical bipolar limb leads show typically a wide S wave and an upright T wave in Lead 1, a wide R wave with inverted T wave in Lead 3, and, like left bundle branch block, a more or less isoelectric Lead 2.

However, again the unipolar precordial leads tell the story best. Over the right ventricle, that is, in Leads V_2 and V_3, there is a wide, notched M-shaped QRS (or RR') complex with inverted T wave, while over the left ventricle there is a wide S wave with upright T wave. (See Figures 136 and 137.)

Here again, however, position of the heart may rarely play an important role, misleading the interpreter if only the classical limb leads are taken. An extremely horizontal heart position may result in limb lead curves that resemble left bundle branch block; the precordial leads at once give the correct answer (see Fig. 138).

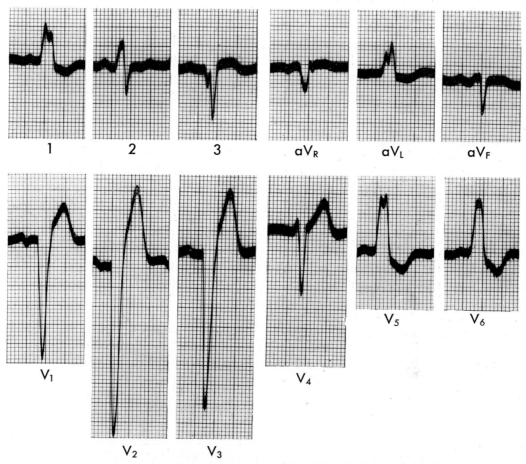

Fig. 133. Left bundle branch block.

Left bundle branch block in a woman of sixty-seven with hypertensive, coronary heart disease, cardiac enlargement, and a history of congestive failure.

INTERPRETATION. Normal rhythm, rate 86, with wide QRS waves (0.14 second), left axis deviation in the limb leads, deep S waves in precordial leads V_1, V_2, and V_3, with little or no R wave, and upright notched R waves in Leads V_5 and V_6.

This record is characteristic of the usual type of left bundle branch block. Lead V_5 is the main clue because of the possibility of mistaking the position of the bundle branch block in the limb lead pattern. The essential absence of R waves in precordial leads over the right ventricle is common and does not indicate complicating myocardial infarction of the anteroseptal region of the heart. However, it must be realized that bundle branch block in older patients is due to infarction, even though microscopic, secondary to coronary occlusion of the vessels supplying the conducting tract.

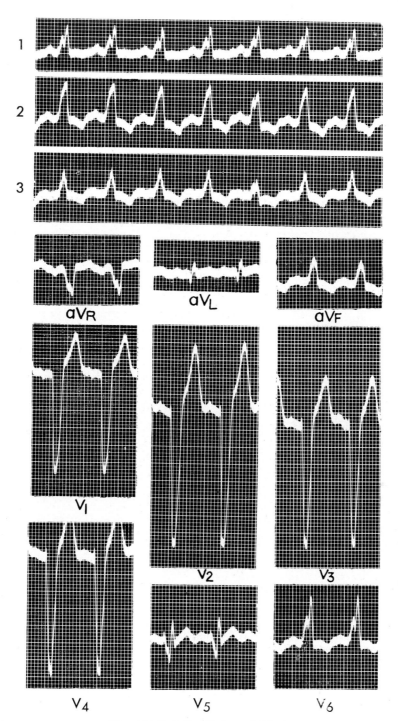

Fig. 134. Left bundle branch block.

Left bundle branch block in a bank teller of fifty-two, following operation for carcinoma of the sigmoid. There was no history of cardiac symptoms and no known heart disease. It was thought that his electrocardiogram probably represented coronary heart disease. Without a clear history of myocardial infarction and with the electrocardiographic pattern obscured by the presence of bundle branch block, it was impossible to determine whether recent injury to the myocardium had taken place. Serial electrocardiograms revealed no changes diagnostic of an acute episode.

The usual cause of bundle branch block is coronary heart disease, which was probably present here, although there was no other indication of heart disease.

INTERPRETATION. Normal rhythm at a heart rate of 110 with normal atrioventricular conduction (P–R interval equals 0.15 second) and left bundle branch block best demonstrated by the wide notched M-shaped R wave in Lead V₆. The wide upright notched R wave in Lead 1 suggests left bundle branch block, but the upright R wave in Lead 3 is unusual. As a rule, there is inversion of the QRS₃ wave in left bundle branch block. The T waves are flat in Lead 1, inverted in Leads 2, 3 and V₆. There are deep wide S waves in the precordial leads V₁ to V₄ inclusive.

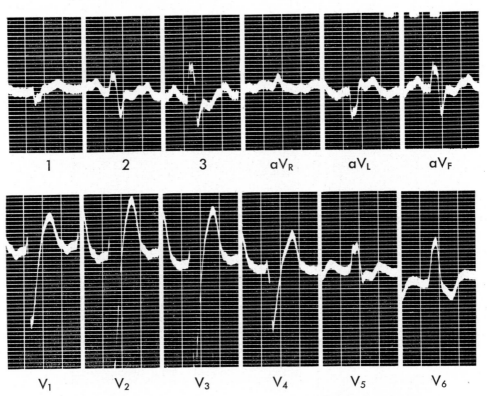

Fig. 135. Left bundle branch block resembling right bundle branch block.*

Left bundle branch block resembling right bundle branch block in the limb leads in a fifty-five year old man with coronary heart disease. This electrocardiogram was taken with the patient lying on his left side. The negative complexes in Lead 1 undoubtedly demonstrate a postural effect, because the QRS complex in this lead became upright, although low, when the position was changed to a fully supine one.

INTERPRETATION. Normal rhythm at a heart rate of 110 and wide QRS waves in all leads, measuring in duration 0.18 second. There is right axis deviation shown in the limb leads, but in the precordial leads there is clear evidence of left bundle branch block shown by deep wide S waves in Leads V_1 through V_4, inclusive, and upright notched R waves in Leads V_5 and V_6.

Thus in the limb leads one might have made a diagnosis of right bundle branch block wrongly. In this case, as in many others, position caused confusion. It was in the left lateral decubitus only that the simulation of right bundle branch block was found.

* Courtesy of Dr. David Littmann, Veterans Administration Hospital, West Roxbury, Massachusetts.

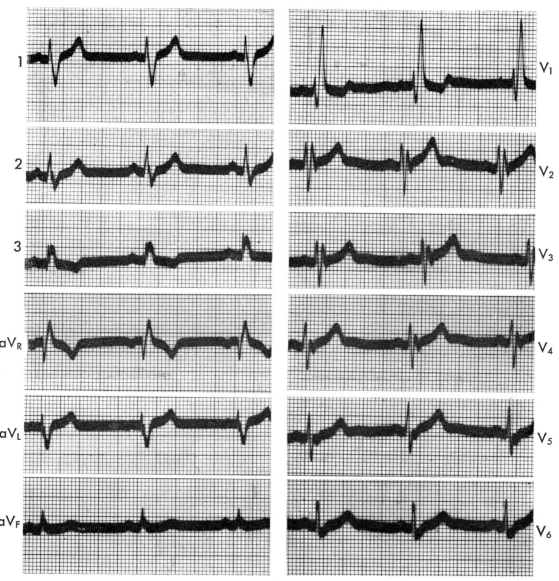

Fig. 136. Right bundle branch block.

Right bundle branch block, an incidental finding in a seventy-two year old farmer with chronic lymphocytic leukemia and diabetes mellitus without cardiovascular complaints. X-ray examination of the chest showed the heart to be rather prominent in the region of the left ventricle, with a slightly tortuous aorta.

INTERPRETATION. Normal rhythm, rate 60. Normal throughout except for wide QRS waves measuring 0.13 second in duration. There is right axis deviation shown in the limb leads with notched M-shaped QRS waves in precordial leads V_2, V_3 and V_4 over the right ventricle and blunt wide S' waves in Leads V_5 and V_6. The T waves are upright in all leads except 3 and aVR.

This record illustrates the common type of right bundle branch block with wide S waves in Lead 1 and M-shaped R waves in the precordial leads over the right ventricle. It is of interest that this was an accidental finding in an old man; such is common and does not indicate a serious cardiac lesion.

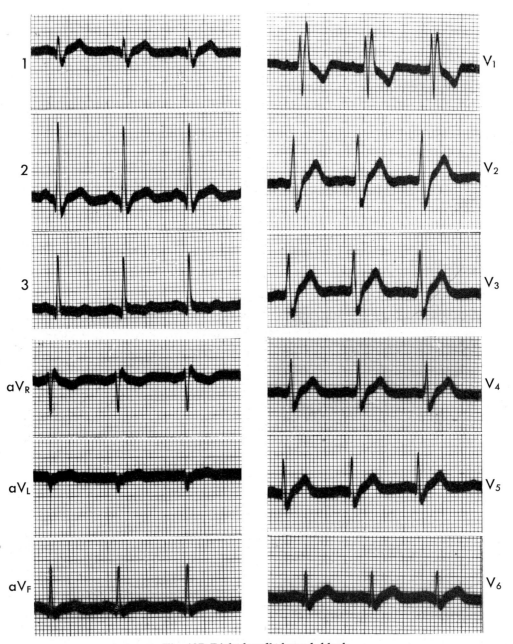

Fig. 137. Right bundle branch block.

Right bundle branch block discovered on routine preoperative examination in a forty-four year old machinist with a diagnosis of a right renal tumor and pulmonary neoplasm.

INTERPRETATION. Normal rhythm at a rate of 90, with wide *QRS* waves in all leads, measuring up to 0.12 second (or a bit more in the precordial leads). There are blunt wide *S* waves in Leads 1 and 2 and in all the precordial leads except V₁, where there are prominent M-shaped QRS waves.

This is a borderline record, but it undoubtedly means the least grade of right bundle branch block that can be diagnosed. Its etiology is not clear in this forty-four year old man. Coronary heart disease is the most likely explanation, but some previous infection may have been the cause.

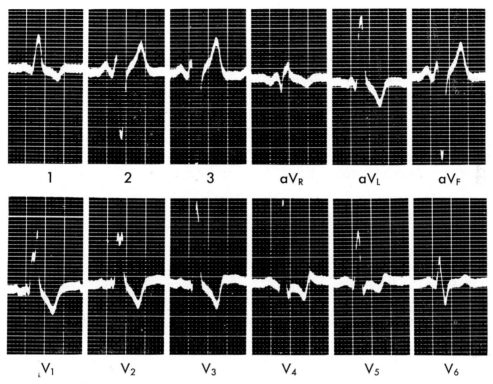

Fig. 138. Right bundle branch block resembling left bundle branch block.*

Right bundle branch block resembling left bundle branch block in the limb leads in a fifty-three year old man who had never had any cardiac complaints and was bothered principally by a lack of pep. Five months before, he had had an abdominal perineal resection for carcinoma of the rectum. On this admission his blood pressure was 100 mm. of mercury systolic and 85 mm. diastolic. There was no clinical evidence of coronary insufficiency. X-ray examination revealed the heart size to be normal, but with an "uptilt" to the left border and, in the left oblique view, a large and rounded left ventricle. The impression from this x-ray film was that this was a vertical heart with clockwise rotation and possibly left ventricular hypertrophy. There was also a slight degree of scoliosis of the spine with convexity to the right.

INTERPRETATION. Normal rhythm at a heart rate of 100, with wide QRS waves in all leads, measuring approximately 0.15 second. There is left axis deviation in the limb leads with inversion of the T waves in Leads 1 and aVR and aVL, but in the precordial leads there is clear evidence of right bundle branch block, as shown by the upright notched R waves in precordial leads V₁, V₂ and V₃ over the right ventricle. In precordial leads V₅ and V₆ there are short wide S waves and upright T waves.

Here, as in Figure 135, in the case of left bundle branch block, the limb leads are misleading, suggesting left bundle branch block when actually right bundle branch block is present. Again, position of the heart doubtless explains this confusion.

* Courtesy of Dr. David Littmann, Veterans Administration Hospital, West Roxbury, Massachusetts.

Bundle Branch Block of Indeterminate Type. Sometimes it is difficult or impossible to determine whether the bundle branch block is right or left (see Fig. 139). This may be due partly to involvement of both bundle branches with slight preponderance of one over the other, or to so-called "arborization block," which is at present a poorly defined condition. In such cases it may be of help to take additional precordial leads below and above the usual positions and possibly from the esophagus too.

Paroxysmal (for Example, 2:1) Bundle Branch Block. Bundle branch block may occur in paroxysms or even every other beat (see Fig. 140). Under such circumstances it has the same significance as constant bundle branch block, which is the ordinary type. The paroxysmal stage, however, may rarely be found during early development of this conduction defect.

The *clinical significance* of bundle branch block is of considerable importance. This finding indicates a pathologic condition of the myocardium of the bundle branches and suggests the possibility, or indeed probability, of more widespread myocardial disease. However, the actual lesions responsible for the electrocardiographic abnormality may be minute, in fact, microscopic, and bundle branch block alone need not often be a cause for anxiety. In the absence of other evidence of heart disease it is compatible with many years of health and full activity, but suggests the advisability of an occasional check-up. Coronary atherosclerosis and infectious scarring are, in that order, the commonest causes of bundle branch block, which, although it is usually constant or permanent, may on occasion be paroxysmal or transient.

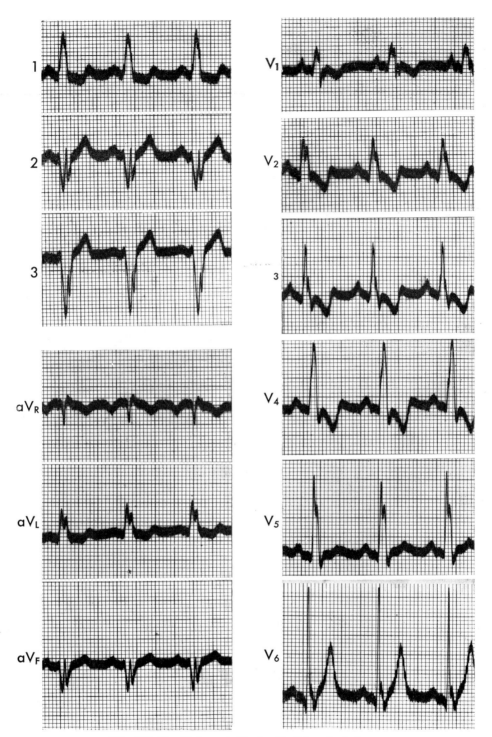

Fig. 139. Bundle branch block of indeterminate type.

Bundle branch block of indeterminate type, looking more like left bundle branch block in the limb leads, like right bundle branch block on the right side of the chest. This electrocardiogram was taken on a twenty-year old man with congenital heart disease, consisting probably of a large high ventricular septal defect. The heart was large, but its shape was nondiagnostic.

INTERPRETATION. Normal rhythm, rate 85, with wide QRS waves in all leads, measuring up to 0.14 second. There is left axis deviation in the limb leads, but a somewhat confusing picture in the precordial leads. Over the right ventricle the record resembles quite clearly that of right bundle branch block, but there is also notching and widening of the QRS waves in Lead V₅ over the left ventricle, the explanation of which is not clear.

Drs. Frank Wilson and Franklin Johnston have suggested that additional leads, including esophageal leads, might be helpful in elucidating this tracing and that an unusual cardiac position may be responsible for the confusion.

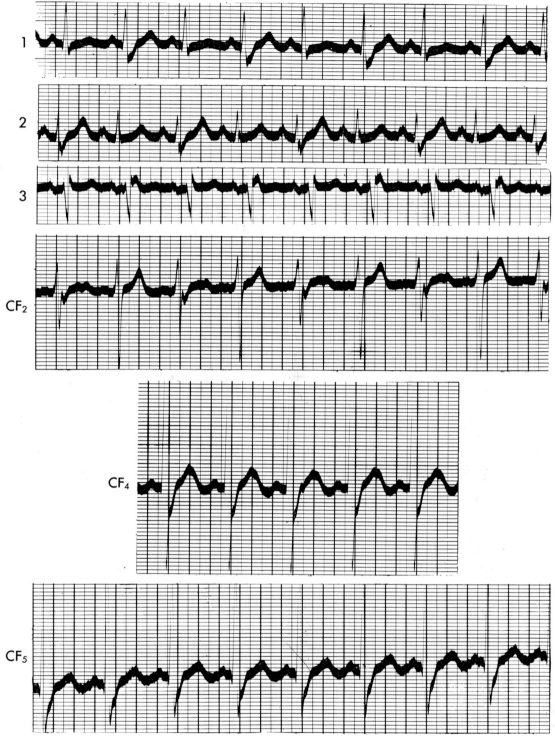

Fig. 140. Bundle branch block, 2:1.

Two-to-one bundle branch block in a man of fifty-nine who had few complaints when examined on February 6, 1945, beyond fatigue and shortness of breath on stairs and hills for a period of one year, without pain. He had had no headaches, but five years previously had been told that his blood pressure was rather high. Three years previously he had been refused life insurance on two occasions because of high blood pressure. Two months before the present visit he had begun to have trouble seeing, and over the last few weeks had noticed drowsiness in the evening and after meals. His father had died at the age of fifty-four of apoplexy.

Physical examination at this time showed his pulse to be regular at a rate of 84. His blood pressure was 230 mm. of mercury systolic and 140 mm. diastolic. The left border of dullness was 12 cm. to the left of the midsternal line, 3

(*Legend continued on facing page*)

MISCELLANEOUS CONDITIONS

Wolff-Parkinson-White Syndrome

There is an interesting variation of the normal cardiac mechanism that has been called the Wolff-Parkinson-White syndrome after the three physicians who first described it. The descriptive label of "short *P–R* interval with wide *QRS* wave" summarizes the electrocardiographic tracing. The time interval from the beginning of the *P* to the end of the *QRS* is equal to that normally, or rather usually, found in a healthy person at the same heart rate, and as a matter of fact is also equal to that found at times in the same person when the *P–R* interval and *QRS* duration change back to a usual timing from that of the short *P–R* interval and wide *QRS*, as may occasionally happen. Thus there is pre-excitation of one ventricle or the other, more commonly of the left, apparently due to atrio-ventricular connections (such as a bundle of Kent) which by-pass the ordinary junctional tissue of atrioventricular node and bundle (of His). (See Figure 141.)

This apparent electrocardiographic anomaly has been on occasion in the past a cause for concern and even alarm on the basis of an erroneous interpretation of bundle branch block or heart disease. Since it is not at all rare and is found in childhood as well as in later life, it should not be a cause for special consideration or treatment which might easily induce a cardiac neurosis. However, a common feature of the syndrome is paroxysmal tachycardia, and this, if frequent or disturbing, should be treated.

Several patients with Wolff-Parkinson-White syndrome have now been carefully followed up for over twenty years and have remained in good health. On the other hand, rare instances are on record of sudden death during tachycardia in persons with the Wolff-Parkinson-White syndrome, an accident that can occur also in paroxysmal tachycardia without the Wolff-Parkinson-White syndrome; the relative frequency of such events we do not know. We have recently encountered such a case for the first time ourselves, a woman aged forty-eight years, who died during or immediately after a paroxysm of extreme tachycardia with heart rate of 300 (Figs. 96 and 141). Further investigation, including especially a long follow-up analysis, of cases with this interesting mechanism is in order.

Electrical Alternans

Mechanical alternation of the arterial pulse (pulsus alternans), most readily identified in brachial or radial pulse, is common, especially in patients with myocardial (left ventricular) insufficiency secondary to hypertension, coronary atherosclerosis or aortic valve disease, but alternation of the amplitude of the ventricular complexes of the electrocardiogram is exceedingly rare. However, such cases are found, and one is shown in Figure 142.

Alternation of shape of successive ventricular complexes occurring at a regular heart rate has already been described as a grave type of ventricular paroxysmal tachycardia (see Fig. 114, p. 124).

Electrical alternans, which, when it occurs, involves as a rule the *R* waves, is, like the mechanical alternans, a serious sign of advanced heart disease with delayed recovery of myocardial function evident on alternate beats. Still more rare is alternans of *P* or *T* waves.

(Legend continued from opposite page, Figure 140)

cm. outside the midclavicular line. The aortic second sound was slightly increased. There was a soft systolic murmur at the apex. There was no edema.

Urine examination revealed a trace of albumin, a few red cells, and many hyalin and granular casts. An x-ray film taken on February 15, the same day as the electrocardiogram shown here, showed cardiac enlargement, principally in the region of the left ventricle, the transverse diameter being 16.5 cm., with an internal thoracic diameter of 30.5 cm. The aorta was tortuous and elongated, but only moderately dilated.

Three months after this examination the patient was admitted to the hospital in an attack of paroxysmal left ventricular failure. His nonprotein nitrogen was 125 mg. per 100 cc. the day after entry and higher on subsequent tests. One week afterward he died.

Alternating or paroxysmal or temporary bundle branch block has almost exactly the same significance as permanent bundle branch block, being evidence of coronary heart disease, which need not be of serious degree. Here it is a complication of hypertensive heart disease. Often bundle branch block is the only sign of trouble. The paroxysmal or alternating variety is rare; it may be a transitional development between normal conduction and constant bundle branch block.

INTERPRETATION. Normal rhythm at a rate of 105, with alternating right bundle branch block and normal intraventricular conduction in Leads 1, 2, 3 and CF2. The bundle branch block is constant in Leads CF4 and CF5. The *P–R* intervals are normal throughout, and the *T* waves are upright in all six leads.

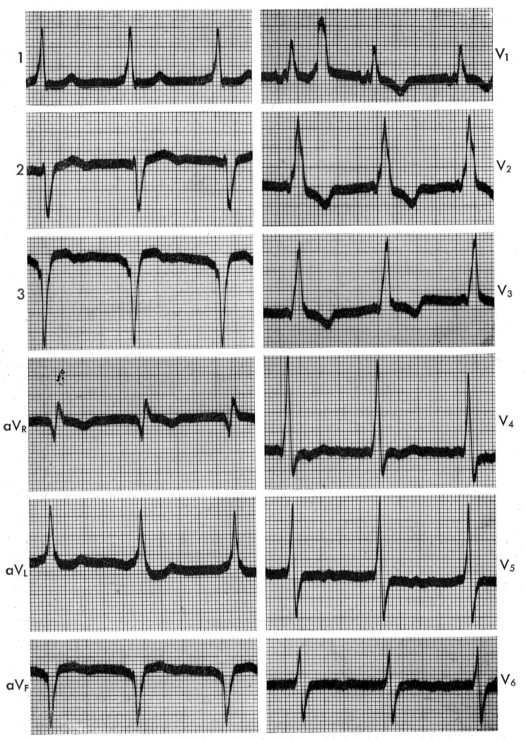

Fig. 141. Wolff-Parkinson-White syndrome.

Wolff-Parkinson-White syndrome in a woman of forty-five subject to attacks of atrial paroxysmal tachycardia (see Fig. 96, A, B, C).

INTERPRETATION. Normal rhythm at a rate of 65, with short P–R intervals of 0.08 second and wide QRS waves measuring 0.12 second in duration. There is marked left axis deviation in the limb leads, and there are prominent R waves in all precordial leads with an especial degree of widening and slurring in Lead V_2. The T's are upright in the limb leads, but inverted in the leads taken over the right ventricle, with, in all probability, a short circuit of impulse transmitted to the left ventricle.

Electrocar

L

Ele

The electrocardiogram may be
the administration of certain dru
portant to be aware of these chang
reasons: first, because it is nece
tinguish between changes due t
those due to disease or other fac
because the progressive electro
changes provide a measure of the
drug on the heart, and this ir
helpful in therapy; third, becaus
cardiogram may provide a usefu
diagnosis of certain metabolic disc
terized by disturbances in acid-bas
the chemical constituents of the b
calcium and potassium.

The effect of many different dru
cals may be due to only a few ca
disturbance in the sympathetic a
pathetic nerve tonus, the blood
coronary arteries, acid-base bala
alteration of cellular membrane
The effect also depends on primary
as dosage and individual variation
and on secondary factors such as
congestion, the improvement in ca
or the onset of nausea and vomitii

Although the electrocardiogra
are nonspecific, some are quite
for example, sagging of the *RS–T*
to digitalis and lengthening of the
in hypocalcemia. The most freque
are depression of the *RS–T* segme
ing or inversion of the *T* waves
heart rate and rhythm and in co
tween atria and ventricles are no
However, the *QRS* complex rep
polarization is not often affected.

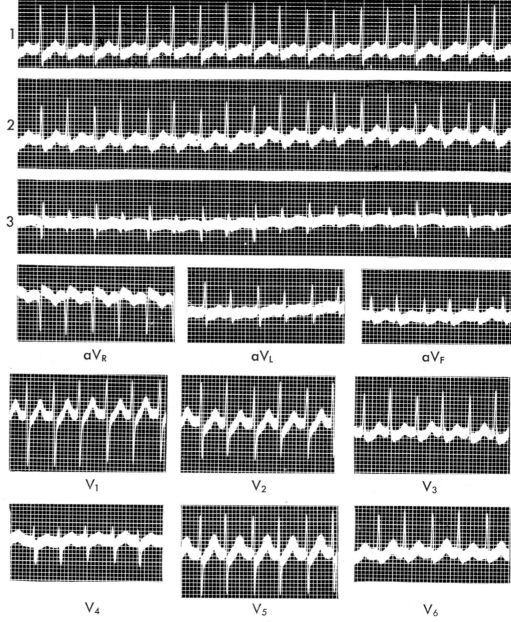

aVR aVL aVF

V₁ V₂ V₃

V₄ V₅ V₆

Fig. 142. Electrical alternans.

Electrical alternans in a woman teacher aged fifty with rheumatoid arthritis, during an attack of atrial paroxysmal tachycardia. Upon the administration of quinidine sulfate the heart rhythm was restored to normal.

INTERPRETATION. Atrial tachycardia at a fast heart rate of 200, with clear-cut alternation of the amplitudes of the *R* waves in Leads 2 and 3. Also, the *T* waves in Leads 2 and 3 alternate a little in amplitude; in Lead 2 the higher *T* waves occur following the shorter *QRS* waves; in Lead 3 the reverse is true. In Lead 2 it is to be observed that the time interval between the peaks of the short *R* waves and the following taller *R* waves is a little less than the succeeding time interval (0.278 versus 0.310). This indicates a slight difference probably in conduction time and may help to explain the alternation, which has the same significance as mechanical alternation of the pulse; both occur more frequently with tachycardia. Electrical alternans is a rare phenomenon, while mechanical alternans is common; they are seldom found in the same person.

obtained from a patient with slight chronic rheumatic heart disease who complained of weakness and anorexia. The electrocardiogram in Figure 144, *A*, shows changes characteristic of digitalization. The drug was omitted and the patient felt much improved, indicating that her symptoms were due in large part to digitalis intoxication. The electrocardiogram obtained after omitting the drug for twenty days is shown in Figure 144, *B*; slight digitalis effects are still present. The electrocardiogram in Figure 144, *C*, was obtained two months later. The digitalis effects have disappeared; there has been a slight shift in the location of the pacemaker after the inscription of Lead 2, and the *P* waves in Leads 3, aV$_R$, aV$_L$ and aV$_F$ have an altered appearance.

The electrocardiogram in Figure 145 was obtained from a patient with chronic rheumatic heart disease who complained of easy fatigability, anorexia and yellow vision. The bigeminal rhythm strongly supports the clinical diagnosis of digitalis intoxication, although other factors might have been responsible.

The electrocardiogram in Figure 146 was obtained from a patient sixty-four years of age who was discovered in her hotel bedroom in a stuporous condition. Several empty medicine bottles were found, including one which had contained digitalis and others a barbiturate preparation. The electrocardiogram, taken soon after admission to the hospital, shows partial atrioventricular block with occasional dropped beats; the atrial rate is 85, and the ventricular rate varies from 85 to 55. There is marked sagging of the *RS–T* segments. This patient died ten days after admission, and autopsy revealed acute terminal thrombosis of the right coronary artery (without infarction), pulmonary edema and hypostatic pneumonia. It was concluded that the chief cause of death was hypostatic pneumonia and that contributing causes included digitalis and barbiturate poisoning.

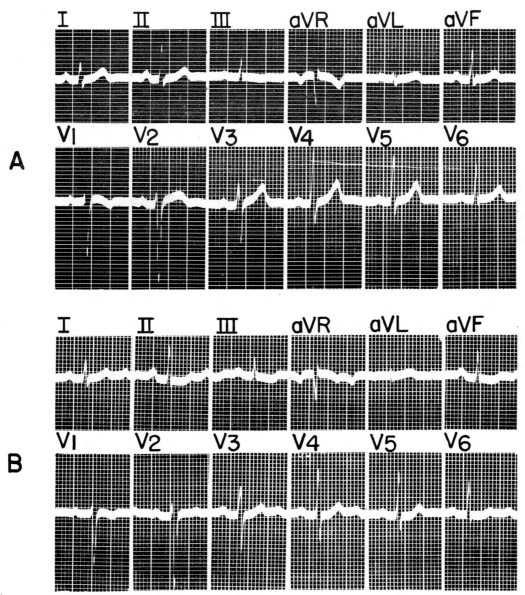

Fig. 143. Electrocardiograms obtained from a young healthy woman. (A) before and (B) after digitalization. The principal alterations are lowering of the RS–T junctions, sagging of the RS–T segments and lowering of the T waves in both the limb and precordial leads. The exception to this generalization is Lead aVR, where, as the result of digitalization, the RS–T segment is slightly elevated and convex and the T wave is less deeply inverted than formerly.

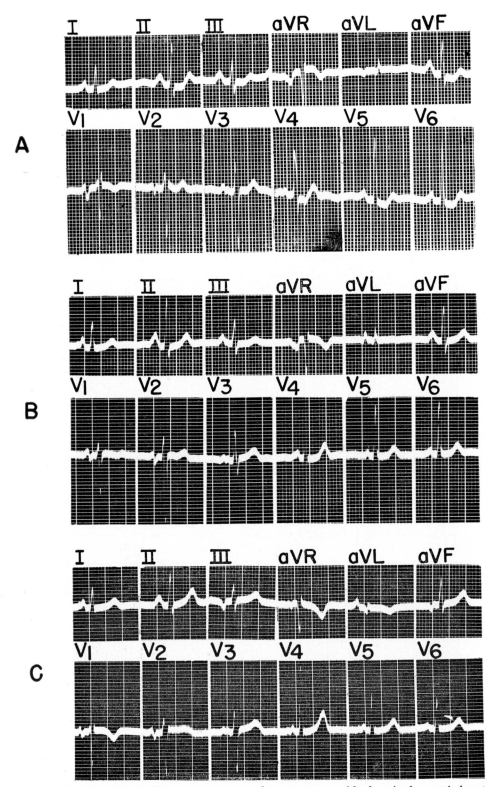

Fig. 144. Electrocardiograms obtained from a woman aged twenty-seven with chronic rheumatic heart disease and mitral stenosis. At the time the electrocardiogram in *A* was obtained, the patient was suffering from digitalis intoxication. This is declared by characteristic changes in the *RS–T* segments and lowering of the *T* waves in both limb and precordial leads. *B* was obtained twenty days after digitalis was omitted. Slight digitalis effects still persist. The electrocardiogram in *C* was obtained nearly three months after digitalis was omitted, and the effects of the drug are no longer evident.

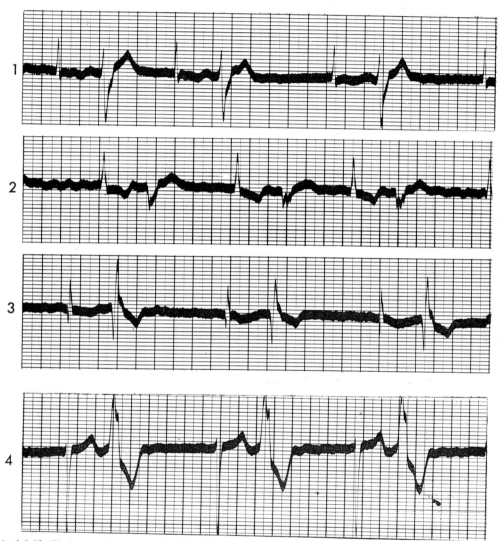

Fig. 145. Atrial fibrillation with bigeminal rhythm due to the occurrence of alternate normal and abnormal (ectopic) ventricular beats associated with digitalis intoxication.

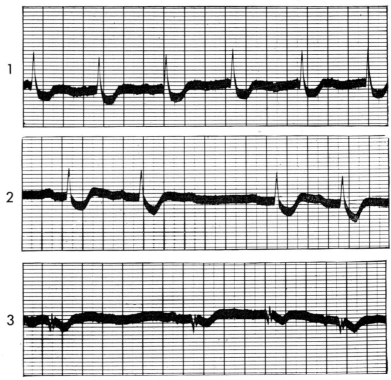

Fig. 146. Digitalis intoxication producing atrioventricular block and deep sagging of the *RS–T* segments.

Quinidine

This drug decreases the relative refractory period of the cardiac musculature, thus tending to reduce rate of atrial flutter or fibrillation in these arrhythmias and to lessen any tendency toward the development of ectopic beats or rhythms. It may transform atrial fibrillation into flutter, and transform flutter with a fast atrial rate to flutter with a much slower rate, eventually abolishing the flutter with restoration of normal rhythm in most cases. However, toxic effects are sometimes evident in the electrocardiogram: marked increase in ventricular rate (associated with a decrease in the grade of atrioventricular block), bundle branch block (which disappears on omitting the drug), depression of either sinoatrial or atrioventricular nodes, with atrial or ventricular standstill, and prolongation of the *Q–T* intervals (duration of systole). Quinidine therapy in full dosage is useful in abolishing atrial fibrillation or flutter, but its action when large amounts are given should be carefully controlled by electrocardiography.

Quinidine sulfate administered in small doses to prevent or reduce the frequency of arrhythmias (premature beats, paroxysmal tachycardia or atrial fibrillation or flutter) affects the electrocardiogram itself very little because of the small amount used.

The electrocardiograms in Figure 147 were obtained from a man fifty-six years of age with hypertensive and probable coronary heart disease, atrial flutter and moderate decrease in cardiac reserve. Strip *A* was obtained before treatment. There is 4 to 1 atrioventricular block; the atrial rate is 280 and the ventricular rate 70 a minute. Strips *B*, *C* and *D* show the progressive slowing of the flutter rate while the patient was receiving 45 grains of quinidine sulfate in divided doses. Strip *E* was obtained shortly after the restoration of normal rhythm. Note the abnormally long *P–R* and *Q–T* intervals. Strip *F* was taken four days later while the patient was ingesting a ration of 3 grains of quinidine every four hours. The *P–R* intervals and *Q–T* durations have shortened.

The electrocardiograms in Figure 148 were obtained from a patient with healed myocardial infarction who was subject to attacks of paroxysmal tachycardia. The record in Figure 148, *A*, was taken after a paroxysm had been in progress for two days. In long strips of the record it was possible to distinguish *P* waves which bore no relation to the ventricular rhythm; hence a diagnosis was made of ventricular tachycardia. Normal rhythm was restored after the administration of 45 grains of quinidine sulfate during a period of six hours. Note the remarkable length of the *Q–T* interval in Figure 148, *B*. The *T* wave changes may be due, in part at least, to the strain induced by the arrhythmia.

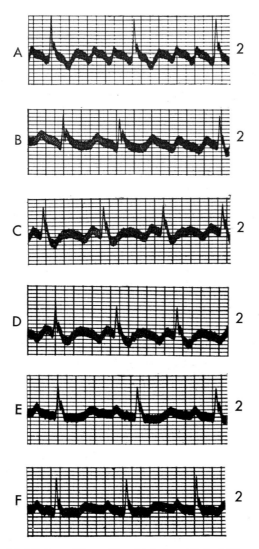

Fig. 147. Action of quinidine on atrial flutter. (From Graybiel, A.: Clinical Electrocardiography in Nelson Loose-Leaf Medicine. New York, Thomas Nelson & Sons, Vol. 4.)

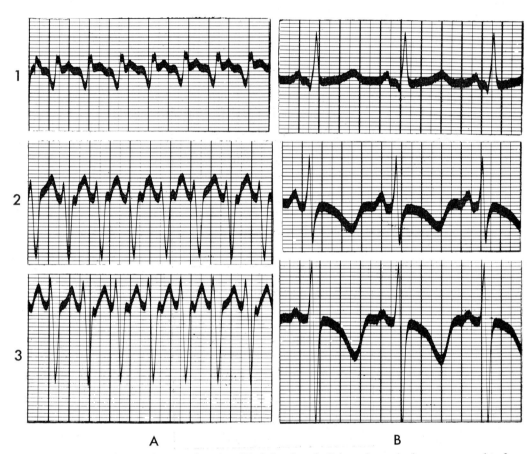

Fig. 148. The effect of quinidine on the $Q-T$ duration (B), following abolition of ventricular paroxysmal tachycardia (A).

Atropine

Atropine paralyzes the vagus nerve action and so removes the inhibition of heart rate. Sinoatrial tachycardia results (with atrioventricular nodal rhythm at times as an intermediate event), and the T waves decrease in amplitude. The electrocardiograms in Figure 149 were obtained from a healthy young woman twenty-four years of age. A is the control record, B was obtained after the injection of 2 mg. of atropine sulfate intravenously. The P waves are somewhat taller, but the T waves are nearly isoelectric. It is noteworthy that the $P-R$ intervals have not shortened; indeed, they appear to be slightly longer. Atropine is sometimes given to determine how much the $P-R$ interval will shorten as the result of release of

vagal tonus. This effect will be discussed later in reference to the electrocardiogram in acute rheumatic fever (p. 221).

Tobacco

Tobacco tends to elevate the heart rate and blood pressure, and, like epinephrine and atropine, to lower (or rarely even to invert) the T waves. The electrocardiograms in Figure 150 were obtained from a healthy young woman twenty-six years of age to test the effect of the inhalation of tobacco smoke. The record in Figure 150, B, was obtained after the inhalation of the smoke from one cigarette. The heart rate has risen to 130, and the T waves have become lower in Leads 1 and 2. This is a striking response observed in only occasional subjects.

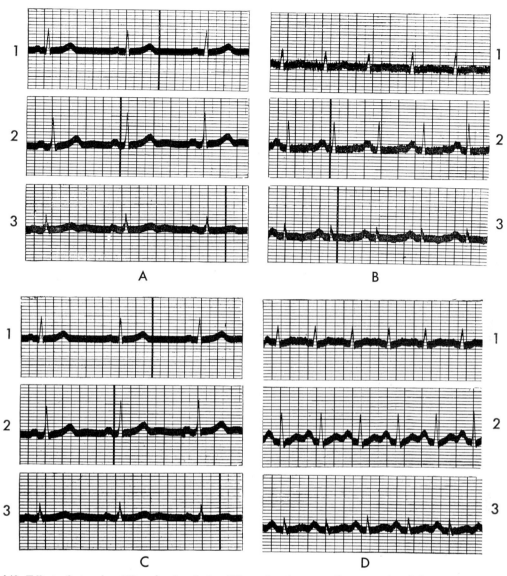

Fig. 149. Effect of atropine (*B*) and epinephrine (*D*) on the electrocardiogram. *A* and *C* are control tracings

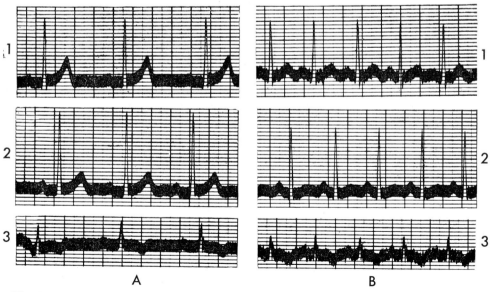

Fig. 150. Effect of tobacco: *A*, before smoking; *B*, after smoking. (Am. Heart J., *15*: 1938.)

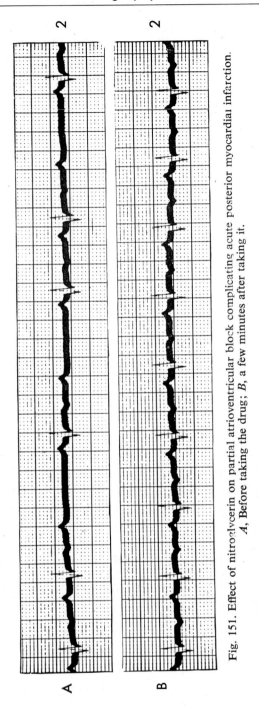

Fig. 151. Effect of nitroglycerin on partial atrioventricular block complicating acute posterior myocardial infarction. A, Before taking the drug; B, a few minutes after taking it.

Nitroglycerin

The electrocardiograms in Figure 151 were obtained from a patient forty-two years of age during his convalescence from myocardial infarction involving the posterior wall of the heart. He was troubled with palpitation due to partial atrioventricular block and dropped beats and by angina pectoris decubitus, but found that he could control both by the use of nitroglycerin and erythrol tetranitrate. In Figure 151 both strips are of Lead 2. Strip A shows partial atrioventricular block and dropped beats. Strip B was obtained shortly after the ingestion of 1/100 grain of nitroglycerin; the atrial rate has increased slightly, the P–R interval is shorter, and there are no dropped beats. This is a good illustration of the beneficial effect of nitrites on coronary insufficiency, which in this case was also responsible for atrioventricular block.

Procaine Amide (Pronestyl)

For a good many years it has been known that cocaine and its derivatives, in particular novocain (procaine), have a quieting effect on the heart in addition to their effects on the central nervous system. Only lately, however, has it been possible practically to utilize this sedative effect through the development of the use of procaine amide (Pronestyl), which, given either parenterally or orally, can abolish ventricular arrhythmias, especially ventricular premature beats and ventricular paroxysmal tachycardia, in a high percentage of cases. Figure 152 is a good example of this specific effect.

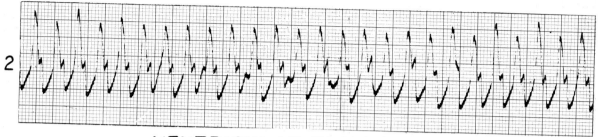

VENTRICULAR TACHYCARDIA

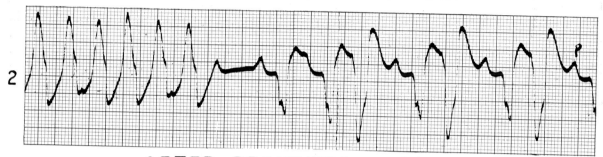

AFTER PRONESTYL — 1000 MG.

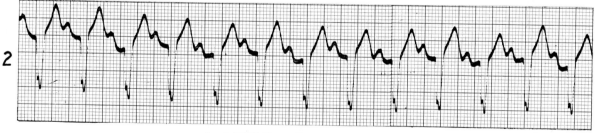

LATER-SAME DAY

Fig. 152. Effect of procaine amide (Pronestyl) on ventricular tachycardia.

Procaine amide and its effect upon ventricular tachycardia in a young man of twenty-one years with myocarditis of unknown etiology. This tracing was obtained shortly after his hospital admission on April 3, 1951. So far as cardiac symptoms were concerned, his past history was essentially negative. He had lost consciousness suddenly while at work and on entry was found to have marked cardiac enlargement, with fever, a gallop rhythm and severe congestive heart failure. It was felt that this was probably on the basis of an idiopathic myocarditis. The loss of consciousness was undoubtedly due to the onset of ventricular tachycardia, which reverted to normal rhythm with bundle branch block after the slow, continuous intravenous administration of 1 gm. (1000 mg.) of Pronestyl (procaine amide).

In addition to digitalis, a low sodium diet, and mercurial diuretics, he was treated with ACTH, with dramatic improvement. However, while he was still receiving this drug the congestive failure again became progressively worse, and he died on April 28 after an episode which appeared to be pulmonary infarction.

Autopsy revealed isolated myocarditis, idiopathic cardiac hypertrophy with mural thrombus of the left ventricle, severe hemorrhagic pulmonary edema, severe chronic passive congestion of lung and liver, and infarcts of the left lung and kidney.

INTERPRETATION. Ventricular paroxysmal tachycardia at a heart rate of 230, stopping after the administration of Pronestyl. The third strip of Lead 2, taken later the same day, shows normal rhythm at a heart rate of 110, with a slightly prolonged P–R interval of 0.21 second and bundle branch block.

COMMENT. This record is an excellent illustration of the favorable and at times life-saving effect of procaine in abolishing ventricular tachycardia. In this case the etiologic factor responsible for the heart disease was myocarditis of unknown cause as identified at autopsy.

Other Drugs and Chemicals

Disturbances of electrolyte balance in the body, in particular those relating to potassium and calcium, are discussed in Chapters 18 and 22. No direct effect on the electrocardiogram is noted from changes in sodium content or has been reported from variations in the content of certain other body chemicals such as phosphorus and sulfur. With acidosis there is usually no change in rhythm, but some slight increase in heart rate, and the *T* waves may become taller. With alkalosis, likewise, there is usually no change in rhythm, a slight increase in rate, and the *S–T* segments and *T* waves may become lower and even inverted and the *Q–T* time (duration of systole) lengthened.

Epinephrine in small dosage has no effect on the electrocardiogram, but in high dosage increases the heart rate, lowers the *S–T* segments and *T* waves (Figure 149, *C*, *D*), and may, in rare instances, cause upright *T* waves to become inverted, especially in Lead 2.

Carbon monoxide in cases of mild poisoning causes no significant changes, but in large dosage there is a tendency to lowering of the voltage of all the complexes with the production of various abnormalities of rhythm and increased heart rate.

Chloroform and *cyclopropane* in the course of induction of anesthesia tend to produce premature beats, paroxysmal tachycardia and, on rare occasions, ventricular fibrillation.

Ergotamine tartrate, through vagal tone, increases the height of the *T* waves and decreases heart rate.

Insulin in high concentration may depress the *S–T* segments and *T* waves in association with the lowering of the blood sugar.

Mecholyl acts favorably in abolishing certain arrhythmias, in particular paroxysmal tachycardia of atrial origin, through its vagal effect.

No significant changes in the electrocardiogram are produced by various other drugs in ordinary dosage: *arsenic, atabrine, barbiturates, benzedrine, bromides, coramine, ether, iodine, ipecac, mercury, morphine, pitressin, physostigmine (prostigmine), salicylates, sulfonamides, thiamine, thyroid* and the *xanthines.*

PART VI

Electrocardiographic Patterns

CHAPTER 11

Electrocardiographic Patterns

Atrial Enlargement

Alterations in the *P* waves may result from hypertrophy and dilatation of the atria. These include (1) an increase in duration, (2) an increase in amplitude, (3) a shift in electrical axis, and (4) peaking or notching of *P*. If the alterations are striking, they may be regarded as reliable signs of hypertrophy, but it should be remembered that a considerable degree of enlargement of the atria may be present before significant changes appear. Serial electrocardiograms are helpful because normally there is pronounced individual variation in the *P* waves.

The electrocardiograms in Figure 153 were obtained from a patient with mitral stenosis and moderate left atrial enlargement. The *P* waves are unusually prominent and sharply peaked, but the *P* wave duration and the electrical axis are normal. The likelihood of finding *P* waves of this sort in the electrocardiogram of a healthy adult is extremely small. Although it may be true that the *P* waves associated with left atrial enlargement tend to be broad and of low amplitude, while in right atrial enlargement they tend to be tall and peaked, there are so many exceptions to this generalization that it cannot be relied upon.

The electrocardiogram in Figure 154 was obtained from a patient with mitral stenosis and great enlargement of the left atrium. The *P* waves are characteristic: note the long duration and rounded contour.

The electrocardiogram in Figure 155 was obtained from a young man with congenital heart disease. The *P* waves are abnormally prominent and peaked in most leads, but the duration and electrical axis are normal. These findings are typical in cases of congenital heart disease with atrial, particularly right atrial, dilatation and hypertrophy.

Ventricular Enlargement and Ventricular "Strain"

Characteristic changes in the electrocardiogram occur with the development of ventricular enlargement. These changes are due in part to the enlargement and in part to associated factors, such as the shift in position of the heart, the development of myocardial ischemia and "strain," and disturbances in intraventricular conduction. Typical patterns have been described for left, right, and combined left and right ventricular enlargement.

As a rule, the greater the degree of enlargement, the more characteristic and the more striking the electrocardiographic alterations. While it is true that a considerable degree of enlargement may be present without producing definite electrocardiographic alterations, it is also true that the electrocardiogram may provide the earliest clue that hypertrophy has occurred. Characteristic changes in the limb leads include (1) a shift of the electrical axis of *QRS*, (2) an increase in voltage of *QRS*, (3) an increase in duration of *QRS*, (4) *RS–T* displacement opposite to the chief *QRS* deflection, and (5) a shift of the electrical axis of the *T* waves. Characteristic changes in the precordial leads include (1) an increase in voltage of *QRS* with a tendency toward the development of large monophasic waves, (2) an increase in the duration of *QRS*, (3) a shift of the transitional zone, usually to the left, for both *QRS* and *T*, and (4) displacement of *RS–T* and *T* in a direction opposite to the chief *QRS* deflection.

The term "ventricular strain" is in common use, but there is no general agreement regarding either its cause or the electrocardiographic criteria on which it is based. It may be used as a convenient term to apply in all instances in which there are *T* wave and *RS–T* changes relating to the ventricular enlargement. These changes may be primary or may be secondary to alterations in *QRS*. The factors responsible for primary changes include absolute or relative myocardial ischemia, increase in intraventricular pressure, and probably other factors as well.

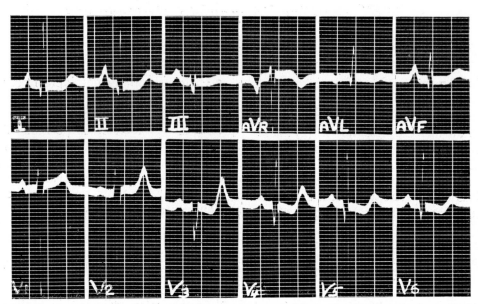

Fig. 153. This electrocardiogram was obtained from a woman aged forty-six with chronic rheumatic heart disease, mitral stenosis, and moderate left atrial and left ventricular enlargement. The P waves are unusually prominent and indicate atrial enlargement. The RS–T segment changes are probably due to left ventricular enlargement and strain. The patient was not receiving digitalis. See text.

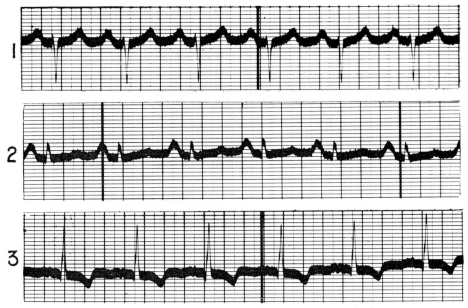

Fig. 154. Prominent P waves associated with mitral stenosis. See text.

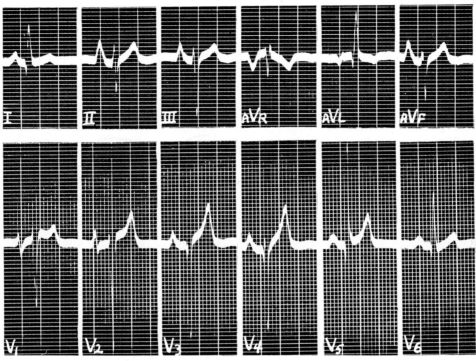

Fig. 155. This record was obtained from a man twenty-one years of age with congenital heart disease, tricuspid atresia and atrial septal defect. The prominent *P* waves indicate atrial enlargement.

Left Ventricular Enlargement

The electrocardiogram in Figure 156 was obtained from a patient of average build with essential hypertension. Roentgenologic examination revealed the size of the heart to be at the upper limit of normal. The limb leads show left axis deviation of *QRS* (approximately −30 degrees), but the electrical axis of *T* points to +30 degrees. In the precordial leads *QRS* complexes, nearly transitional in form, are found in Leads V₃ through V₅, and the transitional zone extends unusually far to the left. The important question is whether these electrocardiographic findings indicate simply a horizontal position of the heart with counterclockwise rotation, or left ventricular hypertrophy. The only evidence possibly suggesting the latter is the fact that the electrical axes of *P* and *T* have not shifted equally with *QRS*. In terms of probability it is more likely that both left ventricular hypertrophy and a shift in position of the heart are responsible for the changes observed, than that they are due solely to a shift in heart position.

The electrocardiogram in Figure 157 was obtained from a patient with essential hypertension and slight left ventricular enlargement. In the limb leads there is left axis deviation of both *QRS* and *T* to an equal degree; this is more indicative of a horizontal position of the heart than of left ventricular hypertrophy. However, the precordial leads are abnormal and clearly indicate left ventricular hypertrophy. The abnormalities are (1) the great amplitude of *S* in V₁ through V₄, and of *R* in V₅ and V₆, (2) the tendency toward monophasic *QRS* waves, and (3) the shift to the left of the transitional zone.

The electrocardiogram in Figure 158 was obtained from a patient with hypertensive and coronary heart disease with well marked cardiac enlargement. Therapy included digitalization at the time this record was obtained. The characteristic findings of left ventricular hypertrophy and strain are present in an extreme degree. Even more striking examples are shown in Figures 197 (p. 231), 211 (p. 250) and 212 (p. 251).

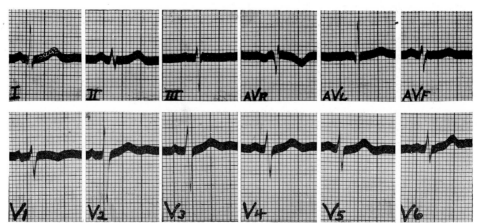

Fig. 156. This electrocardiogram was obtained from a man forty-eight years of age with essential hypertension; the blood pressure was 180 mm. of mercury systolic and 132 mm. diastolic. X-ray examination revealed the heart to be at the upper limit of normal in size. There is a moderate degree of left axis deviation and a rather wide angle (60 degrees) between the electrical axis of QRS and T. This patient died two years later after coronary occlusion. See text.

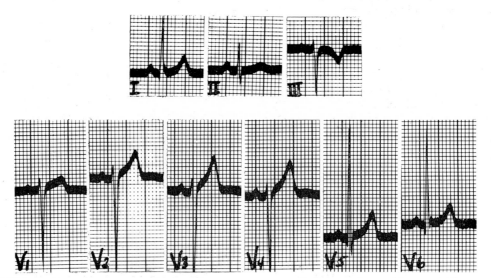

Fig. 157. This electrocardiogram was obtained from a man twenty-five years of age with essential hypertension; the blood pressure was 176 mm. of mercury systolic and 118 mm. diastolic. X-ray examination revealed a moderate degree of left ventricular hypertrophy. In the limb leads the electrical axis of both QRS and T are shifted to the left, and in the precordial leads the S waves are abnormally prominent on the right side and the R waves abnormally prominent on the left. These findings are consistent with left ventricular hypertrophy.

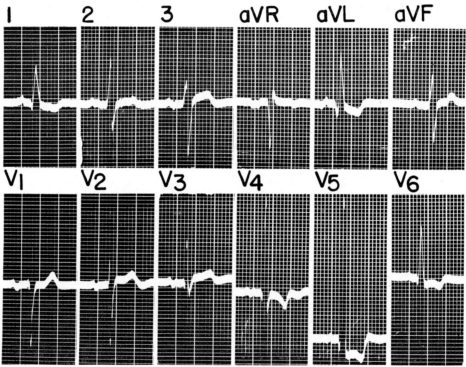

Fig. 158. This electrocardiogram was obtained from a man fifty-six years of age with hypertensive and coronary heart disease; the blood pressure was 180 mm. of mercury systolic and 110 mm. diastolic. X-ray examination revealed moderate left ventricular enlargement. Treatment included digitalization. Limb leads show a moderate degree of left axis deviation, and the precordial leads show prominent R waves in Leads V_4 and V_5 with the T waves oppositely directed. These changes are indicative of left ventricular hypertrophy and strain. Digitalization probably accounts for some of the $RS-T$ segment and T wave alteration. Q waves in Leads aVL, and Leads 1 and V_5 probably result from septal depolarization. They are not prominent enough to suggest myocardial infarction.

Right Ventricular Enlargement

The electrocardiographic findings associated with right ventricular enlargement are not exactly the reciprocal of those described for left ventricular enlargement. This is chiefly because the left ventricle normally predominates in the adult, and a considerable degree of right ventricular hypertrophy must occur before the electrical forces generated by the right ventricle become greater than those generated by the left. This is not so in infants and small children when the right ventricle may normally be preponderant and right ventricular hypertrophy produces striking electrocardiographic changes. Two other points should be mentioned. In right, as contrasted with left ventricular hypertrophy there is a greater tendency toward the development of intraventricular conduction defects and toward the appearance of prominent P waves.

The electrocardiogram in Figure 159 was obtained from a patient twenty-seven years of age with congenital heart disease, moderate right ventricular hypertrophy and probable atrial septal defect. In the limb leads QRS tends to be biphasic, in which case the direction of the mean electrical axis has little significance. However, there is a tendency toward right axis deviation (+120 degrees), although the T waves and the electrical axis of T are normal. In the precordial leads an rR' pattern is observed in V_1 which, in combination with the relatively broad S wave in Lead 1, is consistent with either right ventricular hypertrophy or defective conduction in the right bundle branch, or both. Note the progressive changes in QRS in V_2 through V_6, particularly the notched R in V_2 and the prominent S waves in V_3 through V_6. There is a slight tendency for the RS–T segments to be oppositely directed to the chief QRS component, but the T wave changes are probably primary. The QRS changes in this record resemble those sometimes seen in the electrocardiograms obtained from young apparently healthy persons, and the same thing may be said for the T wave changes in V_4 through V_6.

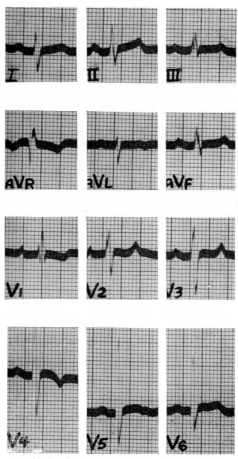

Fig. 159. This electrocardiogram was obtained from a man twenty-seven years of age with congenital heart disease, probable atrial septal defect, and moderate right ventricular enlargement. There are slight alterations in both limb and precordial leads which are consistent with right ventricular hypertrophy. See text.

The electrocardiogram in Figure 160 was obtained from a child five years of age with the tetralogy of Fallot. This diagnosis was later confirmed by postmortem examination. In the limb leads there is marked right axis deviation of QRS (+170 degrees), and the electrical axis of T points to +50 degrees, which is typical of marked right ventricular hypertrophy and strain. Note the prominent, sharply peaked P waves. In the precordial leads an RS pattern is observed in Leads V_1 through V_5. Presumably, leads obtained farther to the right would reveal still taller R waves and inverted T waves. In Lead V_6 an rS pattern is observed, which is typical of right ventricular hypertrophy.

The electrocardiogram in Figure 161 was obtained from a woman forty-three years of age with cor pulmonale secondary to organized emboli of the tertiary pulmonary arteries.*

Postmorten examination revealed marked dilatation and hypertrophy of the right atrium and ventricle. The electrocardiogram was obtained a year before death, at which time she was in congestive failure and was receiving digitalis and diuretics. The limb leads show right axis deviation of QRS (+140 degrees), and the T waves tend to be oppositely directed to the chief QRS deflection, which indicates right ventricular strain. In the precordial leads V_1 and V_2 the S waves are absent and the R waves are abnormally prominent, with associated inversion of the T waves. In Leads V_5 and V_6 the S waves are abnormally prominent. These findings indicate right ventricular hypertrophy and strain.

* Castleman, B., and Bland E. F.: Organized Emboli of the Tertiary Pulmonary Arteries. *Arch. Path.*, *42*:581, 1947.

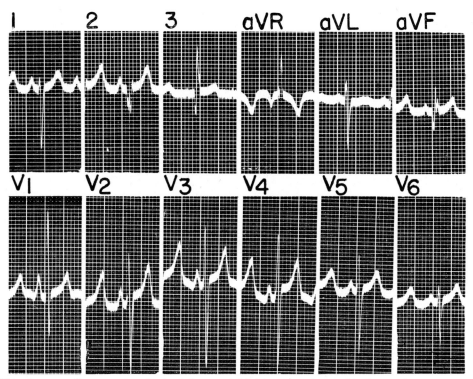

Fig. 160. This electrocardiogram was obtained from a child five years of age with the tetralogy of Fallot. In the limb leads there is marked right axis deviation. In the precordial leads RS complexes are observed in Leads V_1 through V_5 and an rS pattern in V_6. These changes are consistent with right ventricular hypertrophy without strain.

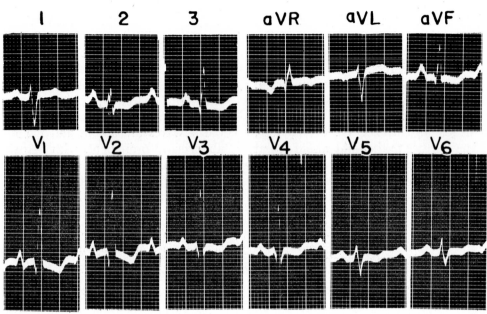

Fig. 161. This electrocardiogram was obtained from a woman forty-three years of age with cor pulmonale and marked right ventricular enlargement. Treatment included digitalization. In the limb leads there is moderate left axis deviation of QRS, and the T waves tend to be oppositely directed to the chief QRS wave in Leads 1 and 3. In the precordial leads the R waves are abnormally prominent in Leads V_1 through V_3 and the T waves are oppositely directed. In Leads V_5 and V_6 the S waves are abnormally prominent. These changes indicate right ventricular enlargement and strain.

Combined Right and Left Ventricular Hypertrophy and "Strain."

Hypertrophy and "strain" of one ventricle may be followed by hypertrophy and "strain" of the other, or they may develop simultaneously in both ventricles. In the former instance, serial electrocardiograms may clearly indicate the change from the left or right to the combined type. The result is usually a curious mixture of signs, some of which suggest left and others right ventricular hypertrophy and "strain." In the absence of serial electrocardiograms, the presence of combined "strain" may still be suspected, but a definite diagnosis cannot always be made with certainty. A chief difficulty rests in the fact that unilateral ventricular hypertrophy and "strain," combined with an unusual position of the heart, may yield electrocardiographic findings which resemble those of combined "strain." Another difficulty is that the $RS-T$ segments and T waves are readily influenced by factors other than hypertrophy and "strain." Nevertheless, combined heart "strain" should always be suspected when some of the electrocardiographic alterations suggest the left and some the right variety. Conversely, electrocardiographic evidence of combined "strain" should be sought when other findings suggest that it may be present.

The electrocardiogram in Figure 162 was obtained from a young man with rheumatic heart disease, free aortic regurgitation and well marked mitral stenosis. There was moderate to great cardiac enlargement involving both right and left ventricles. The patient was not receiving digitalis at the time this record was obtained. In the limb leads the QRS intervals are slightly prolonged; the QRS voltage is large, but the electrical axis is normally directed ($+60$ degrees). There is slight sagging of the $RS-T$ segments in Leads 2 and 3, but the T waves are within the normal limits. The precordial leads reveal an RS pattern with inverted T waves in V_1 through V_4, which is more characteristic of right than of left ventricular hypertrophy. However, the tall R waves and upright T waves in V_5 through V_7 suggest left ventricular hypertrophy.

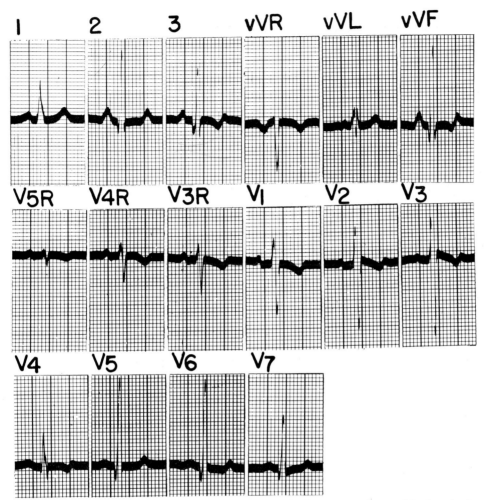

Fig. 162. This electrocardiogram was obtained from a man twenty-four years of age with chronic rheumatic heart disease, aortic regurgitation, mitral stenosis and generalized cardiac enlargement. In the limb leads the *QRS* complexes are slightly prolonged. The electrical axis is normal. The *RS–T* segment is displaced slightly downward in Lead 2, which is indicative of strain. In the precordial leads *RS* patterns are observed in Leads V_{3R} through V_3 and the *T* waves are inverted. The *R* waves are prominent in Leads V_5 and V_6, there is slight downward displacement in *RS–T*, and the *T* waves are low in amplitude. In the presence of cardiac enlargement these electrocardiographic changes are consistent with combined left and right ventricular hypertrophy. In this instance the unipolar limb leads have been equated in magnitude with the bipolar limb leads and have been designated vector unipolar leads (vVR, vVL, and vVF).

Myocarditis

The myocardium may be primarily affected by disease or by some injurious process, or it may be secondarily affected by disease or disorder elsewhere in the body. In most instances the etiologic factors are fairly well known and form the best basis for organizing the descriptions of the associated electrocardiographic findings. These will be found in Part VII.

Pericarditis

The electrocardiogram is of great importance in making the diagnosis of pericarditis and in following the course of this disease. The electrocardiographic alterations, while not pathognomonic, are fairly characteristic and, when they are considered together with the other clinical findings, the diagnosis can usually be made with assurance.

Acute Pericarditis

The electrocardiographic changes are due to inflammation of the subepicardium, inflammation and thickening of the pericardium, pericardial fluid, and shift in position of the heart. The most characteristic changes involve the $RS-T$ segments and T waves. With the onset of acute pericarditis there is elevation of $RS-T$ in several leads. Usually both limb and precordial leads are involved, and reciprocal changes may not be observed if only the standard limb leads and six precordial leads are obtained. The $RS-T$ segment changes are usually transitory and go unobserved unless tracings are taken at an early stage of the disease.

Initially, the T waves may be increased in amplitude, but quickly give way to flattening and inversion. Reciprocal T wave changes in the limb leads, characteristic of myocardial infarction, either are not seen or are ephemeral in nature. Frequently the T waves are low or inverted in all six limb leads and in most, if not in all, of the precordial leads. With recovery the T waves usually revert to their initial form.

In sharp contrast to the regular occurrence of $RS-T$ and T wave changes in pericarditis, QRS changes are of a minor character and conduction disturbances are uncommon. The voltage of QRS is reduced if there is much pericardial fluid or if the pericardium becomes greatly thickened. There is a tendency for the R waves to become relatively small or to disappear in the precordial leads V_1 through V_3. However, the QRS changes resulting from myocardial destruction are not seen in uncomplicated pericarditis. Disturbances in conduction are not due to pericarditis per se; when they are present, they point to some associated or complicating disease or disorder.

The distinction between pericarditis as a complication of disease or injury of the heart and pericarditis as the primary disease must be based on all the available clinical evidence. Serial electrocardiograms should always be taken and may prove helpful. From a practical point of view, the two most frequent problems encountered are the differential diagnosis of acute pericarditis and acute myocardial infarction, and the differentiation between pericarditis and myocarditis. In acute infarction the electrocardiographic signs are those of local ischemia, injury, and death of tissue: typical QRS changes are frequently seen, and $RS-T$ and T wave changes of reciprocal form tend to occur in the standard limb and precordial leads; conduction disturbances are not infrequent, and arrhythmias sometimes occur. The electrocardiographic alterations following myocardial infarction may be permanent, particularly QRS changes.

The differentiation between myocarditis and pericarditis is often difficult or even impossible. In generalized myocarditis without pericardial involvement there may be little change in $RS-T$, or, if change is present, there is sagging and depression. The T waves may become low in amplitude without showing any characteristic form or pattern of change. Conduction disturbances are frequent, particularly atrioventricular delay or block, and arrhythmias sometime occur.

The electrocardiograms in Figure 163 are shown partly to illustrate the difficulty in distinguishing between electrocardiographic alterations due to pericarditis and those due to myocarditis. The tracings were obtained from a man nineteen years of age who entered the hospital March 18, 1947, presenting the classical findings of meningococcal septicemia. He was critically ill for five days, then began to improve rapidly. He was afebrile for three days, but on March 27 slight fever developed without other symptoms or localizing signs. There was no further change, and on April 1 an electrocardiogram was obtained (Fig. 163, A). The only abnormalities are the low or inverted T waves in both the limb and precordial leads. On April 4 cough, chills and high fever developed, and he was severely ill again. The electrocardiogram obtained on that day is shown in Figure 163, B. The T waves in the limb leads have changed only slightly, but in the precordial leads the T waves are now inverted in V_3, taller in V_5 and V_6. The electrocardiogram obtained April 15 (Fig. 163, C) shows T waves which have reverted toward normal, and the record taken on April 30 (Fig. 163, D) shows normal T waves.

It was concluded that the electrocardiographic changes were slightly more characteristic of pericarditis than of myocarditis because of (1) the progressive changes in the precordial leads which are typical of pericarditis, and (2) the absence of conduction defects, particularly the failure of P–R to lengthen. The other clinical findings were consistent with either pericarditis or myocarditis, but not definitely diagnostic of one to the exclusion of the other. Lastly, the diagnosis of pericarditis was favored because the time-course of the T wave changes did not coincide well with the time-course of the symptomatology; that is, further inversion of the T waves occurred during a period when the patient was obviously getting better.

The electrocardiograms in Figure 164 were obtained from a Negro woman forty-five years of age who entered the hosptial complaining of severe pain in the left side of the chest. For the past three weeks she had been treated for "pericarditis" in another hospital. Examination revealed the heart to be enlarged, and a friction rub was heard over the precordium. The rhythm was normal and no murmurs were heard. The blood pressure was 90 mm. of mercury systolic and 50 mm. diastolic. The neck veins were distended, rales were heard over both lung bases, and the liver was greatly enlarged and tender. X-ray examination revealed considerable enlargement of the cardiac silhouette and congestive phenomena in the lungs.

The initial electrocardiogram (Fig. 164, A) showed elevation and convexity of the RS–T segment in Lead 2 and deep inversion of the T waves in Leads 1 and 2. The T waves were also inverted in precordial leads V_2 through V_6. The patient received digitoxin and mercurial diuretics and, one week later, aureomycin. She improved rapidly and was discharged three weeks after entry with a diagnosis of acute pericarditis and acute myocarditis. An electrocardiogram obtained four days before discharge (Fig. 164, B) revealed striking improvement. The slight sagging of the RS–T segments and the rather low T waves could be explained entirely or in part by the digitalization.

The electrocardiograms in Figure 165 were obtained from a schoolgirl thirteen years of age who entered the hospital July 6, 1944, complaining of pain of two days' duration in both shoulders and in the upper portion of the chest on the left side. The body temperature was 102°F. Examination of the heart and lungs revealed no abnormality. The white blood count on the day prior to admission was 22,000 cells per cubic millimeter. An x-ray film of the chest on the day of admission showed the cardiac silhouette to be slightly larger than normal. Two days later the enlargement was greater. A diagnosis was made of acute pericarditis with effusion.

The electrocardiogram in Figure 165, A, was obtained on July 14, 1944, at which time mild chest pain was still present. It shows moderate left axis deviation of the QRS complexes (0 degrees) and low diphasic T waves in all three leads. The T wave changes are consistent with the diagnosis. The electrocardiogram in Figure 165, B, was obtained on August 1, at which time the patient was much improved; the pain had disappeared, and the heart shadow as revealed by roentgenogram was no longer enlarged. In the limb leads the T waves have become deeply inverted in Lead 1 and upright in Lead 3; these reciprocal changes are noteworthy because they are not often seen in the standard leads. In the precordial leads the T waves were inverted in CF_2, CF_4 and CF_5. It is noteworthy that the electrocardiogram showed a greater degree of abnormality at the time when the patient was improving; this is observed not infrequently. The curves in Figure 165, C, were obtained three months later and are normal; the left axis deviation of QRS and T is due to a horizontal position of the heart associated with obesity.

The electrocardiograms in Figure 166 were obtained from a woman fifty-eight years of age who was suffering from tuberculous pericarditis with effusion. The cardiac silhouette was greatly enlarged. The venous pressure was increased, and there was congestion of the lungs and fluid in the left pleural cavity. She was receiving digitalis and antibiotic drugs. The striking feature of this record is the low voltage of the QRS and T waves in all the leads. Records similar to this may be obtained from patients with myxedema, beriberi, severe congestive failure or Pick's disease.

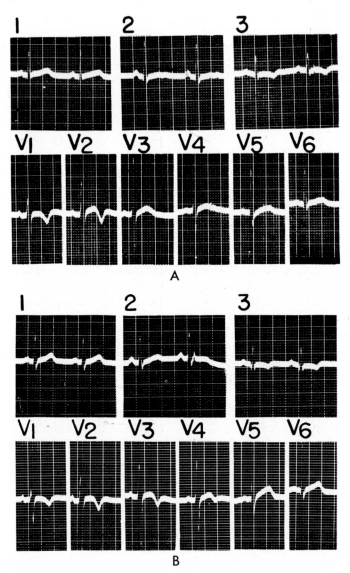

Fig. 163. The electrocardiograms obtained from a young man nineteen years of age who was suffering from meningo-coccal septicemia. *A* shows abnormally low or inverted *T* waves in both limb and precordial leads. *B* was obtained three days later. In the limb leads *T* waves have reverted toward the normal, and in the precordial leads *T* is inverted in Leads V_1 through V_4. (*Legend continued on facing page.*)

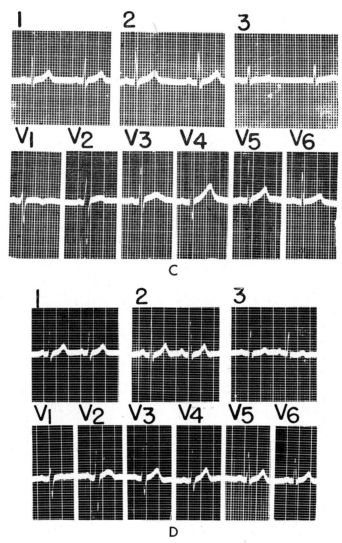

C

D

(*Legend continued from opposite page, Figure 163.*)

C was obtained fifteen days later. Both limb and precordial leads are within the normal range. D was obtained thirty days later and shows no abnormality. These changes are consistent with the diagnosis of acute pericarditis with recovery.

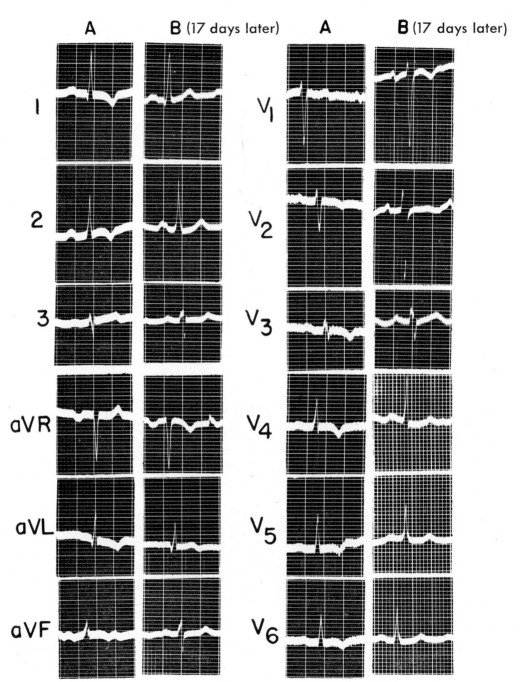

Fig. 164. This electrocardiogram was obtained from a Negro woman forty-five years of age with acute benign pericarditis complicated by cardiac tamponade. The electrocardiogram in *A* shows elevation and convexity of the *RS-T* segment in Lead 2 and inversion of the *T* waves in Leads 1 and 2. In the precordial leads the *T* waves are low or inverted in all leads. The electrocardiogram in *B* was obtained seventeen days later, at which time she was greatly improved. Treatment included digitalization. The only abnormalities are sagging of the *RS-T* segments and rather low *T* waves in some of the limb and precordial leads, but these effects might be explained by digitalization.

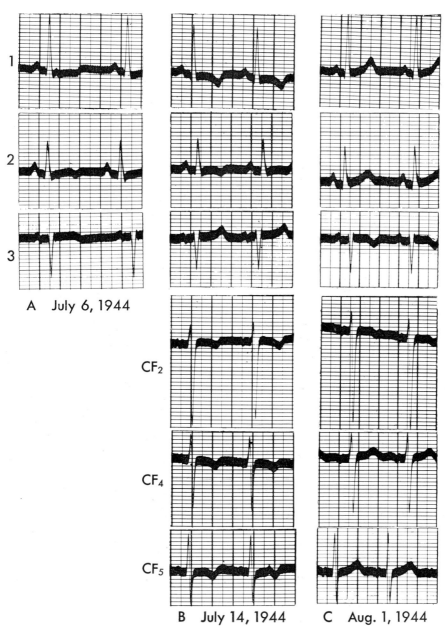

A   July 6, 1944

CF₂

CF₄

CF₅

B   July 14, 1944   C   Aug. 1, 1944

Fig. 165. Evolutionary electrocardiographic changes in acute pericarditis. See text.

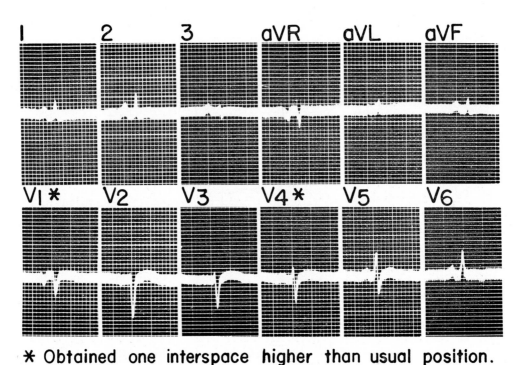

✳ Obtained one interspace higher than usual position.

Fig. 166. This electrocardiogram was obtained from a woman fifty-eight years of age with tuberculous pericarditis and effusion. Treatment included digitalization. There is low voltage of *QRS* and *T* waves in both limb and precordial leads. These changes are consistent with the diagnosis of pericarditis. See text.

Chronic Pericarditis

The electrocardiogram in Figure 167 was obtained from a woman thirty-nine years of age who twenty years previously had undergone an operation for constrictive pericarditis. Prior to operation she had generalized anasarca and was unable to walk more than a few steps. At operation a large area of thick pericardium was removed, including a band constricting the inferior vena cava. She made a remarkable recovery and eleven years later married and subsequently gave birth to two children, without cardiac difficulty. At the time this record was obtained (March, 1950) she looked well; her blood pressure was 140 mm. of mercury systolic and 90 mm. diastolic, pulse 72, color normal. The neck veins were not pulsating. The chest was clear. The heart was not enlarged. Sounds were of good quality with A-2 greater than P-2. There were no murmurs. The rhythm was regular. There was no enlargement of the liver, although it was slightly tender in the right upper quandrant. There was no edema. A few months later a total hysterectomy and appendectomy were performed, with uneventful convalescence, and in June, 1950, her condition was reported as excellent.

In the limb leads the *QRS* voltage is low, but the duration and axis are normal. The *T* waves are also of low amplitude; they are nearly isoelectric in Lead 2 and inverted in Lead 3. The precordial leads show no definite abnormality. The alterations in the limb leads are characteristic.

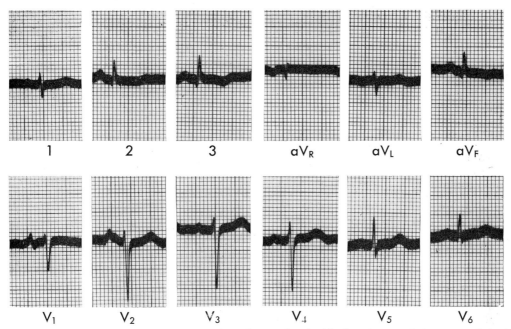

Fig. 167. Low voltage of *QRS* and *T* waves in limb leads associated with chronic constrictive pericarditis. See text.

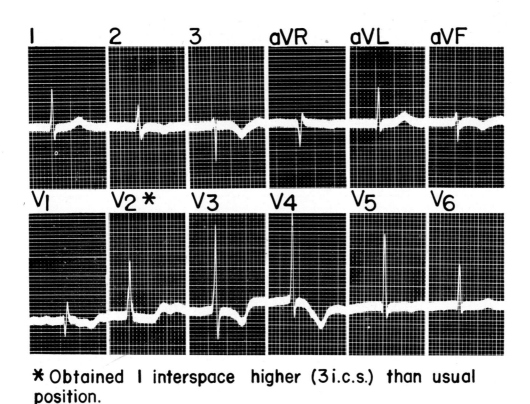

✱ Obtained I interspace higher (3 i.c.s.) than usual position.

Fig. 168. This electrocardiogram was obtained from a man fifty-one years of age with chronic constrictive pericarditis. Pericardiolysis had been performed nine months previously with moderate improvement. Treatment included digitalization. In addition to atrial fibrillation there is moderate left axis deviation of both *QRS* and *T* in the limb leads. In the precordial leads the *QRS* complexes are essentially normal, but there is downward displacement of the *RS–T* segments and inversion of the *T* waves in Leads V₁ through V₅. The left axis deviation of *QRS* and *T* in the limb leads may be due in large part to the anatomic position of the heart. The *RS–T* segment and *T* changes in the precordial leads may be attributed to pericarditis.

The electrocardiogram in Figure 168 was obtained from a man fifty-one years of age with chronic constrictive pericarditis. He had had a pericardiolysis performed nine months previously which had resulted in much improvement, but he was still limited in his activity and required digitalis and mercurial diuretics. The electrocardiogram shows atrial fibrillation; the ventricular rate, determined from a long strip of the record, averaged 75. There is normal voltage of the QRS complexes and the T waves in both limb and precordial leads. In the limb leads there is moderate left axis deviation of both QRS and T waves, suggesting that heart position may be a factor. The inversion of the T waves in the precordial lead is abnormal and attributable to the pericarditis.

The electrocardiogram in Figure 169 was obtained from a man forty-seven years of age with chronic constrictive pericarditis. Again atrial fibrillation is present. There is right axis deviation of QRS in the limb leads, and the maximal amplitude of QRS is unusually great. The inverted T waves in both limb and precordial leads are not typical of right or left ventricular strain and are probably due solely to the pericarditis. This combination of atrial fibrillation and right axis deviation strongly points to preponderant constriction of the left heart chambers obstructing the circulation. Thus it resembles the mechanical obstruction associated with mitral stenosis, and the similarity between this record and those obtained from certain patients with mitral stenosis is readily apparent.

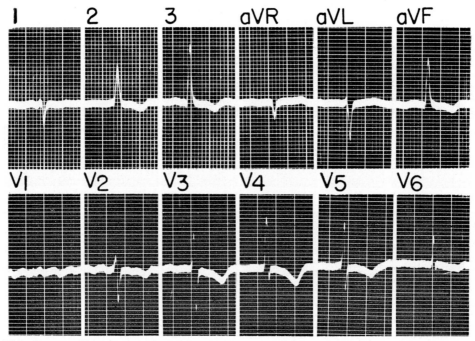

Fig. 169. This electrocardiogram was obtained from a man forty-seven years of age with chronic constrictive pericarditis. In addition to atrial fibrillation there is considerable right axis deviation of QRS in the limb leads. The T waves are low and inverted in both limb and precordial leads. The combination of atrial fibrillation and right axis deviation may be due to constriction of the left heart chambers which resembles the mechanical obstruction associated with mitral stenosis. See text.

CHAPTER 12

Congenital Heart

Not infrequently the electrocardiogram is normal in the less grave types of congenital defects. These include *patency of the ductus arteriosus* (see Fig. 170), *ventricular septal defect* (see Fig. 172), a *vascular ring* (see Fig. 173) and *coarctation of the aorta* (see Fig. 174). When such defects are of high degree (except in the case of a vascular ring), electrocardiographic abnormalities are likely to occur. In extensive patency of the ductus arteriosus both ventricles tend to be enlarged, with left ventricular hypertrophy predominating (sometimes with a little right as well) (Fig. 171). With coarctation of the aorta, when the electrocardiogram is abnormal, the pattern is that of left ventricular enlargement (see Fig. 175).

In cases of the morbus caeruleus (*maladie bleue*), that is, congenital cardiac defects with cyanosis, the pattern is more often that of right ventricular and atrial enlargement than of left. This is true of the *tetralogy of Fallot* (see Fig. 176), of *pulmonary stenosis with atrial septal defect* (see Fig. 177) and of *Eisenmenger's complex*, in which there is a high degree of right ventricular enlargement. However, in the cyanotic type of heart disease due to *tricuspid atresia* (see Fig. 178) the left ventricle is enlarged and the electrocardiogram shows that pattern. This differentiation can be very helpful.

Transposition of the great arteries (see Figs. 179, 180), which is an uncommon congenital anomaly, is attended as a rule by enlargement of both ventricles and so shows an electrocardiographic pattern indicating such a finding. However, the pattern is nondiagnostic.

In the rare cases with a single ventricle, either *cor triloculare biatriatum* (see Fig. 181) or *cor biloculare*, the electrocardiogram tends to show

large *[...]*
is not *[...]*
one.

With *[...]*
sis or v *[...]*
patterr *[...]*
right v *[...]*
is char *[...]*
namely *[...]*
with o *[...]*
monary *[...]*
Fig. 18. *[...]*
find the *[...]*
ponder: *[...]*
times ir *[...]*
block, *[...]*
dilatati *[...]*
sponsib *[...]*

With *[...]*
lum bel *[...]*
cardiog *[...]*
left vent *[...]*

Rare *[...]*
of the co *[...]*
teristic *[...]*
abnorma *[...]*
in partic *[...]*
example. *[...]*
from the *[...]*

Also, *[...]*
atrioveni *[...]*
usually a *[...]*

Finally *[...]*
other car *[...]*
situs inve *[...]*
inversion *[...]*
2 and 3, *[...]*
(see Fig. *[...]*

PART VII

Etiologic Types

Introduction

Some years ago (1940) an important and useful book concerning electrocardiographic patterns was published by Arlie Barnes.* This led the way to the practical utilization of the form of the electrocardiogram in its various leads in the etiologic and structural diagnosis of heart disease. Although emphasis has often been placed on electrocardiographic patterns as applied to the various etiologic types of heart disease and their subdivisions, it is important first to recognize, as emphasized in Part VI of this book, that there are general patterns that apply to several different etiologic groups. There is rarely any specific etiologic pattern. Not infrequently the general patterns described in Part VI are combined in various degrees and forms in the different etiologic types of heart disease which are discussed in Chapters 12 through 22.

* Barnes, A. P.: Electrocardiographic Patterns. Springfield, Illinois, Charles C Thomas, 1940.

Summary of Electrocardiographic Patterns to Be Expected in Individual Congenital Cardiovascular Anomalies

Patency of the Ductus Arteriosus (Uncomplicated)

The electrocardiogram is found in general to be within normal limits, but there are instances in which the ductus is large and the strain on the ventricular musculature considerable. In a series[1] of twenty-four cases, the QRS progression in the precordial leads suggested predominance of the left ventricle in fifteen instances, and indicated left ventricular enlargement in six and combined ventricular hypertrophy in the remaining three. The rhythm was regular in twenty-three of the twenty-four cases, the exception showing frequent ventricular premature beats.

Coarctation of the Aorta (Uncomplicated)

The electrocardiogram may be within normal limits, but there are instances of markedly high blood pressure in which the strain on the ventricular musculature is considerable. In a series[2] of twenty-one cases, five were found to have normal electrocardiograms, while sixteen showed abnormalities, consisting in the main of left ventricular hypertrophy, but with right bundle branch block in two.

Atrial Septal Defect

The electrocardiogram almost always shows right ventricular preponderance. In a series[3] of fifty-three cases of atrial septal defect, of which four of ten autopsied cases had mitral stenosis, forty-one showed right ventricular hypertrophy (twenty-one suggesting incomplete right bundle branch block), five showed complete right bundle branch block, and seven were within normal limits. The rhythm was normal in forty-seven, while atrial fibrillation was present in six. In another series[4] of sixty-five cases, there was either right ventricular preponderance or a partial or complete right bundle branch block in all tracings; eleven cases showed prolonged P–R intervals.

Ventricular Septal Defect (Uncomplicated)

There may or may not be a normal electrocardiogram. Of ten autopsied cases from the literature summarized by Selzer,[5] normal tracings were reported in two, right axis deviation in three, high voltage diphasic QRS complexes in four, and right bundle branch block in one. Four of the last mentioned five cases showed large defects at autopsy.

Pulmonary Stenosis (Uncomplicated)

The great majority of these cases show right ventricular hypertrophy. In a series[1] of eight cases, five showed definite right ventricular preponderance, and a sixth was suggestive of this; the rhythm was normal in all eight cases. Right bundle branch block may also occur in this defect.[6]

Aortic or Subaortic Stenosis (Uncomplicated)

The majority of the relatively few cases of these defects that have been noted have shown evidence of left ventricular enlargement. In a series[1] of four probable cases, all the electrocardiograms were consistent with some left ventricular preponderance (in the precordial leads), but in only one was the fully characteristic left ventricular hypertrophy or "strain" pattern seen. The rhythm was normal in all four cases.

Tricuspid Atresia

This defect produces, as a rule, left ventricular hypertrophy. In a series[7] of six cases, electrocardiograms were recorded in four, all of which showed left ventricular preponderance. However, two out of three cases reported elsewhere[8,9] failed to show left axis deviation, and large peaked P waves were present in the standard leads in one of these two.

Tetralogy of Fallot

Electrocardiographic evidence of much right ventricular hypertrophy is present in almost all cases. For example, twelve of fifteen cases of one series[1] showed clear evidence of right ventricular preponderance in the precordial leads, one demonstrating right bundle branch block. The rhythm was normal in thirteen cases; one showed a wandering atrial pacemaker, and in one there was atrial fibrillation (thyrotoxicosis was suspected clinically). In another series[2] of thirty-four cases the electrocardiogram presented typical right ventricular hypertrophy in thirty-three instances and right bundle branch block in the remaining case.

Eisenmenger's Complex

Electrocardiographic evidence of right ventricular hypertrophy is present in almost all cases. In a series[10] of twelve electrocardiograms reported in the literature, there was electrocardiographic evidence of right ventricular enlargement in eight and left ventricular hypertrophy in one while two were tabulated as showing respectively "no axis deviation, notched QRS" and "no axis deviation," and there was one normal tracing. In another series[1] of four cases, three showed right ventricular enlargement in the precordial leads and the fourth showed a mixed progression of QRS complexes over the chest, suggesting combined ventricular hypertrophy; the rhythm was normal in all but one of these cases, which demonstrated a variable atrioventricular block and occasional nodal rhythm.

Trilogy of Fallot (Pulmonary Stenosis, Atrial Septal Defect, and Right Ventricular Enlargement)

Right ventricular hypertrophy is shown regularly in the electrocardiogram. In a series[1] of seven cases of pulmonary stenosis with atrial septal defect, four showed characteristic and one suggestive evidence of right ventricular preponderance in the precordial leads; the rhythm was normal in all seven cases. In another series[11] of three cases, the electrocardiogram manifested either right bundle branch block or right ventricular hypertrophy in all three. Atrioventricular block and high peaked P waves are also noted in this defect.[11]

Transposition of the Great Vessels

In five cases reported severally, the electrocardiogram was consistent with right ventricular enlargement with normal rhythm in two,[1] there was marked right axis deviation in a patient who lived to the age of thirty-eight with this anomaly in a third instance,[12] a fourth case presented normal rhythm with right ventricular hypertrophy, and in only one was there no definite evidence of right ventricular strain, although atrial hypertrophy was present.[14]

Triloculate Heart (Cor Triloculare Biatriatum)

The electrocardiogram is apparently always abnormal. In all of four cases, tall wide diphasic QRS complexes were found. In another series[1] of three cases the electrocardiogram showed increased voltage of the QRS complexes in two, and in addition, in one each, right ventricular preponderance, complete right bundle branch block, and probable incomplete left bundle branch block.*

---

* We are indebted to Dr. Gordon S. Myers of the Cardiac Department of the Massachusetts General Hospital for his aid in the preparation of this chapter.

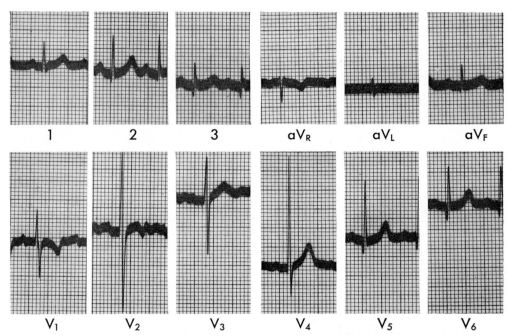

Fig. 170. Patent ductus arteriosus.

Patent ductus arteriosus in a little girl of six whose mother had had German measles in the first month of pregnancy. Congenital heart disease was first discovered in this child when she was one year old. She had had no cardiac symptoms, but in her fifth year it had become apparent that her hearing was somewhat impaired and that she tired too easily.

Physical examination on November 28, 1949, revealed a thin, pale, rather poorly developed child. There was a prominent arterial pulsation in the suprasternal notch, and a systolic thrill was felt in this region and to right and left of the upper sternum. The typical machinery murmur of patent ductus arteriosus was audible in the pulmonary area, widely transmitted to the neck, back and precordium with systolic accentuation. P_2 was plus, A_2 well heard. An inconstant third heart sound was present at the apex in recumbency. At rest her blood pressure was 120 mm. of mercury systolic and 60 mm. diastolic; with exercise it was 130 mm. systolic and 58 mm. diastolic. There were good arterial pulsations in both legs. An x-ray film of the chest at this time showed the heart to be within normal limits with no evidence of congenital heart disease. The electrocardiogram is shown here.

The possibility of a complicating aortic valve defect was raised by the finding of the thrill, but this did not affect the advisability of ligation of her patent ductus, and the patient underwent this operation on December 7. Postoperatively no continuous or diastolic murmurs were audible, but a Grade 2 systolic murmur transmitted to the back and neck could be heard at the base of the heart and, faintly, at the apex, and a pulsation in the suprasternal notch could still be seen and palpated.

INTERPRETATION. Normal rhythm, rate 120, with normal complexes and time intervals in all twelve leads. There are prominent R waves throughout the precordial leads, especially in V_4, and inverted T waves in V_1 and V_2 in keeping with the age of this child.

COMMENT. There is nothing in this record to indicate the presence of congenital patency of the ductus arteriosus, which has not yet caused severe enough strain on the heart to produce an abnormal pattern. Despite the apparent normality of the heart by x-ray film and electrocardiogram, the operative closure of the patent ductus was advisable for two reasons: first, to prevent the serious complication of subacute bacterial endocarditis, which is common with this deformity, and second, to get rid of the strain, even though not great, of the shunt of a certain amount of blood from the aorta to the pulmonary circulation.

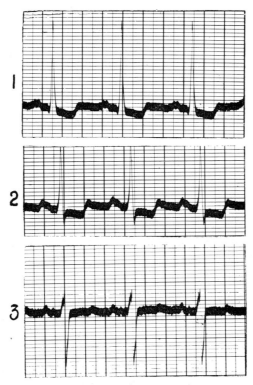

Fig. 171. Patent ductus arteriosus.

Patent ductus arteriosus with cardiac enlargement in a young woman aged twenty-seven. This patient had remained well despite the finding of cardiac abnormality from birth until tonsillectomy at the age of twenty-one, after which she noted shortness of breath and a throbbing in the neck. For two years prior to our examination she had had rather frequent attacks of palpitation.

Upon physical examination on June 30, 1944, there was found to be a notable increase in arterial pulsation in the neck. The heart was enlarged, and a Grade 3 continuous murmur was heard at the base, particularly at the upper end of the sternum and over the pulmonary area. Slight Grade 2 systolic and mid-diastolic rumbling murmurs were audible at the apex. There was a pulmonary systolic thrill. Except for occasional premature beats the heart rhythm was regular at a rate of 88. The blood pressure was 140 mm. of mercury systolic and 80 mm. diastolic in both arms. Fluoroscopic examination revealed a big left ventricle; the left atrium was only slightly enlarged. The electrocardiogram is shown here.

One month later ligation of the patent ductus was undertaken. The ductus was found to be wide and long, anteriorly placed, easily reached and dissected. Unfortunately, the heart was unable to maintain its tone in the course of this procedure, and death occurred within two hours of the opening of the chest wall, despite such measures as cardiac massage and therapy with digitalis intravenously. Autopsy showed a large ductus, marked hypertrophy and dilatation of the left ventricle, moderate congestion and edema of the lungs, and considerable congestion and enlargement of the liver. The mitral and aortic valves were normal, and there was no septal defect.

INTERPRETATION. Normal rhythm at a rate of 85, with considerable left axis deviation, inverted *T* waves in Lead 1 and diphasic *T* waves in Lead 2.

COMMENT. The pattern shown in the limb leads is clearly that of left ventricular enlargement, such as one finds especially in hypertensive heart disease or in aortic valve disease. In occasional instances of congenital defects giving rise to strain, especially on the left ventricle, this same pattern is observed. In this case there had been a large shunt of blood from the aorta into the pulmonary circulation over a period of a good many years. This had precipitated considerable left ventricular enlargement and such limited reserve that the myocardium was not able to support the strain of the operative procedure and the closure of the shunt which required the left ventricle to put all the blood into the aorta; the aorta distal to the arch is not infrequently less capacious than is the rule in persons with normal circulation.

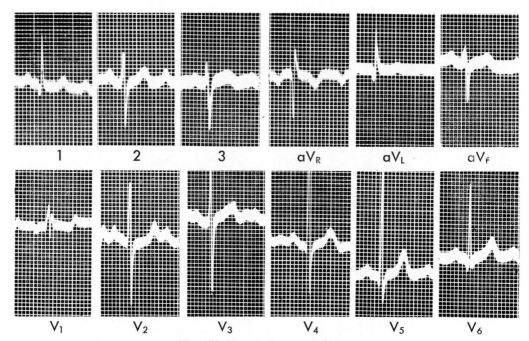

Fig. 172. Ventricular septal defect.

Ventricular septal defect in a little girl aged nine. In her infancy this child had been cyanotic upon crying, and a heart murmur had been observed when she was six months old. When she was four or five years old, her exercise tolerance seemed to improve.

Physical examination on May 9, 1949, revealed a thin child with moderate depression of the sternum. A systolic thrill was palpable over the entire precordium, and a loud, Grade 4 harsh systolic murmur could be heard over this area, loudest along the left sternal border. This could be heard, although poorly, at the neck and was present also in the axilla and over the back bilaterally, especially on the right. P_2 was greater than A_2. The liver was not enlarged. The blood pressure was 100 mm. of mercury systolic and 65 mm. diastolic in the right arm, 96 mm. systolic and 60 mm. diastolic in the left arm.

An x-ray film demonstrated enlargement of the left atrium and of both ventricles; its appearance was thought to be consistent with a ventricular septal defect and/or patent ductus arteriosus.

The findings on cardiac catheterization, performed May 9, were compatible with the presence of an uncomplicated ventricular septal defect with slight pulmonary and right ventricular hypertension. Her electrocardiogram is shown here.

INTERPRETATION. Normal rhythm, rate 100, with slight left axis deviation shown by the limb leads and high R waves in precordial leads V_2 and V_5 over the right and left ventricles respectively. The T waves are within normal limits throughout.

COMMENT. As shown by other evidence than the electrocardiogram, the ventricular septal defect in this case had produced evident cardiac enlargement and probably some strain upon both ventricles. The prominence of the R waves in the leads over both ventricles is in support of x-ray evidence, although in a child the relative thinness of the chest wall allows the electrodes to be close to the heart and may itself be responsible for some increase of amplitude of the complexes in the chest leads.

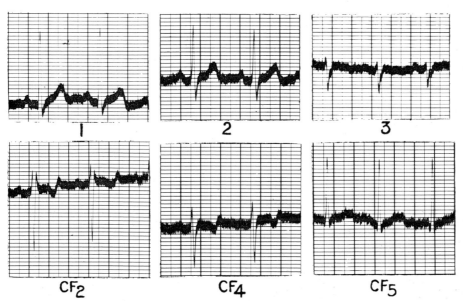

Fig. 173. Vascular ring.

Vascular ring in a boy of five, who had had nine previous hospital admissions between 1942 and 1947 for treatment of acute bronchitis and pneumonia. His tenth admission in February, 1947, followed an upper respiratory infection of five weeks' duration.

On physical examination he was small for his years and underweight, and appeared to be chronically ill, with an intermittent cough. Tonsils and adenoids were present. The heart was of normal size, the blood pressure was 120 mm. of mercury systolic and 65 mm. diastolic, and there were no murmurs. A_2 equaled P_2. An x-ray film of the chest with barium swallow on February 2 revealed a defect on the posterior margin of the aorta such as would be produced by a right-sided aorta crossing the esophagus; the pulmonary markings were prominent. The electrocardiogram was taken on February 7.

A pneumothorax developed with collapse of the left lung as a complication of bronchoscopy, which was performed on February 24. When this had subsided, fluoroscopy was done with barium swallow on March 15, and at this time it was apparent that there was unquestionable indentation of the esophagus posteriorly and from the right side. After this x-ray confirmation of the diagnosis of a vascular ring about the trachea and esophagus in conjunction with a right-sided aorta, and as soon as his condition had improved sufficiently, a division of the vascular ring was accomplished on April 23.

At operation it was evident that the vascular ring consisted of a double aortic arch. The anterior smaller portion which caused the constriction was severed. After this procedure the esophagus and trachea were released from the constriction.

The patient was discharged home on May 8, and when seen again in November of that year he had been eating well, had been free of wheezing, and had had only one cold since he had left the hospital.

INTERPRETATION. Normal rhythm, rate 105, with normal complexes and time intervals in all six leads. There are prominence of the S waves and inversion of the T waves in precordial leads CF_2 and CF_4.

COMMENT. This electrocardiogram is perfectly normal. Lead CF_4 with prominent S and inverted T waves is undoubtedly located over the right ventricle and is normal for a child of this age. Thus the vascular ring has apparently produced no abnormality of the heart or of the electrocardiogram.

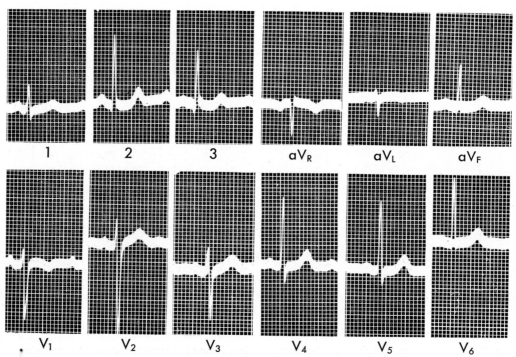

Fig. 174. Coarctation of the aorta.

Coarctation of the aorta in a girl of fifteen. There were no maternal complications during pregnancy. This patient developed normally after a normal delivery until, at the age of seven, a high blood pressure was first detected. The following year a diagnosis of coarctation of the aorta was made, later confirmed by diodrast studies. She had no complaints other than fatigue in the early morning; moderate restriction of such activities as swimming and dancing had been voluntary.

On physical examination she appeared well. She weighed 135 pounds and was 5 feet 7 inches tall. There was no pulse deficit. The blood pressure was 145 mm. of mercury systolic and 75 mm. diastolic in both arms. The heart sounds were normal. There was a moderate, rather harsh systolic murmur heard at the base, less well in recumbency, clearly audible along the upper thoracic vertebrae. No diastolic murmurs were heard, and there was no thrill. The lungs were clear. Dorsalis pedis and posterior tibial pulsations were absent.

Surgical correction of the coarcted aorta was advised, and three months later her local doctor reported that she was getting along nicely after this procedure, although she continued to have a mild hypertension.

INTERPRETATION. Normal rhythm at a rate of 95, with normal complexes and time intervals in all twelve leads. There is a tendency to right axis deviation, as indicated by the limb leads, which is probably in keeping with her build.

COMMENT. This record is completely normal and is an example of many instances of coarctation of the aorta where the strain of hypertension has not yet interfered with the heart itself.

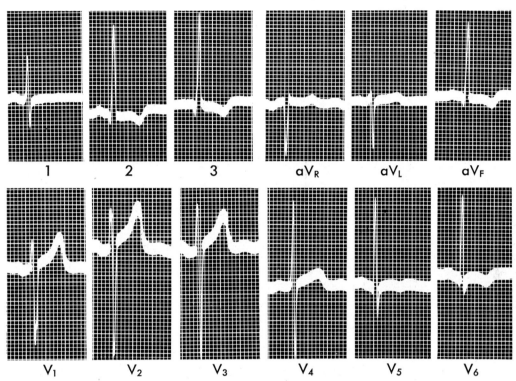

Fig. 175. Coarctation of the aorta.

Coarctation of the aorta in a boy of seventeen. At the age of six he had had a tonsillectomy, and at that time a heart murmur was first discovered. His activities were moderately restricted thereafter, but it was not until ten years later, upon routine school examination, that his blood pressure was found to be "over 200." Urine examination showed no abnormalities. He had headaches rarely.

Upon physical examination at this time (November, 1948) he looked well. There was no cyanosis and no clubbing. Arterial pulsations in the neck were more than normally vigorous. Pulsations of the abdominal aorta, the femoral, popliteal and ankle vessels could not be felt. The subscapular arteries pulsated and were easily palpable. The blood pressure was 210 mm. of mercury systolic and 110 mm. diastolic in both arms. A rather loud Grade 3 systolic murmur was heard at the base of the heart to the right and left of the upper sternum, was well heard in the third left interspace in recumbency, and was also audible, although less well heard, in the upper back over the spine.

By fluoroscopy the heart was slightly enlarged in the region of the left ventricle and rather globular in shape. The aortic knob was diminished. The cardiothoracic ratio was 12:24 cm. An x-ray film confirmed these findings and demonstrated in addition slight notching of the lower borders of the seventh and eighth ribs. Small cervical ribs were also evident bilaterally.

It was hoped that a surgical resection of the coarcted aorta might offer some relief, and in June, 1949, an exploratory thoracotomy was performed. Unfortunately, the tubular-like narrowing of the aorta was found to be so long and extended so high that it was impossible to proceed with the operation.

On June 3, 1950, at which time the electrocardiogram shown here was obtained, the patient had recovered from the operative procedure and was in good health, but without change in his cardiac findings. His blood pressure was 200 mm. systolic and 100 mm. diastolic. He was last seen during his college vacation in December, 1950, and appeared well without symptoms. He was studying hard, but engaged in no competitive sports. His blood pressure was 190 mm. systolic and 110 mm. diastolic in both arms.

INTERPRETATION. Normal rhythm, rate 67, with abnormality of the T waves as shown particularly by flat T's in Lead 1, inverted T waves in Leads 2, 3, V_5 and V_6 and upright T waves in Lead aV_R. There is large amplitude of the R waves in Leads 2 and 3, V_4, V_5, and V_6, and of the S waves in Leads V_2 and V_3.

COMMENT. In this case the sustained hypertension due to coarctation of the aorta over a period of some years had resulted in definite enlargement of the heart, with preponderant left ventricular strain. The pattern in the limb leads is somewhat unusual, but an alteration in position of the heart can explain this finding.

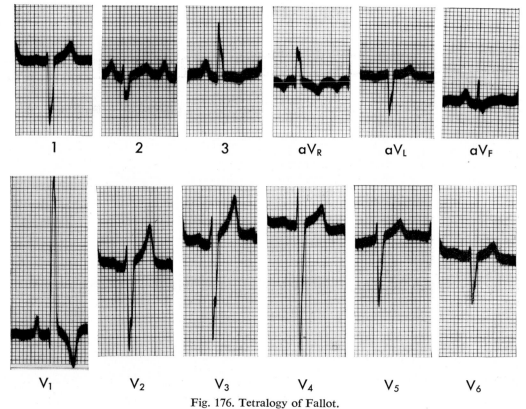

Fig. 176. Tetralogy of Fallot.

Tetralogy of Fallot in a boy of eighteen. A murmur had been noted since the age of eighteen months, and his history included exertional dyspnea to a greater degree than that experienced by his playmates. He was first seen in our clinic at the age of twelve, at which time he appeared rather small for his age, with slight cyanosis of lips and fingernails. There was moderate finger clubbing. Pulsations of the neck were normal. The pulse was regular at 80. The heart by percussion seemed to be of full size or slightly enlarged. Heart sounds were good. A_2 was greater than P_2, which was diminished. There was a Grade 4 systolic murmur along the left sternal border, maximal in the second and third intercostal spaces and transmitted to the upper back.

An x-ray film at this time revealed a cardiothoracic ratio of 10.7:22.9 cm. The left ventricle appeared to be slightly elevated and rotated; in the lateral view there was definite right ventricular enlargement. The aorta appeared normally wide and normal in contour. There was no evidence of pulsation in the hilar vessels and no evidence of enlargement of the left atrium. These findings were thought to be confirmatory of the clinical impression that the patient had the tetralogy of Fallot.

He was only moderately limited by his congenital defect, but a consideration of the possibility of surgical relief led to his admission to the hospital in January, 1951, for cardiac catheterization. This procedure proved the presence of pulmonary stenosis and right ventricular hypertension. A blood sample from high in the right ventricle revealed a significantly increased oxygen content compatible with a ventricular septal defect. A blood sample from high in the atrium likewise showed high oxygen content, which raised the question of a possible aberrant pulmonary vein draining into the right atrium. Accordingly, a diodrast study was carried out, which demonstrated prompt filling of the aorta, apparently from the right ventricle, with the appearance of a small amount of dye in the left ventricle, probably through the high ventricular septal defect. The pulmonary arteries were poorly visualized, but appeared small.

The electrocardiogram shown here was taken in February, 1951. A few days later the Blalock operation with left end-to-side subclavian to pulmonary anastomosis was successfully performed. He was last seen on April 5, one and a half months postoperatively, and the results seemed to be excellent. A Grade 4 systolic murmur could be heard in the fourth intercostal space to the left of the sternum, and a continuous murmur was heard best in the second left intercostal space. He was able to walk as much as he liked without dyspnea.

INTERPRETATION. Normal rhythm at a rate of 110, with a high degree of right axis deviation as shown by the limb leads, prominent R waves in Lead aV_R, high R waves in Lead V_1, and exaggerated S waves in Leads V_2 to V_6 inclusive. The T waves are upright throughout except for Leads 3, aV_R, and V_1. There is slight widening of the QRS waves to 0.11 second. The P waves are high in Leads 2, 3 and V_1.

COMMENT. This record is characteristic of a high degree of right ventricular enlargement, as is seen particularly with congenital heart disease in the form either of the tetralogy of Fallot, as here, or of atrial septal defect.

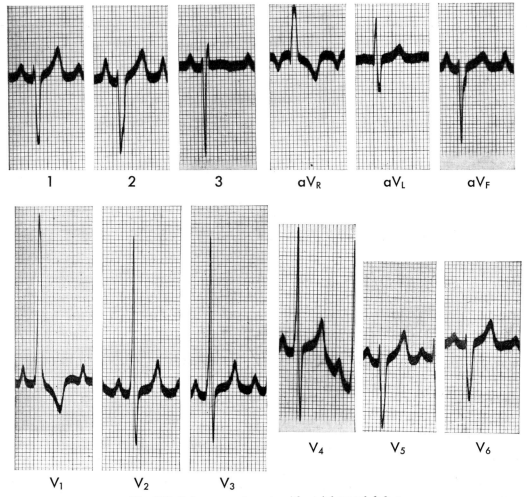

Fig. 177. Pulmonary stenosis with atrial septal defect.

Pulmonary stenosis with atrial septal defect in a mentally retarded boy of nine. This child of a feeble-minded mother and an alcoholic father (who had died of pneumonia) had been cyanotic since birth, dyspneic on exertion, and a "squatter" when he walked.

On physical examination his appearance was Mongoloid, with evident cyanosis of lips and nailbeds and notable clubbing of the fingers and toes. The heart appeared to be enlarged. A high-pitched murmur of Grade 2-plus intensity was heard in the pulmonary area, transmitted to the back on the left. This murmur, although faint, seemed to be continuous. There was slight reduplication of the first sound at the apex. A_2 was slightly greater than P_2. There was increased pulsation over the right ventricle at the lower end of the sternum. The blood pressure was 90 mm. of mercury systolic and 60 mm. diastolic. The electrocardiogram shown here was taken just prior to hospital admission for further study.

An x-ray film of the chest revealed the heart to be enlarged, with a cardiothoracic ratio of 11:20.5 cm. and prominence chiefly to the left, probably as a result of right ventricular enlargement. The pulmonary artery did not appear unduly prominent. The aortic arch was on the left. There was a slight increase in vascular prominence of the lung fields, considered possibly due to collateral circulation. Congenital fusion anomalies of the right eighth, ninth and tenth ribs posteriorly were evident. The cardiac findings were thought to be consistent with those of the tetralogy of Fallot.

Cardiac catheterization was performed shortly after his admission to the hospital. The data recorded therefrom, in conjunction with the clinical story, the electrocardiogram and the x-ray findings, were consistent with the presence of pulmonary stenosis and an atrial septal defect with right to left shunt predominant. An exercise test demonstrated restriction of the pulmonary blood flow, and the operative procedure of either Blalock or Potts was recommended at that time (early in 1949); pulmonary valvulotomy would now (1951) be the measure of choice. One week after entry an exploratory thoracotomy was done. The pulmonary artery was discovered to be only 3 mm. in diameter and not adequate for anastomosis. His condition was unchanged upon discharge.

INTERPRETATION. Normal rhythm at a rate of 100, with an electrocardiographic pattern of marked right ventricular enlargement, as shown by deep S waves and small R waves in Leads 1 and aV_F, high wide R waves in Lead aV_R, high R waves in precordial leads V_1 to V_4, inclusive, and prominent wide S waves in Leads V_5 and V_6. Also, the P waves are prominent throughout, indicative of atrial hypertrophy evidently involving the right atrium in this case.

COMMENT. This record shows an extreme degree of right ventricular perponderance, one of the most striking ever noted by the authors of this volume. It is in complete accord with the diagnosis otherwise established of pulmonary stenosis with atrial septal defect, but it is not specifically diagnostic thereof.

Page 209

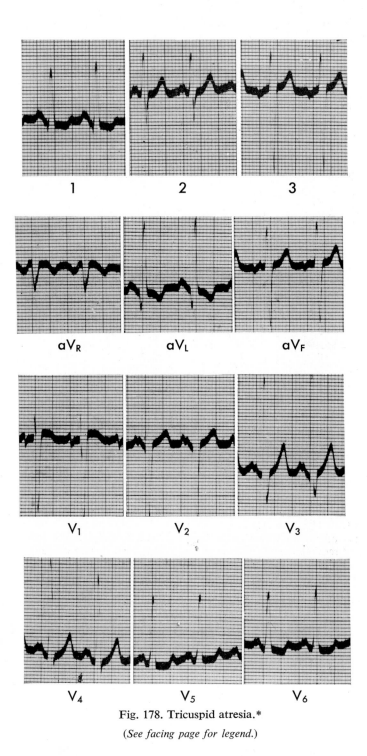

Fig. 178. Tricuspid atresia.*

(*See facing page for legend.*)

* We are indebted to the House of the Good Samaritan of Boston for the summary of this patient's hospital record, to Dr. Sidney Davidson of Lake Worth, Florida, for his clinical follow-up of the case, for the electrocardiogram shown in this figure, and for the postmortem findings, and to the pathologists of the Children's Hospital in Boston for their postmortem examination of the thoracic vessels which were sent to them by Dr. Davidson for this purpose.

(Legend continued from opposite page, Figure 178.)

Tricuspid atresia in an eight year old boy whose parents had both died of tuberculosis when he was nine months old. It is reported that his mother's pregnancy was uneventful and the delivery normal. At birth he weighed 3 pounds, and his subsequent development was slow. After the death of his parents, about which time cyanosis and clubbing of the fingers were observed, the diagnosis of primary tuberculosis was made on this infant, and he remained at a sanatorium for four years before his transfer to the House of the Good Samaritan in Boston for cardiac evaluation. When he was two years old there had been a single attack of extreme cyanosis followed by unconsciousness which lasted about two hours. Clubbing and cyanosis, as well as shortness of breath on walking short distances, had continued.

Upon physical examination in June, 1947, at the time of his transfer to the hospital, the child (then four years of age) was cyanotic and of slender build, with pronounced clubbing of the fingers and toes. The heart was moderately enlarged. There were no murmurs. His blood pressure was 84 mm. of mercury systolic and 60 mm. diastolic. Laboratory tests showed a red blood cell count of 6.6 million per cu. mm., hemoglobin of 19.2 gm., hematocrit 75 per cent. Electrocardiographically there was extreme left axis deviation, with depression of $S-T_1$ and inversion of T_1, and upon fluoroscopy the heart was found large with a full left border and a large aorta. In the right anterior oblique view the heart encroached upon the retrosternal and retrocardiac areas, displacing the esophagus posteriorly. An angiocardiogram demonstrated free passage of the blood through the superior vena cava into the heart, with almost immediate diffuse distribution throughout both right and left sides. The arterial oxygen content of arterial blood was 30.17 volumes per cent, corresponding to 20.5 gm. of hemoglobin. Resting arterial saturation was about 70 per cent, with moderate exertion producing a fall to 64 per cent. The pulmonary flow was calculated at about 2 liters. A diagnosis of congenital heart disease with tricuspid atresia had been made upon entry.

The patient underwent, in November, 1948, a modified Potts procedure, with end-to-side anastomosis of the left pulmonary artery to the aorta. The small caliber of the pulmonary artery made it impossible to accomplish a side-to-side anastomosis. After four months of convalescence he had improved somewhat with respect to his cyanosis and easy fatigability.

After discharge in April, 1949, the boy was sent to Florida, where the electrocardiogram shown here was taken in June of that year. He did well for some time, in fact, had no therapy, gained weight, and lived a fairly normal life, playing and going to school with other children until the summer of 1950, when he began to lose ground. That fall he showed evidences of apparent heart failure, with shortness of breath, increased cyanosis, pulmonary hemorrhages, and upon one occasion a nasal hemorrhage. In January, 1951, he had an acute upper respiratory infection, from which he failed to recover satisfactorily and so was admitted to a hospital in Florida, where he was placed in an oxygen tent. Despite oxygen, digitoxin, a salt-free diet and occasional mercuhydrin, his course was steadily downhill. No peripheral edema or enlargement of the liver was observed at any time. In March he complained of severe and increasing headaches, pains in the legs, inability to eat, and occasional vomiting. Rales at both lung bases became especially prominent posteriorly. He died on April 4, 1951.

Postmortem examination revealed a large heart with abnormalities as follows: (1) a large patent ostium primum 3.2 by 1.5 cm.; (2) *tricuspid atresia;* (3) a small hypoplastic right ventricle located transversely across the anterior surface of the heart just inferior to the right atrium, and 5 cm. long with an average circumference of 1.8 cm., without interventricular septum; (4) a patent left pulmonary-aortic surgical anastomosis 0.8 by 0.4 cm. located 6.5 cm. distal to the aortic ring (the right pulmonary artery was 1 cm. in caliber and normally distributed, and the branches of the pulmonary artery were distal to the anastomosis and distended); (5) a left ventricular wall 2.3 cm. thick.

The lungs showed extensive tuberculosis throughout their entire substance. There were multiple tubercles, a cavity in the right upper lobe, atelectatic right middle lobe, and involvement of bronchiolar walls.

The child probably died as a result of the pulmonary tuberculosis as much as from the serious congenital heart defect.

INTERPRETATION. Normal rhythm at a heart rate of 110 with left axis deviation and depressed $S-T$ segments in the limb leads, high R waves in precordial leads V_3 to V_6 inclusive, with low T waves in Leads V_5 and V_6.

COMMENT. This electrocardiogram, indicating preponderant enlargement of the left side of the heart, is characteristic of tricuspid atresia. When, in a baby or young child with cyanosis and clubbing of the fingers, the electrocardiogram shows left ventricular enlargement, as in this case, tricuspid atresia is to be strongly suspected.

(For another case of tricuspid atresia, see page 181, Figure 155.)

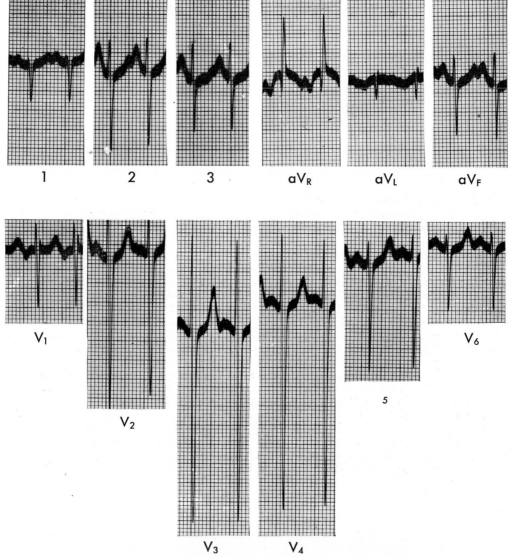

Fig. 179. Transposition of the great arteries with ventricular septal defect.

Transposition of the great arteries with ventricular septal defect in a boy aged eight who was believed ante mortem to have Eisenmenger's complex. He had been a blue baby from birth, and congenital heart disease had been diagnosed when he was one week old. There was no history of maternal rubella during pregnancy. Despite frequent colds, easy fatigue, many nosebleeds and a tendency to squat when playing or walking, this child had done fairly well until, in December, 1949, at the age of seven, he had become seriously limited by severe pains in his legs, to a point where he had been unable to play and had practically dropped out of school. The soreness had extended over his arms and trunk, but was particularly distressing in his legs, preventing him from walking more than a few steps in comfort. The cyanosis had increased somewhat, and he had had severe nosebleeds of viscous blood.

Upon physical examination on February 14, 1950, cyanosis of the lips and fingers was striking, and there was severe clubbing of his fingers and toes. The blood pressure was 100 mm. of mercury systolic and 65 mm. diastolic. The neck veins were normal, and the chest was clear. The ankles were prominent with some tenderness of the joints. The heart rhythm was regular at a rate of 130. There was a Grade 1 pulmonary systolic murmur. P_2 was greatly accentuated. The liver edge could be felt about 1 cm. down and was nontender. There was no edema. The hemoglobin was 16 gm., and the red cell blood count was 9,140,000 per cu. mm. An electrocardiogram taken at this time is shown here.

X-ray examination revealed no enlargement of the heart, but a large pulmonary artery was viewed from both sides. Angiocardiography in July, 1947, had demonstrated an overriding aorta, a high septal defect, and a definite pulmonary artery, the appearance of the pulmonary tree favoring a diagnosis of tetralogy of Fallot. The exploratory thoracotomy performed shortly thereafter had confirmed the presence of a large pulmonary artery, which was believed to be under high pressure (close to 500 mm. of water), and the pressure determinations had made further operation seem inadvisable. The diagnosis of Eisenmenger's complex with possible additional pulmonary arteriolar disease was believed to be most likely.

(*Legend continued on facing page.*)

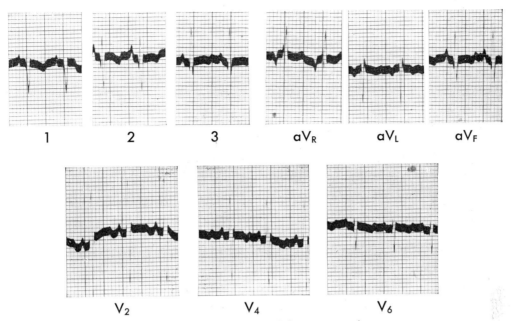

Fig. 180. Transposition of the great arteries.

Transposition of the great arteries in a male infant of two weeks. He was cyanotic from birth, but there were at that time no other evident abnormalities. The lungs were clear. The heart was not enlarged. The sounds were of good quality, and there were no murmurs. The rhythm was regular at a rate of approximately 150, and there was no evidence of congestive failure. He was hypertonic and restless, however, with spells of irregular respiration. Despite morphine and digitalization subsequently, his course was progressively downhill, and he died on the forty-fourth day after birth, with the diagnosis of his congenital heart lesion still unclassified (tetralogy of Fallot or a similar defect seemed probable).

A chest x-ray film taken one month before death, when he was two weeks old, and a few days after the electrocardiogram shown here demonstrated increase in heart size over a previous examination, with greater congestion of the pulmonary vascular tree radiating from the hila than had been seen before. The transverse diameter of the base in the anteroposterior view appeared small and narrower than usual and in the lateral view somewhat wider than usual. The possibility of transposition of the great vessels was suggested in view of these findings. This diagnosis was confirmed at autopsy.

INTERPRETATION. Normal rhythm, rate 150, with considerable right axis deviation, inversion of the T waves in Leads 1, V_4 and V_6, and upright T waves in aV_R. There are prominent R and S waves in Leads V_2 and V_4 and small R and prominent S waves in Lead V_6.

COMMENT. This record, so far as the QRS waves are concerned, is within normal limits for this infant's age of a few weeks. The T waves, however, especially in Leads 1, 2 and V_6, are abnormal and suggest inadequate oxygenation of the myocardium, doubtless dependent here on the supply of venous blood to the coronary arteries from the aorta, which rises at the base of the right ventricle. However, this pattern is not diagnostic. Inversion of the T waves in Leads 1 and 2 has been noted with origin of the left coronary artery from the pulmonary aorta (see Fig. 185).

(*Legend continued from opposite page, Figure 179.*)

In April, 1950, cardiac catheterization was performed, but after this procedure the diagnosis was still in doubt. It showed an increase in pressure in the right ventricle and evidence of a large ventricular septal defect; the pulmonary artery was not intubated. In October of that year the patient died suddenly. Autopsy findings included the following: enlargement of both ventricles, particularly the right (thickness of the wall equaled 0.8 cm.), transposition of the great arteries, and ventricular septal defect. There was potential patency of the foramen ovale. The heart weighed 310 gm., more than twice the normal for this age.

INTERPRETATION. Sinoatrial tachycardia, rate 140, with deep S waves in the classical limb leads and in all the precordial leads, especially in V_3 and V_4, and prominent R waves in Leads aV_R, V_2, V_3 and V_4. The T waves are not remarkable.

COMMENT. This electrocardiogram is in keeping with the autopsy findings of enlargement of both ventricles (particularly the right) as shown by the deep S waves in most leads and the right axis deviation in the limb leads. The absence of high R waves in Leads V_5 and V_6 would seem to indicate no enlargement of the left ventricle, but it is probable that the left ventricular enlargement would have become apparent if further leads had been taken beyond the left axilla toward the back, as is suggested by the deep S waves in V_3 and V_4. However, it would not seem possible to be able to diagnose transposition of the great vessels from this electrocardiographic pattern. Close proximity of the chest electrodes to the heart in a young child like this can account for some, but probably not all, of the amplitude of the R and S waves.

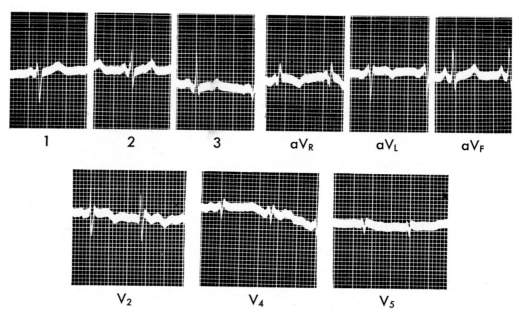

Fig. 181. Cor triloculare biatriatum.

Cor triloculare biatriatum in a male infant who was born August 27, 1948, and died August 31. Save for the finding of cyanosis at birth, continuing thereafter with little clearing despite oxygen therapy and intensified by crying, there were no definite cardiac signs or symptoms. The heart was not enlarged to percussion, the rate was slow, and the rhythm was regular. There were no murmurs. The lungs were clear.

An x-ray film on August 30 revealed the lung fields to be bright; the lungs were symmetrically aerated, and the diaphragm moved freely and equally on both sides. The vascular lung markings were less prominent than was customary, and the site of the main pulmonary artery appeared more than usually concave. The aortic arch could not be identified and was thought possibly to lie on the right. X-ray findings were consistent with congenital heart disease and probable diffuse emphysema of the lungs. The tetralogy of Fallot was mentioned as a possible cause of these abnormalities.

On the evening of August 30, because of irregular and gasping respirations and the finding of a palpable liver 1½ fingersbreadth below the costal margin, digitalization was begun, but in spite of this measure the infant died early in the morning of the following day. The pathologic report described the finding of congenital heart disease with cor biatriatum triloculare, anoxia, left-sided inferior vena cava, left-sided gallbladder, right-sided aorta, splenic agenesis. A more detailed description of the pathologic findings in the heart is as follows:

"The inferior vena cava and superior vena cava open into the right auricle which communicates freely through two defects with the left auricle. . . . Both auricles empty into a common ventricle posterior to a single valve flap measuring 2.0 by 0.6 cm. The wall of this common ventricle measures 0.3 cm. thick. The outflow tract is anterior and both the aorta and pulmonary artery leave from it. The aorta measures 2.5 cm. in circumference and has a three cusped valve. No cusps are recognizable in the pulmonary cavus and it is only 0.1 cm. in diameter. The pulmonary artery beyond this is grossly normal. The left coronary artery passes anterior to the pulmonary artery. On the wall of the large ventricle on the left side below the auriculoventricular groove is a vestige of a ventricle measuring 0.7 by 0.2 by 0.2 cm. At its upper border is the vestige of a valve with chordae attached. The descending aorta is right-sided."

INTERPRETATION. Normal rhythm, rate averaging about 100, with right axis deviation in the limb leads and small complexes in precordial leads V_4 and V_5, possibly due to the emphysema of the lungs.

COMMENT. This record is not diagnostic of the pathologic condition that was found. In fact, it is essentially within normal limits for a newborn baby. Here the clinical and x-ray evidence were much more important than the electrocardiogram.

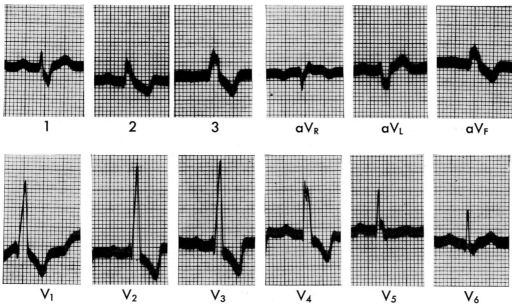

Fig. 182. Atrial septal defect.

Atrial septal defect in a forty-eight year old machinery maintenance man who entered the hospital for cardiac catheterization studies to determine the cause of his chronic pulmonary disease. Three months before, he had come to the hospital complaining of morning fatigue over the past year and rapid heart action following an episode of "pneumonia." X-ray films of the chest had revealed considerable enlargement of the pulmonary artery and of its branches, and an electrocardiogram had demonstrated right bundle branch block. His symptoms of wheezing and a mild cough had been unaccompanied by definite asthma or troublesome dyspnea, although he had always led an active life.

On physical examination he did not appear ill. His blood pressure was 130 mm. of mercury systolic and 80 mm. diastolic. His neck veins were flat. There was no edema. A few scattered rales were heard throughout the chest. The heart rhythm was regular at 90. There was reduplication of the second sound at the apex, and reduplication of the first sound upon exercise. A Grade 1 to 2 high-pitched systolic murmur was heard, loudest at the third sternocostal junction on the left. P_2 was greater than A_2.

The x-ray changes were similar to those reported fourteen years before, and further x-ray films of the chest indicated that the cardiac enlargement with pronounced increase in both hilar regions was probably congenital in origin.

After cardiac catheterization the conclusions were that an atrial septal defect was present, as evidenced by 3.1 volumes per cent increase in oxygen content between the blood in the superior vena cava and that in the right atrium, and passage of the catheter into the left atrium. There was pulmonary hypertension of moderate degree due to pulmonary arteriolar changes (normal left atrium and pulmonary capillary pressures). There was no evidence of pulmonary stenosis, since the right ventricular and pulmonary artery systolic pressures were equal. A small right to left shunt was evidenced by lower oxygen content of arterial than of left atrial blood. There was no evidence of right or left ventricular failure, as demonstrated by normal right and left atrial pressures. It was observed that these findings are frequently seen in patients with atrial septal defects who have pulmonary hypertension with a resultant decrease in the volume of the left to right shunt, a subsequent development of right to left shunt, and the ultimate occurrence of visible cyanosis and polycythemia.

INTERPRETATION. Normal rhythm, rate 86, with right bundle branch block as evidenced by wide *S* waves in Lead 1 and *R* waves in Lead 3, and wide slurred *R* waves in Leads V_1 to V_4 inclusive over the right ventricle.

COMMENT. With atrial septal defects two electrocardiographic patterns are commonly seen: either marked right axis deviation in the limb leads, with right ventricular hypertrophy shown by the precordial leads, or right bundle branch block, as here. The latter probably signifies a higher degree of abnormality.

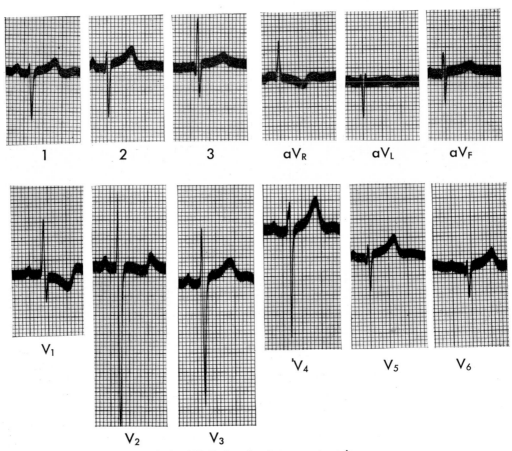

Fig. 183. Isolated pulmonary stenosis.

Isolated pulmonary stenosis in a boy of fifteen who had been a blue baby and in whom a heart murmur was discovered in 1936 at the age of two, at which time the diagnosis of congenital heart disease was made. His activities had been somewhat limited because of this, and his development, although apparently normal, had been marked by general weakness, failure to gain weight, and frequent colds, with slight retardation in his school work.

Upon physical examination in March, 1948, no dyspnea, clubbing or cyanosis was apparent. There was no definite arachnodactylia, although his fingers and hands were rather long. The neck veins were distended and pulsating about 2 cm. above the clavicle at a 45 degree angle. The chest was clear, but presented a deformity of the pigeon-breast type with prominence at the right costochondral junction: this somewhat obscured the degree of cardiac enlargement (1.5 cm. to the left of the midclavicular line in the fifth interspace and enlargement to the right). A long, harsh, Grade 5 systolic murmur was heard, loudest in the second and third left interspaces, but transmitted widely over the anterior and posterior chest walls, heard less well along the spine and also audible over the upper arms. There were no diastolic murmurs. A_2 and P_2 were not heard. The blood pressure was 110 mm. of mercury systolic and 50 mm. diastolic in both arms. Neither liver nor spleen was palpable. The femoral pulses were well felt.

Cardiac catheterization was carried out at this time and confirmed the clinical impression of isolated pulmonary stenosis (by the finding of pulmonary arterial hypotension and right ventricular hypertension).

The electrocardiogram shown here was taken on December 14, 1949, and an x-ray examination was obtained the same day. By fluoroscopy the right ventricle appeared to be rather prominent; the diaphragm moved normally. X-ray films of the chest revealed that the retrosternal area was encroached upon in the lateral view by the enlarged right ventricle. The right ventricular outline was prominent in the left anterior oblique view. The sternum appeared to be asymmetrical. These findings were considered strongly suggestive of a high degree of right ventricular hypertrophy.

When last seen in the clinic, in February, 1951, the patient had been feeling well.

INTERPRETATION. Normal rhythm with a heart rate of 67, with considerable right axis deviation shown best by the limb leads, prominent R waves in Leads aV_R, V_1, V_2 and V_3, and deep S waves in chest leads V_2, V_3 and V_4. The T waves are inverted in chest lead V_1 and diphasic in V_2.

COMMENT. This record is characteristic of preponderant enlargement of the right ventricle and is in full accord with the clinical diagnosis of pulmonary stenosis, whether isolated or not. It is of interest that here, as in other patients with pronounced right ventricular hypertrophy, the RS pattern across the chest is the reverse of the usual normal.

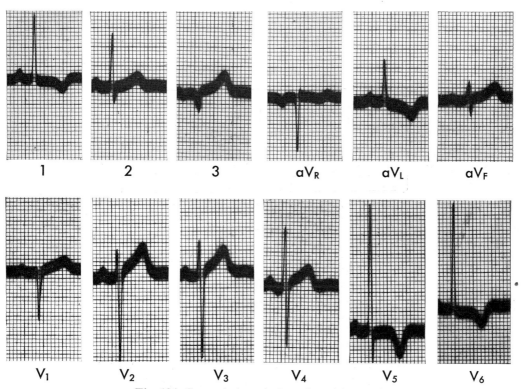

1   2   3   aV$_R$ aV$_L$ aV$_F$

V$_1$ V$_2$ V$_3$ V$_4$ V$_5$ V$_6$

Fig. 184. Congenital aortic (or subaortic) stenosis.

Congenital aortic (or subaortic) stenosis in a young man twenty-eight years old who had been followed in our clinic for ten years (since 1939). At the age of seven this boy had been seen in another hospital because a "leaky heart valve" had been diagnosed at school. At that time there was a loud systolic murmur with a questionable aortic diastolic murmur, and there was also a questionable story of joint pains. X-ray films showed moderate enlargement of the cardiac shadow, with prominence in the right supracardiac region, which was interpreted as enlargement of the great vessels and was thought to be on a congenital basis. His family included a younger brother said to have congenital heart disease and a sister who died in 1939 at the age of fourteen with the diagnosis of acute cardiac failure in chronic valvular disease (presumed to be congenital, and no definite diagnosis ever made of rheumatic heart disease).

Upon x-ray examination of the chest here in 1939, the findings of left ventricular hypertrophy and dilatation of the ascending aorta were suggestive of aortic valve disease.

The electrocardiogram shown here was taken on the occasion of the patient's last visit to the hospital, August 18, 1949. Upon physical examination he was overweight (201 pounds). A basal systolic thrill could be felt over the aortic area and into the neck. A Grade 4 systolic murmur was audible over the entire precordium, loudest over the second right interspace. The aortic diastolic murmur was Grade 1 to 2 in intensity. There was a third heart sound at the apex. A$_2$ was not heard. His blood pressure was 116 mm. of mercury systolic and 80 mm. diastolic.

The examiner's impression upon this occasion was that a considerable degree of aortic stenosis was present, as well as slight aortic regurgitation.

INTERPRETATION. Normal rhythm at a heart rate of 65, with left axis deviation in the limb leads and enlargement of the left ventricle indicated in the precordial leads by deep S waves in V$_2$ and V$_3$ and high R waves in Leads V$_5$ and V$_6$. The inversion of the T waves in Leads 1, V$_5$ and V$_6$ is confirmatory of the diagnosis of left ventricular enlargement.

COMMENT. The physical findings are practically pathognomonic of aortic stenosis. X-ray and electrocardiographic examinations are in accord. Since the prominent systolic murmur in the aortic valve area was heard at the age of seven, it is probable that this defect was congenital.

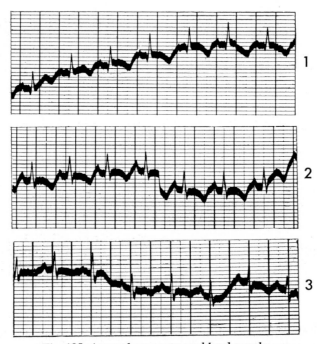

Fig. 185. Anomalous coronary blood supply.

Anomalous coronary blood supply in a three months old male infant who had been apparently healthy until two weeks before admission to the hospital, when he began to suffer recurring attacks of dyspnea, pallor and sweating. These episodes were brought on by the exertion of nursing and were sometimes accompanied by transient loss of consciousness. Upon physical examination he was found to be well developed. There was no cyanosis or clubbing. The heart was greatly enlarged. The rhythm was normal, and there were no murmurs.

The baby died in one of his attacks a few days after admission. Postmortem findings revealed an abnormal origin of the left coronary artery from the pulmonary artery, which had resulted in marked increase of the heart size and extensive degenerative change in the left ventricular myocardium supplied by the malposed vessel.

INTERPRETATION. Sinoatrial tachycardia (normal rhythm) is present at a rate of 150, with low voltage of the QRS waves in the three limb leads ($QRS_1= -1, +3$ to 4; $QRS_2= +4, -1$; $QRS_3= +3, -2$), and sharp late inversion of the T waves in Leads 1 and 2 (characteristically "chronic coronary T's"). The P–R interval, QRS duration, and length of systole (beginning of QRS to end of T) are all brief, as is to be expected in the case of tachycardia in an infant.

COMMENT. The coronary T waves, associated with the deficient circulation to the major part of the myocardium, make probable the interpretation of this baby's attacks as angina pectoris. Other cases with left coronary artery rising from the pulmonary artery have been encountered, both with and without such so-called coronary T waves.

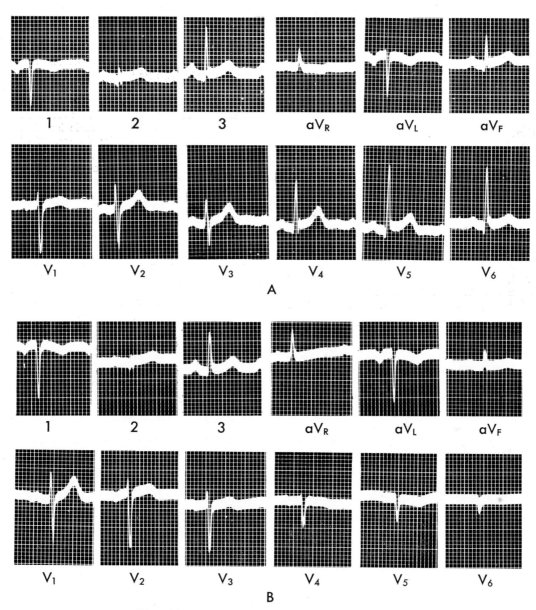

Fig. 186. Dextrocardia with complete situs inversus.

Dextrocardia with complete situs inversus in a man of fifty-two years who had known of this finding since the age of fifteen. He had been referred here from Cuba for study of a tumor in the chest which had been diagnosed as possible aneurysm. X-ray films of the chest had revealed complete situs inversus of the thoracic and abdominal viscera with enlargement of what appeared to be the main pulmonary artery shadow. Careful study pointed to the presence of tumor rather than of aneurysm, and on June 10, 1949, a mediastinal tumor was removed. He has been in excellent health since.

INTERPRETATION. *A,* Normal rhythm at a rate of 85, with complete inversion of the complexes in Leads 1 and aV$_L$. The precordial leads taken over the anterior wall of the right side of the chest show normal complexes throughout.

B, The routine left chest precordial leads in congenital mirror-type dextrocardia show right ventricular complexes of diminishing amplitude; this is the most important clue in distinguishing such dextrocardia from the technical error of reversal of arm wires.

COMMENT. This record is characteristic of congenital dextrocardia of the "mirror image type" (as a rule uncomplicated by other cardiac anomalies). An error in the application of the electrodes to the arms (the right and left arm wires reversed) would simulate congenital dextrocardia in the limb leads, but not in the precordial leads. (See Figure 37, *B.*)

References

1. Paul, O., Myers, G. S., and Campbell, J. A.: The Electrocardiogram in Congenital Heart Disease: A Preliminary Report. Circulation, *3:* 564, 1951.
2. Sokolow, M., and Edgar, A. L.: A Study of Unipolar Precordial and Limb Lead Electrocardiograms in Congenital Heart Disease. Am.J.Med., *8:* 528, 1950.
3. Bedford, D. E., Papp, C., and Parkinson, J.: Atrial Septal Defect. Brit.Heart J., *3:* 37, 1941.
4. Barber, J. M., Magidson, O., and Wood, P.: Atrial Septal Defect, with Special Reference to the Electrocardiogram, the Pulmonary Artery Pressure and the Second Heart Sound. Brit.Heart J., *12:* 277, 1950.
5. Selzer, A.: Defect of the Ventricular Septum. Summary of 12 Cases and Review of the Literature. Arch.Int.Med., *84:* 798, 1949.
6. Greene, D. G., and others: Pure Congenital Pulmonary Stenosis and Idiopathic Congenital Dilatation of the Pulmonary Artery. Am.J.Med., *6:* 24, 1949.
7. Sommers, S. C., and Johnson, J. M.: Congenital Tricuspid Atresia. Am.Heart J., *41:* 130, 1951.
8. Kroop, I. G.: Congenital Tricuspid Atresia. Am. Heart J., *41:* 549, 1951.
9. Ebel, E. H., Lynxwiler, C. P., and Moragues, V.: Tricuspid Atresia with a Rudimentary Right Ventricle. Case Report. J.Pediat., *39:* 211, 1951.
10. Selzer, A., and Laqueur, G. L.: The Eisenmenger Complex and Its Relation to the Uncomplicated Defect of the Ventricular Septum. Arch. Int. Med., *87:* 218, 1951.
11. Engle, M. A., and Taussig, H.B.: Valvular Pulmonic Stenosis with Intact Ventricular Septum and Patent Foramen Ovale; Report of Illustrative Cases. Circulation, *2:* 481, 1950.
12. Messeloff, C. R., and Weaver, J. C.: A Case of Transposition of the Large Vessels in an Adult Who Lived to the Age of 38 Years. Am.Heart J., *42:* 467, 1951.
13. Taussig, H. B., and Bing, R. J.: Complete Transposition of the Aorta and a Levoposition of the Pulmonary Artery. Am.Heart J., *37:* 551, 1949.
14. Goodwin, J. F., Steiner, R., and Wayne, E. J.: Transposition of the Aorta and Pulmonary Artery Demonstrated by Angiocardiography. Brit.Heart J., *11:* 279, 1949.

CHAPTER 13

Rheumatic Heart Disease

The electrocardiographic method is of value throughout the long natural history of rheumatic heart disease. Although frequently the electrocardiographic alterations are nonspecific, yet when they are considered along with the other clinical findings, the resulting conclusion may be of a definitive nature.

Acute Rheumatic Heart Disease

The electrocardiogram is often helpful in the diagnosis of the initial attack, particularly of the mild form when other signs may be few and indefinite. Involvement of the myocardium may be declared by prolongation of the conduction time between atrium and ventricle or, rarely, by lowering or inversion of the T waves. These changes are usually ephemeral, and it may be necessary to obtain records at frequent intervals in order to detect them.

In the more severe attack the electrocardiographic findings may provide some indications of the degree of involvement of the myocardium and of the presence or absence of pericarditis as a complication. Serial electrocardiograms may aid in following the course of the carditis and in making a decision as to the termination of rheumatic activity. Also, after the initial attack the electrocardiogram may be helpful in the diagnosis of recurrence of such activity.

The involvement of the myocardium by the rheumatic process may be indicated by sinus bradycardia, sinus tachycardia, and conduction defects, particularly prolongation of the $P–R$ interval. The electrocardiogram in Figure 187 was obtained from a boy eleven years of age shortly after the onset of the initial attack of rheumatic fever. There is considerable variation in heart rate, probably related to respiration, and occasionally there is sinoatrial block. At relatively fast heart rates the $P–R$ interval is abnormally prolonged, while at relatively slow heart rates or after a pause the $P–R$ interval is normal or nearly so. In other words, at a heart rate of 80 or above there is insufficient time for com-

plete recovery, and conduction between atrium and ventricle is delayed. Note the notched T waves in Leads V_2 and V_3; these are sometimes observed normally.

An electrocardiogram obtained on the same patient one day later showed partial heart block with dropped beats. The record in Figure 188, A, was obtained two days later and shows sinoatrial bradycardia at a rate of 60, which is abnormal during acute rheumatic fever and has much the same significance as prolongation of the $P–R$ interval. Later during convalescence, when the patient was improved, the heart rate nevertheless was much more rapid (Fig. 188, B). Rarely in acute rheumatic fever the patient may have complete atrioventricular block and Adams-Stokes attacks.

Ordinarily the atrioventricular block observed during the acute attack is transitory, but sometimes it persists as a permanent residuum. The electrocardiogram in Figure 189 was obtained from a female patient forty-three years of age with chronic rheumatic heart disease and mitral stenosis. She complained of vague aches and pains, and the question arose, whether or not she had a mild recrudescence of rheumatic activity. None of the clinical findings suggested active rheumatism except the long $P–R$ interval in the electrocardiogram, which became normal after the administration of 1.3 mg. of atropine sulfate intravenously. In view of this finding, a definite decision could not be reached and further observation was advised. It may be mentioned in passing that this test is not a reliable indicator of rheumatic activity.

The electrocardiogram in Figure 190 was obtained from a male patient twenty-four years of age with acute rheumatic pericarditis. Note the inversion of the T waves in both limb and precordial leads.

The electrocardiograms in Figure 191 were obtained from a male patient twenty years of age. The tracing in Figure 191, A, was taken November 29, 1950, at which time he had acute rheumatic fever and pericarditis. There is rather low voltage of QRS in the limb leads and inversion of the T waves in all leads shown. He appeared to convalesce uneventfully, and on January 4, 1951, the only abnormal finding was in the electrocardiogram (Fig. 191, B). Sometimes long periods are required before the QRS and T waves return to their initial form, or they may even fail to do so.

Chronic Rheumatic Heart Disease

The electrocardiogram here provides exact information concerning the arrhythmias and conduction defects and is of value in the detection of atrial and ventricular hypertrophy and "strain" resulting from valvular damage. In addition to evaluation of the cardiovascular status, the electrocardiogram is also helpful in directing therapy, particularly during the administration of digitalis and quinidine.

In chronic rheumatic heart disease the aortic or mitral valve, or both, may be involved. Involvement of the mitral valve alone, with resulting insufficiency, may lead at first to left atrial and ventricular enlargement, but as stenosis develops, the strain becomes less on the left ventricle, greater on the left atrium and right ventricle. Arrhythmias, especially atrial fibrillation, are prone to develop and may remain as a permanent functional disorder.

The electrocardiogram in Figure 192 was obtained from a female patient with chronic rheumatic heart disease and mitral stenosis. There was no reason whatever to suspect rheumatic activity. The P–R interval is abnormally prolonged and did not shorten appreciably after atropine. This record illustrates the permanent character of partial heart block in some patients with chronic rheumatic heart disease.

The electrocardiogram in Figure 193 was obtained from a woman forty-six years of age with chronic rheumatic heart disease, left atrial and slight left ventricular enlargement, mitral stenosis and insufficiency, but fairly good reserve. An additional diagnosis was funnel chest, which was thought to be of sufficient degree to influence the shape of the heart. She was not receiving digitalis or other medication. In the limb leads the QRS axis points toward 0 degrees, which is consistent with the finding of slight left ventricular enlargement. The RS–T segments are depressed in Leads 1 and 2 and in precordial leads V_3 through V_6; this is con-

sistent with a diagnosis of left ventricular "strain." The prominent P waves are related to the enlargement of the left atrium.

The electrocardiogram in Figure 194 was obtained from a woman twenty-six years of age with moderate cardiac enlargement, considerable mitral stenosis and greatly decreased reserve. The pulmonary second sound was accentuated. An additional diagnosis was funnel chest, which was thought to be sufficient to displace the heart to the left. She was digitalized at the time the electrocardiogram was obtained. In the limb leads the QRS axis points toward +120 degrees and the axis of the T waves toward 0 degrees; the resulting angle is abnormally large. In Lead V_2 there is a qR complex with T inverted, and in V_4 also T is deeply inverted. These findings indicate preponderant enlargement and "strain" of the right ventricle. The prominent P waves indicate atrial enlargement.

The electrocardiogram in Figure 195 was obtained from a woman thirty-seven years of age with considerable cardiac enlargement, an extreme degree of mitral stenosis, and congestive failure. Enlargement involved, mainly, the left atrium and the right ventricle. Cardiac catheterization revealed abnormally high pressures in the pulmonary artery, 100 mm. of mercury systolic and 50 mm. diastolic at rest, and 140 mm. systolic and 70 mm. diastolic after slight exercise. She was receiving digitalis at the time the electrocardiogram was taken. In the limb leads the QRS axis points toward +130 degrees. The RS–T segments are depressed and the T waves low or inverted. In the precordial leads R in V_1 is abnormally tall, and the S waves are abnormally prominent in V_4 through V_6. The RS–T segments are depressed and the T waves abnormally low in V_4 through V_6. The QRS changes in this record are consistent with right ventricular hypertrophy, and the RS–T and T wave changes are due to digitalis or right ventricular "strain," or both.

Involvement of the aortic valve leading to aortic regurgitation or stenosis throws an extra burden primarily on the left ventricle which leads eventually to preponderant enlargement and "strain" of this chamber.

The electrocardiogram in Figure 196 was obtained from a male patient forty-one years of age with chronic rheumatic heart disease, free aortic regurgitation and slight left ventricular enlargement. The slight sagging of the *RS–T* segments in Leads 2 and V₅ and the rather low *T* waves in these leads suggest early left ventricular "strain."

The electrocardiogram in Figure 197 was obtained from a patient fifty-five years of age with aortic stenosis, marked cardiac enlargement and slight congestive failure. The blood pressure was 130 mm. of mercury systolic and 72 mm. diastolic. Treatment included digitalization at the time the tracing was taken. In the limb leads the QRS axis points toward -10 degrees, and in Leads 1 and 2 QRS is essentially monophasic in form with the *RS–T* segments and *T* waves oppositely directed. In the precordial leads also the QRS complex is essentially monophasic in form, directed downward in Leads V₁ through V₃ and upward in V₄ through V₆ with the *T* waves pointing in the opposite directions. These changes are typical of left ventricular hypertrophy and "strain."

Frequently in chronic rheumatic heart disease both aortic and mitral valves are affected. This leads to hypertrophy of the ventricle under the greater strain and then of both ventricles.

The electrocardiograms in Figure 198 were obtained from a man twenty-one years of age with chronic rheumatic heart disease, slight cardiac enlargement, aortic regurgitation and slight mitral stenosis. The electrocardiogram in Figure 198, *A*, was taken before the patient arose in the morning. The prominent *S* waves in Leads V₂ and V₃ and prominent *R* waves in V₅ strongly suggest left ventricular hypertrophy. The sagging of the *RS–T* segments and the low *T* waves in Leads 2, V₄, V₅, and V₆ in the absence of digitalis therapy suggest left ventricular "strain." The tracing in Figure 198, *B*, was obtained on the same day after moderate exercise and the "strain" pattern is more evident, especially in the limb leads.

The electrocardiogram in Figure 199 was obtained from a man thirty-eight years of age with chronic rheumatic heart disease, aortic and mitral stenosis, and generalized cardiac enlargement. Treatment included digitalization at the time this record was taken. In the limb leads the electrical axis of QRS is shifted to the right ($+120$ degrees); the *RS–T* segment changes are characteristic of digitalization rather than of ventricular "strain," and the *T* waves are nearly isoelectric. In the precordial leads the *S* waves are abnormally prominent in Leads V₂ through V₅ and the *T* waves are upright. These findings are not characteristic of either right or left ventricular hypertrophy, but rather are a mixture of both. The right axis deviation in the limb leads is consistent with right ventricular hypertrophy, but the findings in the precordial leads are somewhat more suggestive of left-sided enlargement.

The electrocardiogram in Figure 200 was obtained from a patient with chronic rheumatic heart disease, great cardiac enlargement and marked aortic and mitral stenosis. The patient was digitalized. In the limb leads there is a tendency for the QRS complexes to have a monophasic form with the *T* waves oppositely directed. Because of the great magnitude of the waves the precordial leads were obtained using one half the customary sensitivity. The alterations are consistent with left ventricular hypertrophy and "strain."

It is worth emphasizing that in some patients with chronic rheumatic heart disease the electrocardiogram is not appreciably altered. The record in Figure 201 was obtained from a man fifty-five years of age with considerable mitral stenosis, which had developed after an attack of rheumatic fever at the age of twenty-five. X-ray examination revealed the heart to be full-sized with moderate enlargement of the left atrium, but there is no definite abnormality in the electrocardiogram.

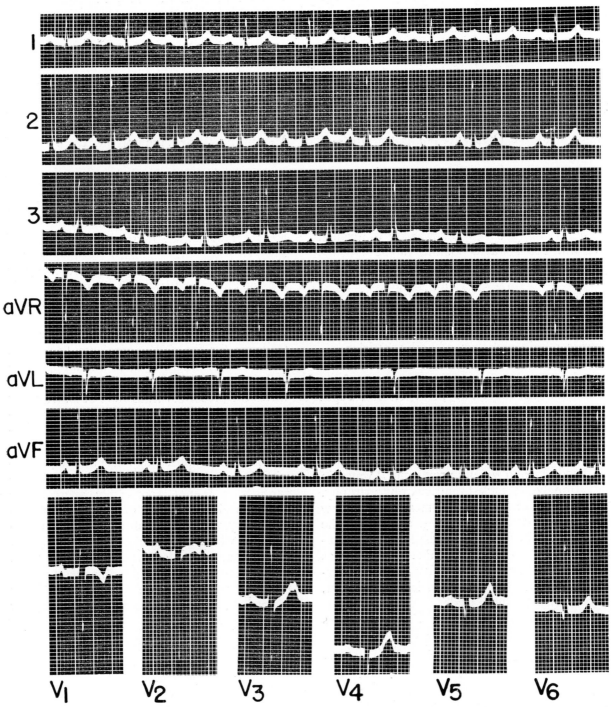

Fig. 187. This electrocardiogram was obtained on a boy aged eleven, shortly after the onset of an initial attack of rheumatic fever. The *P–R* intervals are abnormally prolonged, but this prolongation shows a dependence on heart rate. Thus in Lead 2, following a relatively long pause which may be due to sinoatrial block, the *P–R* interval is only 0.15 second, whereas in Lead 1 the *P–R* interval is as long as 0.22 second.

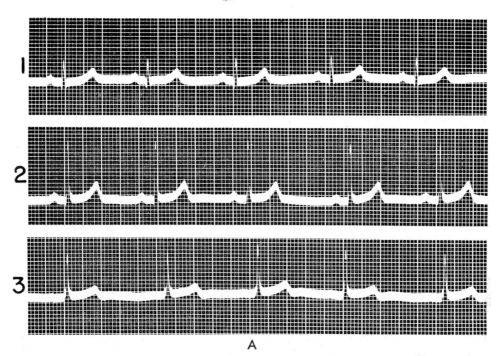

Fig. 188. *A*, Same case as in Figure 187, but electrocardiogram obtained two days later. It shows an abnormally slow heart rate for a patient with acute rheumatic fever. See text.

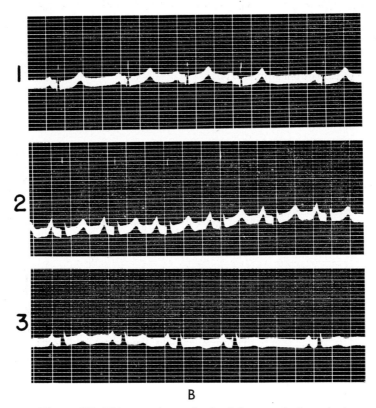

Fig. 188. *B*, Same case as in Figure 187. This record was obtained three weeks later during convalescence. The heart rate is more rapid despite the fact that the patient was better. See text.

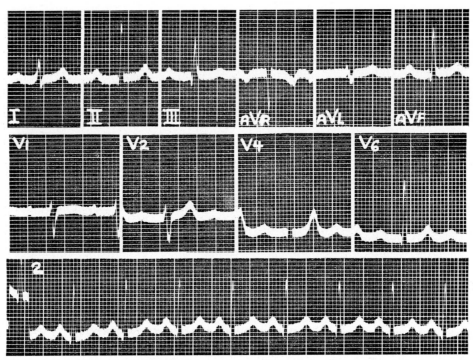

Fig. 189. This electrocardiogram was obtained from a woman forty-three years of age with chronic rheumatic heart disease and mitral stenosis. The *P–R* interval is abnormally prolonged (0.28 second), but shortens after the administration of atropine, as shown in the bottom strip. See text.

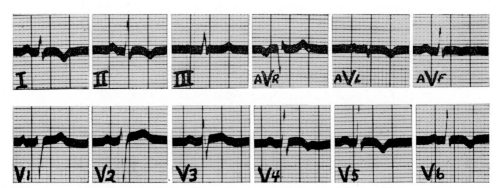

Fig. 190. This electrocardiogram was obtained on a man twenty-four years of age with acute rheumatic fever complicated by rheumatic pericarditis. In addition to the clinical findings, the diagnosis of pericarditis was supported by the low or inverted *T* waves observed in both limb and precordial leads.

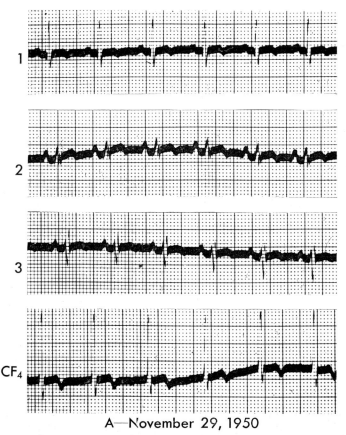

A—November 29, 1950

Fig. 191. *A,* This electrocardiogram was obtained on a young man twenty years of age who was suffering from an initial attack of acute rheumatic fever complicated by pericarditis. The *RS–T* segments are slightly elevated in Lead 2, and the *T* waves are inverted in all four leads.

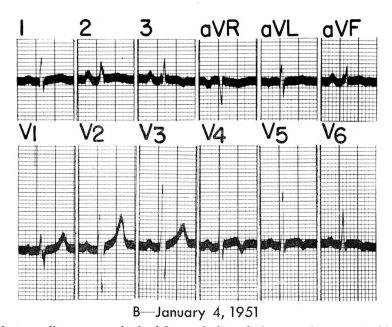

B—January 4, 1951

Fig. 191. *B,* This electrocardiogram was obtained five weeks later during convalescence, at which time there was no evidence of active infection. Nevertheless the *T* waves are still abnormally low in some of the limb leads and are abnormally prominent in precordial leads V_1 and V_2, and inverted in V_4 through V_6. As a rule the *T* wave changes resulting from rheumatic pericarditis do not remain for a long time, but in some instances the *T* waves never return to their original form.

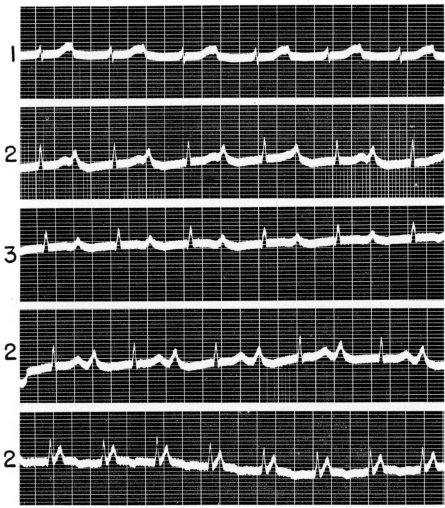

Fig. 192. This electrocardiogram was obtained from a woman forty-one years of age with chronic rheumatic heart disease and mitral stenosis without any evidence of active rheumatic infection. The P waves are 0.47 second long ard are superimposed on the descending limb of the T waves. The fourth strip shows Lead 2 when the heart rate was relatively slow, and both P and T are clearly defined. The fifth strip was obtained soon after the administration of 2 mg. of atropine sulfate intravenously. The heart rate has increased, as have the P–R intervals, which are now about 0.51 second long; the resulting QRS occurs immediately prior to the next succeeding P wave. This record illustrates the permanent character of partial atrioventricular block in some cases of chronic rheumatic heart disease.

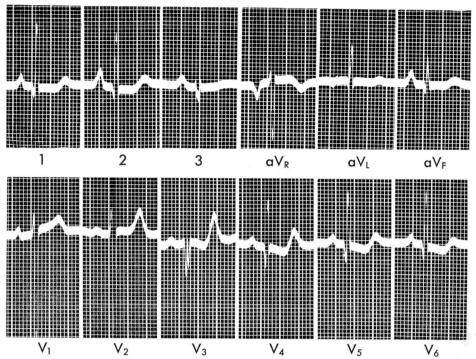

1   2   3   aV$_R$ aV$_L$ aV$_F$

V$_1$ V$_2$ V$_3$ V$_4$ V$_5$ V$_6$

Fig. 193. This electrocardiogram was obtained from a woman forty-six years of age with chronic rheumatic heart disease, mitral stenosis and regurgitation, and left atrial and ventricular enlargement. In addition to the prominent P waves which indicate left atrial hypertrophy, there is a tendency toward left axis deviation of QRS, and there is slight downward displacement of the $RS-T$ segments in some of the limb leads and in precordial leads V$_3$ through V$_6$. These changes in the absence of digitalis administration were thought to be due to left ventricular "strain" and hypertrophy.

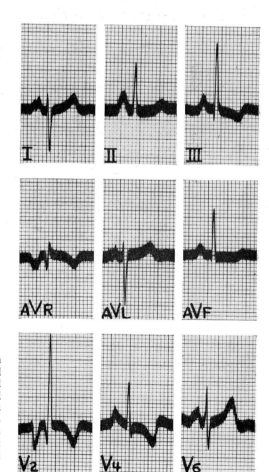

Fig. 194. This electrocardiogram was obtained from a woman twenty-six years of age with chronic rheumatic heart disease, mitral stenosis, and moderate cardiac enlargement. She was digitalized at the time the record was taken. In the limb leads the electrical axis of QRS points to the right. In the precordial leads the R waves are abnormally prominent in Lead V$_2$, and the S waves are abnormally prominent in Lead V$_6$. The T waves are inverted in Leads V$_2$ through V$_4$. These changes indicate a high degree of right ventricular hypertrophy. It is unusual for normal rhythm to persist in mitral stenosis with so much right ventricular enlargement.

Page 229

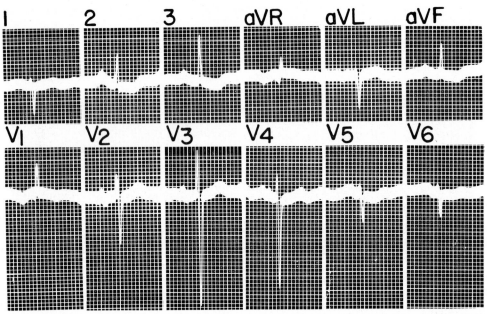

Fig. 195. This electrocardiogram was obtained from a woman thirty-seven years of age with chronic rheumatic heart disease, a high degree of mitral stenosis, and congestive failure. She was receiving digitalis at the time this record was made. In the limb leads the electrical axis of QRS is shifted to the right, and in the precordial leads the R wave is abnormally prominent in V₁, and the S waves are abnormally prominent in V₄ through V₆. These changes are characteristic of right ventricular hypertrophy. The changes in the RS–T segments and T waves in both limb and precordial leads are probably due, in large part at least, to digitalis.

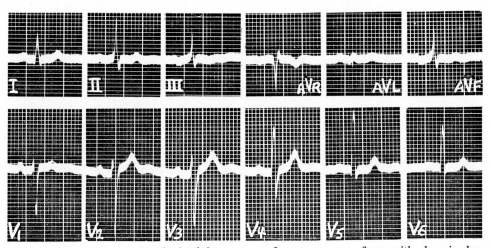

Fig. 196. This electrocardiogram was obtained from a man forty-one years of age with chronic rheumatic heart disease, slight left ventricular enlargement and free aortic regurgitation. He was not receiving digitalis at the time this record was made. The slight sagging of the RS–T segments in some of the limb leads and in precordial leads V₅ and V₆ suggests slight left ventricular "strain."

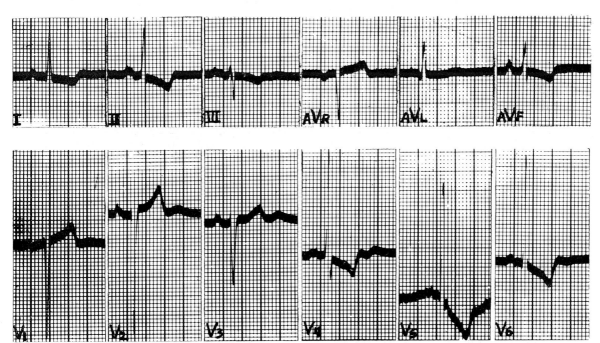

Fig. 197. This electrocardiogram was obtained from a man fifty-five years of age with marked aortic stenosis, presumably rheumatic in origin. The heart was greatly enlarged in the region of the left ventricle. Treatment included digitalization at the time this record was taken. In the limb leads the *QRS* complexes tend to be monophasic in form and the *T* waves are usually oppositely directed. In the precordial leads the *S* waves are abnormally prominent and the *QRS* complexes tend to be monophasic in form, being downwardly directed in Leads V_1 through V_3 and upwardly directed in V_4 through V_6. The *T* waves are oppositely directed to the chief *QRS* deflection. These changes are consistent with marked left ventricular hypertrophy and "strain."

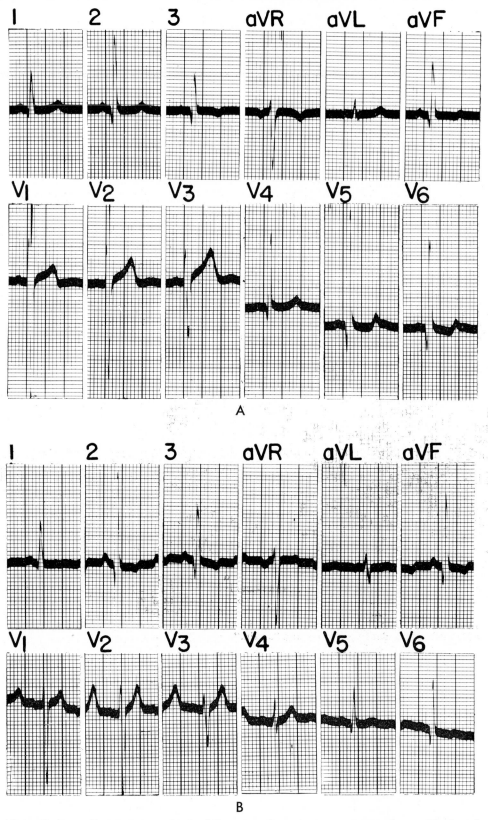

Fig. 198. These electrocardiograms were obtained from a patient twenty-one years of age with chronic rheumatic heart disease, slight cardiac enlargement, aortic regurgitation and slight mitral stenosis. *A*, At rest; *B*, after mild exercise. The changes in these records were considered to indicate left ventricular hypertrophy and "strain."

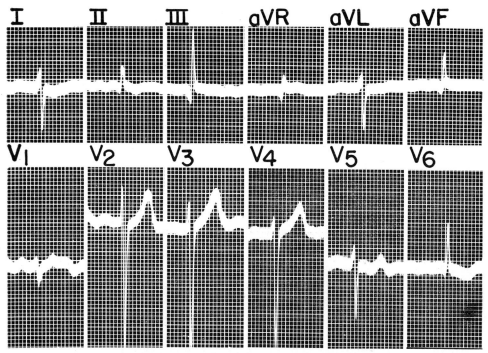

Fig. 199. This electrocardiogram was obtained from a man thirty-eight years of age with chronic rheumatic heart disease, aortic and mitral stenosis, and generalized cardiac enlargement. The electrocardiographic alterations indicate combined left and right ventricular enlargement, though the latter is preponderant. See text.

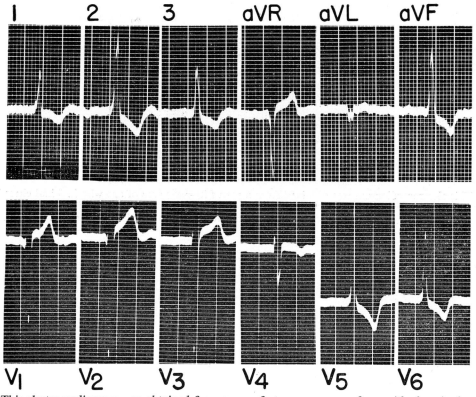

Fig. 200. This electrocardiogram was obtained from a man forty-seven years of age with chronic rheumatic heart disease, aortic and mitral stenosis, marked cardiac enlargement, and congestive failure. He was digitalized at the time this record was obtained. The changes are typical of left ventricular hypertrophy and "strain."

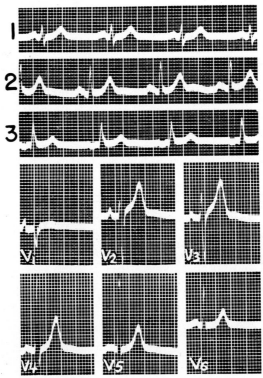

Fig. 201. This electrocardiogram was obtained from a man fifty-five years of age who had had chronic rheumatic heart disease with considerable mitral stenosis since the age of twenty-five. X-ray examination revealed a full-sized heart with moderate enlargement of the left atrium. This record shows no definite abnormality. See text.

CHAPTER 14

Subacute Bacterial Endocarditis

There is no characteristic electrocardiogram in subacute bacterial endocarditis. Indeed, not infrequently, with slight cardiac defects, congenital or rheumatic, the electrocardiogram may be quite normal. It is also true that many patterns of abnormality may be encountered in association with endocarditis lenta, depending upon the underlying developmental faults or valvular lesions, and the presence of active rheumatic fever, focal embolic myocarditis, uremia and other disorders. Rarely, embolism from valvular lesions to a coronary artery may produce the characteristic pattern of myocardial infarction.

CHAPTER 15

Cardiovascular Syphilis

Abnormal electrocardiographic patterns seen in association with syphilitic aortitis depend chiefly on two pathologic alterations. Free aortic regurgitation leads to left ventricular hypertrophy and the classical electrocardiographic pattern thereof. Narrowing of the coronary ostia may produce electrocardiographic evidence of myocardial involvement due to interference with the coronary circulation; thus bundle branch block and *T* wave inversion are occasionally encountered in patients with syphilitic aortitis. It should also be emphasized that the electrocardiogram may be quite normal in this disease, especially when there is no aortic regurgitation or involvement of the coronary ostia. Combinations of patterns representing left ventricular hypertrophy and coronary insufficiency may also be expected.

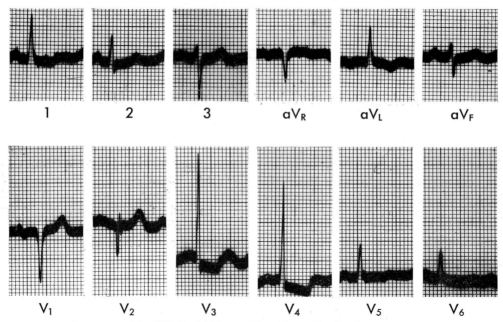

Fig. 202. Syphilitic aortitis with cardiac involvement.

Syphilitic aortitis with cardiac involvement in a fifty-eight year old painter who was first seen on September 15, 1950, with typical angina pectoris which had been present for at least four years. There had been no episode of prolonged substernal pain and no history of paroxysmal nocturnal dyspnea. Thirty years before, the patient had had a penile chancre treated with mercury pills; no parenteral therapy was given at that time.

Physical examination in 1950 showed a slightly obese man who looked well. The pulse was regular at 75. The blood pressure was 140 mm. of mercury systolic and 60 mm. diastolic. The patient was barrel-chested, and the cardiac impulse was not felt. The heart sounds were well heard, with a loud aortic second sound of tambour quality. A mid-diastolic gallop was present at the apex. No diastolic murmur was heard.

Fluoroscopy showed slight cardiac enlargement, the transverse cardiac diameter being 14 cm., in comparison with an internal diameter of the thorax measuring 27 cm. The aorta was dilated in its proximal portion and showed "Corrigan" pulsations. A blood Hinton reaction was positive.

INTERPRETATION. Normal sinus rhythm at a rate of 90, with $P–R$ interval of 0.16 second; T_1 inverted, T_2, T_3 upright; moderate left axis deviation. There is an inverted T in aV_L. The chest leads show T waves upright in V_1 and V_2, with prominent Q waves in V_2 (there is also an R in this lead). The T waves in V_3 and V_4 are inverted, with sagging of the $S–T$ segments; the QRS complexes are of high amplitude in these leads. The T waves in V_5 and V_6 are low to slightly inverted.

COMMENT. Syphilitic aortitis may be silent so far as any clinical manifestations are concerned, or there may be dilatation of the aorta without symptoms, or there may be aortic regurgitation producing strain and enlargement of the left ventricle, with or without myocardial failure. Finally, there may be coronary insufficiency, due chiefly to the narrowing of the coronary ostia from the aortitis itself. It seems likely that the last-mentioned complication of syphilitic aortitis was present in this case, giving rise to the angina pectoris and the dilatation of the left ventricle, along with the electrocardiographic changes that have been described. It is possible also that some aortic regurgitation may have been present, not, however, diagnosable in the absence of a diastolic murmur.

(*Legend continued from facing page, Figure 203.*)

INTERPRETATION. *A, December 30, 1947.* Sinus arrhythmia at a rate averaging 100, with varying degrees of atrioventricular block; QRS complexes of low amplitude in the classical leads, and inverted T waves in all leads; moderate right axis deviation.

B, January 16, 1948. Sinus or atrial tachycardia at a rate of 150, with 2:1 heart block, QRS complexes of normal duration; T waves upright, but low in Lead 1 and in the chest leads, and inverted in Leads 2 and 3; moderate right axis deviation.

COMMENT. Electrocardiograms taken almost daily on this patient showed persistent abnormality. In addition to the changes seen in these tracings, complete heart block and atrial fibrillation were recorded. The two tracings illustrate the marked degree of electrocardiographic abnormality sometimes encountered in diphtheritic heart disease. Bundle branch block was not recorded in this case. The right axis deviation found in *A* was confirmed in *B*, although at first glance it seemed possible that there might have been an artifact due to error of technique with reversal of the two arm electrodes.

CHAPTER 16

Diphtheria

Heart damage in diphtheria is effected by the action of potent circulating bacterial toxins on the heart muscle and on the conduction system. If the resulting myocarditis is mild, electrocardiographic changes in the form of conduction defects, low voltage of *QRS* complexes, and low to inverted *T* waves may be the only evidence of cardiac involvement. In the more severe cases, cardiac dilatation and, rarely, failure and death may complicate the course of the disease. Conduction defects include bundle branch block and atrioventricular block in all grades of severity from slight prolongation of the *P–R* interval to complete heart block. (See Figure 203.)

If diphtheritic involvement does not end in death, functional recovery of the heart muscle is complete. However, conduction defects in the form of atrioventricular block and bundle branch block may persist in rare cases for years

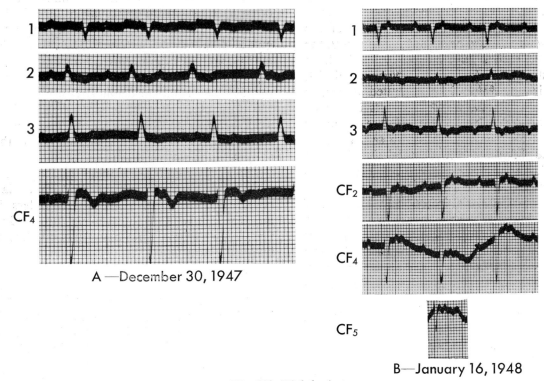

A —December 30, 1947

B—January 16, 1948

Fig. 203. Diphtheria.*

Diphtheria in a nine year old girl who was admitted to the hospital on December 14, 1947, five days after the onset of a sore throat. A throat culture taken the day before admission was reported positive for diphtheria. Physical examination revealed an acutely ill, emaciated girl with cervical adenopathy and edematous tonsils and pharynx covered with an adherent grayish membrane. The heart size was normal, and no murmurs were heard.

Despite treatment with antitoxin, penicillin and streptomycin, heart block was evidenced on the second hospital day and persisted throughout the illness; palatal paralysis set in on the ninth day, and cardiac failure, which appeared on the thirteenth day, remained resistant to therapy until death five weeks after admission. An autopsy confirmed the clinical impression of diphtheritic myocarditis. (*Legend continued on opposite page.*)

* We are indebted to Dr. Louis Weinstein, Medical Director of the Haynes Memorial Hospital, Boston, for the privilege of reproducing these data.

CHAPTER 17

Other Infections

Many other infections besides those noted in previous chapters (rheumatic fever, subacute bacterial endocarditis, diphtheria and syphilis) can cause heart disease, but they do not in this part of the world—that is, in the United States—to an extent that requires special chapters here. The miscellaneous infections to which we refer are either rare in themselves, or they infrequently affect the heart to any appreciable degree (and then, as a rule, only in patients seriously or fatally ill with the disease in question). Thus echinococcus disease is uncommon in this country; even in certain parts of the world where it does occur not infrequently, the heart and pericardium are rarely involved. In contrast, Chagas' disease (trypanosomiasis), which is not found in the United States, is common in Brazil, where it results in a high percentage of cases of heart disease, in many of which electrocardiograms are said to show evidence of diffuse myocardial involvement (arrhythmias, long $P-R$ intervals and abnormalities of QRS and T waves).

Virus and rickettsial infections, which are, of course, common diseases, have of late years been identified as causing in rare instances heart disease and abnormal electrocardiograms. For example, epidemic parotitis (mumps) is said to have caused heart block, and influenza can initiate serious myocarditis in rare cases.

Most bacterial diseases have no specific effect on the heart, but they can in fatal cases produce terminal pathologic changes in the cells of the myocardium, and, of course, bizarre electrocardiograms are not infrequently obtainable in patients dying of any infection.

Parasitic diseases encountered in the United States—in particular, trichinosis—may involve the heart importantly in a small minority of cases. Malaria can act either directly or through the consequent anemia, but usually the heart

escapes. Trypanosomiasis and echinococcus disease have already been mentioned.

Finally, there is heart disease extensive in degree and evidently infectious in origin, but of unknown etiology. We suspect an unidentified virus in the majority of such cases.

Myocarditis of Unknown Etiology

There is a large group of exudative and destructive lesions of the myocardium commonly termed "myocarditis of unknown etiology." Usually there is no evidence of infection elsewhere in the body; when this is the case, the myocarditis is sometimes classified as "Fiedler's" or "interstitial" or "isolated" myocarditis, a designation without specificity so far as the etiology or histologic detail is concerned and less satisfactory than the term used here. Much work remains to be done in the direction of resolution of confusion pertaining to this subject.

The electrocardiographic changes are protean and cannot be considered specific from a diagnostic viewpoint. They include disorders in atrioventricular and intraventricular conduction, low voltage of QRS complexes and low or inverted T waves.

Trichinosis

As a rule, cardiac involvement in trichinosis is unimportant, and the electrocardiographic changes are of little significance. Minor T wave changes, prolongation of the $P-R$ interval and other nonspecific changes have been reported. Rarely, infestation of heart muscle with the trichina organisms assumes clinical significance, and then cardiac dilatation with or without congestive heart failure may supervene. It is well known that no encysted forms of the organism are found in heart muscle even when damage has been severe.

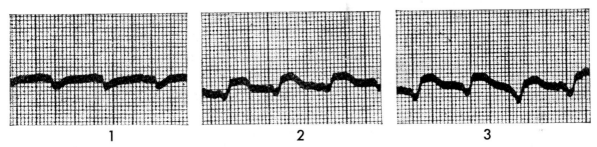

Fig. 204. Myocarditis in influenza.*

Acute myocarditis in influenza in a woman who was in good health until 1942, when at the age of thirty-four she had a respiratory infection diagnosed as "flu." After several months of malaise and cough, fever developed and she was admitted to the hospital with a diagnosis of pneumonia.

Physical examination on admission revealed an extremely ill young woman with a temperature of 102.2° F. Blood pressure was 80 mm. of mercury systolic and 70 mm. diastolic. Dullness, bronchial breathing and moist rales were heard at the right lung base, while at the left lung base breath sounds were suppressed. The heart was not enlarged clinically, but heart sounds were distant. Examination of the abdomen was negative except for slight distention. She was restless and complained of substernal constriction and at the same time was quite dyspneic. A bedside chest film taken several hours after admission showed fine mottling of both lungs with irregular consolidation through most of the left lung.

The patient failed rapidly and died the same day. An electrocardiogram was taken two hours before death. Postmortem examination revealed bloody exudate in the lungs and bilateral hydrothorax. The heart was not especially remarkable on gross examination except for slight dilatation of the chambers. However, microscopic examination of the myocardium showed marked necrosis of muscle fibers and infiltration with lymphocytes and plasma cells. Influenza A was isolated from the lungs. The organism was not isolated from the heart, but the relationship between the two lesions seemed more than coincidental.

INTERPRETATION. Sinus tachycardia, rate 105, with P–R interval of 0.08 second. QRS and T complexes are of low amplitude; there appears to be some sagging of the S–T interval in Lead 1. Serious elevation of the S–T interval is seen in Leads 2 and 3.

COMMENT. This electrocardiogram suggests widespread damage to heart muscle, but it is not specific for any given lesion. Undoubtedly in this case the cause of death was involvement of the heart by an acute process.

* This case has been previously published in the American Journal of Medical Science, 209: 455, 1945. We are indebted to the publishers, Lea & Febiger of Philadelphia, and to Dr. Maxwell Finland, Boston, for permission to reproduce this information and the electrocardiogram.

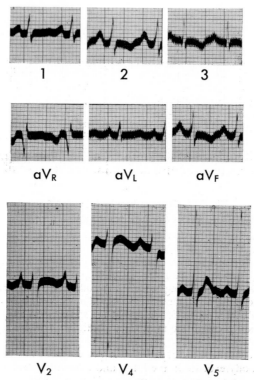

Fig. 205. Myocarditis of unknown etiology.

Myocarditis of unknown etiology in a six year old schoolboy who entered the hosptial on June 11, 1948, because of persistent vomiting and abdominal pain. Physical examination revealed dyspnea and considerable cardiac enlargement, with gallop rhythm at the apex. No murmurs were heard. A chest film showed moderate cardiac enlargement without characteristic configuration. The electrocardiogram was obtained three days after admission. On the sixth hospital day a right hemiplegia occurred. In spite of treatment, congestive heart failure persisted, and the patient died on June 27, shortly after a second cerebrovascular accident.

Postmortem examination revealed cardiac enlargement with hypertrophy of both ventricles and mural thrombi in both ventricular cavities. Microscopic sections showed areas of focal tissue reaction and necrosis with little cellular reaction interspersed among hypertrophied heart muscle fibers.

INTERPRETATION. Rapid sinus rhythm at a rate of 130; P–R interval of 0.12 second; T waves low in Lead 1, inverted in Leads 2 and 3. The chest leads show inverted T's in V_2 and V_4, upright T's in V_5.

COMMENT. The changes seen in this electrocardiogram, taken three days after admission, are nonspecific, but are consistent with some degree of myocardial damage. This was really a focal myocarditis of unusual kind and unknown etiology associated with idiopathic hypertrophy. The episodes of hemiplegia were undoubtedly embolic in origin, arising from mural thrombi. This is often encountered in "nonspecific" myocarditis.

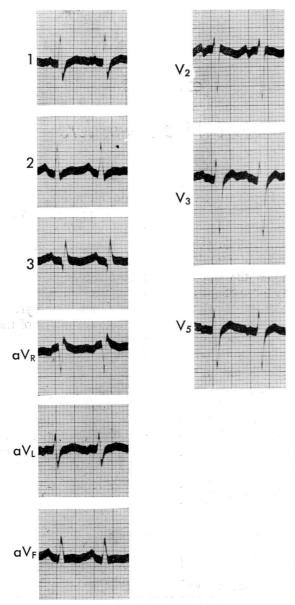

Fig. 206. Trichinosis.*

Trichinosis in a twenty-eight year old male machinist admitted to the hospital on February 12, 1948 The illness began three weeks before admission, with malaise and weakness, and was characterized by progression of these symptoms, with occasional bouts of vomiting. On admission he appeared weak and ill and was barely able to move his extremities. No periorbital edema was seen. Pain was slight. His temperature on admission was 104° F., and it remained elevated until his death on February 23. The patient was examined by one of us (C. W.) on February 19, at which time no cardiac involvement was evident clinically. The electrocardiogram shown here was obtained on that day. Two days before death congestive failure with dyspnea developed and there was a rise in pulse rate to 130. The congestive failure did not respond to therapy.

Autopsy revealed massive infestation with trichinae, involving the extremities, diaphragm and heart muscle. No encysted forms were found in the heart muscle, but destruction of the muscle fibers in characteristic fashion was extreme.

INTERPRETATION. Sinus tachycardia at a rate of 120; *P-R* interval of 0.16 second; low *T* waves in chest and extremity leads.

COMMENT. At the time this tracing was taken, five days before the patient's death, cardiac involvement must have been proceeding, although no definite clinical evidence had yet appeared. The electrocardiogram is abnormal, without specific pattern, but is consistent with early myocardial damage. It is likely that tracings taken later, just before death, would have shown a much more abnormal pattern.

* We are indebted to Dr. Leslie S. Joliffe, Pathologist, Lawrence General Hospital, Lawrence, Massachusetts, for permission to include this case.

CHAPTER 18

Endocrine Disorders

Except for thyroid disease of both toxic and deficient types, the relationship of endocrinopathy to the electrocardiogram has been an obscure and neglected subject. Of late years, however, there has developed a new interest in the effect on the heart and on the electrocardiogram of such diseases as those of the adrenals (Addison's and pheochromocytomas), the parathyroids (hyperparathyroidism and hypoparathyroidism), and the pituitary (acromegaly and Cushing's syndrome). Much of such effect is due to the influence of the hormones on the electrolyte (especially potassium, sodium and calcium) and water balance of the body, some is due to intermediary effects such as the hypertension of Cushing's disease and of pheochromocytomas, but some remains obscure. Ovarian and testicular diseases seem per se to have little or no effect on the electrocardiogram. Much research remains to be done in this field.

Thyroid Disease

Hypothyroidism

Hypothyroidism, when present in significant degree (myxedema or cretinism), produces significant alterations in electrocardiographic pattern. *P* and *QRS* waves usually diminish in amplitude; *T* waves may be low to inverted. In some instances, when *T* waves are inverted abnormally or even normally (as in Lead 3) before the onset of myxedema, these may become flat or slightly upright with the development of the hypothyroid state. Thyroid therapy corrects deviations of the electrocardiogram toward the pattern which existed prior to the onset of myxedema, in degree parallel to the basal metabolic rate.

Hyperthyroidism

The most striking electrocardiographic changes seen in thyrotoxicosis are associated with the effect of the thyroid hormone on heart rate and irritability of the atrial muscle. Sinoatrial tachycardia is the commonest finding, but atrial fibrillation and flutter are frequently seen, especially in the older age groups. Minor changes in *P* and *T* waves are often observed, but these constitute no specific diagnostic pattern. The faster the heart rate, the lower are the *T* waves, a sympathetic effect, as in normal health.

(*Legend continued from facing page, Figure 207.*)

Myxedema in a sixty-seven year old janitor who showed the classical signs of this disease at the time of his first admission to the hospital in 1937. His basal metabolic rate was −30. He responded well to thyroid, but stopped taking it at least two years before hospital re-entry on March 24, 1951, when he again showed dry skin, a puffy face, a hoarse voice, slow speech and mental retardation. His blood pressure was 114 mm. of mercury systolic and 82 mm. diastolic. His basal metabolic rate was −40. Thyroid was again administered in small doses, and he showed gradual clinical improvement. On May 4, 1951, his basal metabolic rate was −20.

INTERPRETATION. *A, March 26, 1951.* Slow sinus rhythm at a rate of 65 (rate determined from complete tracing). The *P* waves and the *QRS* complexes appear to be within normal limits. The *T* waves are of low amplitude throughout.

B, May 4, 1951. Greatly increased amplitude of *QRS* and *T* waves in most leads in comparison with record *A*; low *T* waves in Leads 2 and in V$_6$, with slight sagging of the *S–T* segment. There is a slight artifact due to overshooting in this record (see standardization).

COMMENT. These changes illustrate the effect of thyroid treatment on the electrocardiogram in myxedema. Increase in amplitude of *QRS* and *T* waves is the most striking feature. It is interesting to observe that *T* waves which are inverted in the first tracing are more so in the second. The pattern of the latter tracing rather suggests left ventricular hypertrophy (high *QRS* and low *T* waves with sagging *S–T* segments in Lead V$_6$), although there was no apparent cause in this case. Coronary artery disease may contribute to the patterns. Overshooting may add a little to the height of *QRS* and depth of *S* waves in the second tracing, but the chief factor responsible is treatment with thyroid hormone. Overshooting of this degree does not affect *T* waves significantly. The striking serial changes in V$_5$ and V$_6$ in the two records are probably due mostly to changes in position of the recording electrode in successive tracings.

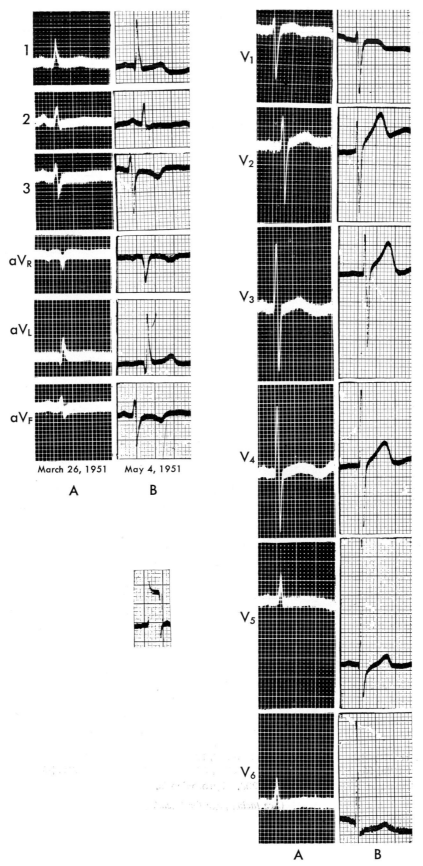

1

2

3

aV_R

aV_L

aV_F

March 26, 1951   May 4, 1951

A   B

V_1

V_2

V_3

V_4

V_5

V_6

A   B

Fig. 207. The effect of treatment of myxedema on the electrocardiogram.

(*See opposite page for legend.*)

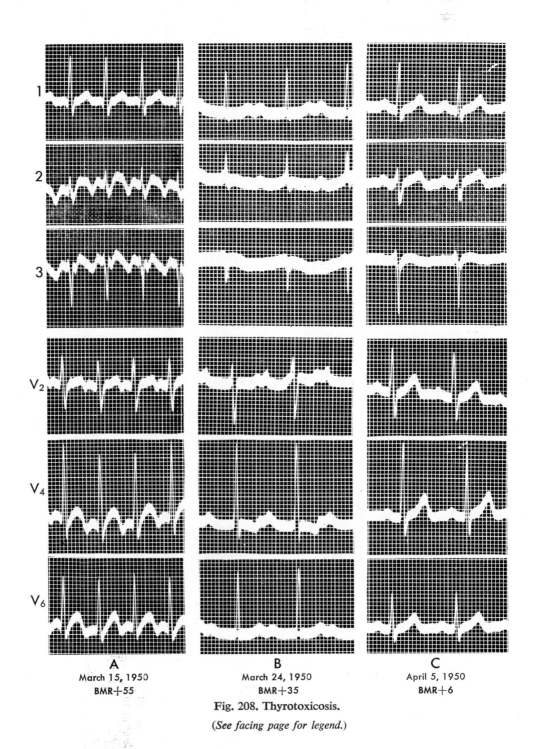

A
March 15, 1950
BMR+55

B
March 24, 1950
BMR+35

C
April 5, 1950
BMR+6

Fig. 208. Thyrotoxicosis.

(*See facing page for legend.*)

(*Legend continued from opposite page, Figure 208*)

Thyrotoxicosis in a fifty-two year old bookkeeper who was admitted to the hospital on March 14, 1950, with a diagnosis of thyrotoxicosis. Over a period of four years he had noticed increased appetite, tremor and sweating. Exophthalmos had become apparent, and he had lost 15 pounds in weight. Two years before admission a course of thiouracil therapy had produced some remission in his symptoms, but they had again become well established by the time of this admission to the hospital.

Physical examination revealed a flushed and nervous man, with a heart rate of 160. Tremor and exophthalmos were present, and the thyroid was diffusely enlarged. No heart murmurs were audible. There was questionable cardiac enlargement by x-ray examination. The basal metabolic rate was plus 55.

Treatment was instituted with thiouracil, iodine and digitalis. On the sixth hospital day the heart rate dropped suddenly to 100. Sub-total thyroidectomy performed three weeks after admission was followed by uneventful recovery.

INTERPRETATION. *A, March 15, 1950.* Atrial flutter at a rate of 300, with 2:1 heart block; ventricular rate 150. The *T* waves are obscured by flutter waves, the combination producing a curve resembling the "cove-plane" contour of recent myocardial infarction.

B, March 24, 1950. After restoration of normal rhythm. The heart rate is 100. The *P–R* interval is prolonged to 0.3 second. The *T* waves are low to inverted in all leads.

C, April 5, 1950. This tracing is within normal limits except for the degree of left axis deviation. However, the horizontal position of the heart shown in the x-ray film may explain this.

COMMENT. The first tracing shows atrial flutter, a common complication of thyrotoxicosis. The artifact produced by blending of flutter waves with *T* waves might well lead to a mistaken diagnosis of myocardial infarction.

After the restoration of normal rhythm (tracing *B*), the prolonged *P–R* interval and low to inverted *T* waves, with short *Q–T* duration, suggest the possibility of digitalis effect. Coronary artery disease, in the presence of previous sustained tachycardia, may have been a contributing factor, although this tracing was taken four days after the restoration of normal rhythm.

Digitalis was stopped four days before the final tracing (*C*). It is interesting to speculate on the direct effect exerted by excess of thyroid hormone on the heart in the first two tracings. No conclusions are permissible in this complex situation.

Adrenal Disease

Addison's Disease

The complicated disturbances in electrolyte balance, circulatory function, and nutrition associated with adrenal hypofunction and its treatment in Addison's disease may produce abnormalities in the electrocardiogram. It is well known that levels of serum potassium tend to rise above the normal in the untreated case, while sodium and chloride serum levels fall below the normal, especially in crises. On the other hand, treatment of this disease with desoxycorticosterone acetate and cortisone may result in abnormally low potassium levels as a result of increased urinary excretion of that ion. The use of testosterone as an adjunct in the treatment of this disease also lowers serum potassium and is thought to favor migration of potassium into the cells.

It is evident that abnormal electrocardiographic patterns encountered in the course of this disease must be interpreted with caution in view of the complexity of factors determining the clinical course and influencing the electrocardiogram. In general, in Addison's disease there tends to be, during periods of hyperpotassemia, elevation and sharpening of the T waves along with shortening of the duration of systole; while in its treatment, when the potassium and calcium levels are much reduced, the opposite takes place, with flattening of T waves and prolongation of systole.

Parathyroid Disease

The electrocardiographic pattern associated with low levels of serum calcium, as in hypoparathyroidism and other disorders, is characterized by prolongation of the Q–T duration. As a rule, this pattern differs from that produced by hypopotassemia, which also is characterized by a long Q–T duration, in one important respect: in hypocalcemia, prolongation seems to affect principally the S–T interval, which becomes long without important alteration of its position, that is, elevation or depression, and without production of significant T wave change. In many electrolyte disturbances the electrocardiogram may be affected by the combination of altered concentrations of both ions.

Hyperparathyroidism is said to shorten the Q–T duration, but this results in a less distinctive pattern. Of course it is well known that not all important alterations in serum calcium levels are associated with disease of the parathyroid glands.

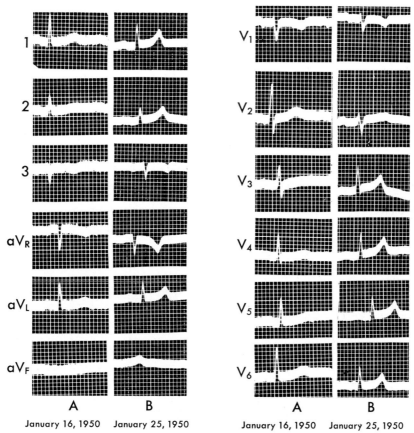

Fig. 209. Addison's disease.

Addison's disease in a housewife who began to exhibit the classical symptoms of this disorder in 1946 at the age of fifty-two. These included vomiting, weight loss, progressive weakness, and pigmentation. Physical examination at the time of her first hospital admission May 7, 1946, showed malnutrition, a blood pressure of 98 mm. of mercury systolic and 70 mm. diastolic, and considerable brownish pigmentation of the skin, especially marked in the creases and over the elbows and knuckles. After treatment with DOCA (desoxycorticosterone acetate) she responded very well and was discharged on July 5, 1946.

She was then maintained with implantation of DOCA pellets and the administration of testosterone. In December, 1949, she was readmitted after development of a psychosis six months before, but was discharged two months later after unsuccessful attempts to alter the psychosis by hormone and electrolyte manipulation.

INTERPRETATION. A, *January 16, 1950.* Sinus rhythm at a rate of 100; low T waves in Leads 1 and 2 and in precordial leads V_2 through V_6; $Q-T$ duration of 0.36 second (the upper limit of normal for this heart rate is 0.35 second). The QRS complexes are rather low in amplitude.

B, *January 25, 1950.* Sinus rhythm at a rate of 75 (heart rate obtained from complete tracing). The T waves are sharp and peaked, the QRS complexes rather low in amplitude. The $Q-T$ duration measures 0.32 second (upper limit of normal 0.39 second for this heart rate).

COMMENT. Tracing A, which is consistent with low potassium effect, but not diagnostic of it, was taken seventeen days after admission, after a long period of treatment with DOCA and testosterone. The serum sodium level on that day was 130.3 milliequivalents per liter; the serum potassium 3.7 milliequivalents per liter. The latter was questioned because the patient had been taking potassium chloride by mouth for ten days; however, it was later thought to represent a true value. Tracing B, taken nine days after A, shows the changes of early hyperpotassemia. The serum potassium level on January 23, 1951, two days before B was taken, was 5.7 milliequivalents per liter.

This series of changes is strongly suggestive of what might be expected with the emergence of the patient from a low, or low normal, potassium state to levels above the normal. The evidence is not conclusive, and it should be remembered that serum levels are only rough indicators of potassium distribution through the body. Thus it is perfectly possible that the patient was in low potassium balance at the time tracing A was taken, although the serum level was at a low normal. In any event, the changes seen in record B suggest that serum potassium levels were rising above the normal, and that caution must be used in the further administration of potassium. It should be remembered also that other factors may have been important in producing the pattern seen in A. These electrocardiograms illustrate the limitations as well as the usefulness of the electrocardiogram in the treatment of Addison's disease.

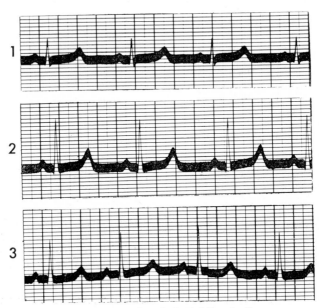

Fig. 210. Hypocalcemia in Addison's disease.

Hypocalcemia of obscure endocrine origin in a nine year old schoolgirl who was hospitalized at the age of seven with classical symptoms and findings of Addison's disease. She responded well to treatment with DOCA and cortical extract. On March 3, 1942, at the age of nine, she was admitted to this hospital for re-evaluation of therapy after a weight loss of 5 pounds in two weeks.

Physical examination revealed further spread of pigmentation. The serum sodium was 143 milliequivalents per liter, the serum chloride 99.2 milliequivalents per liter, and sugar 45 mg. per cent. A low level of serum calcium was first suspected from an electrocardiogram taken April 27. Serum levels on May 19 were as follows: potassium 3.6 milliequivalents per liter, calcium 6.9 mg. per cent. The electrocardiogram shown here was taken on July 21, 1942, at which time the calcium was 7.9 mg. per cent, phosphorus 11 mg. per cent. Several potassium determinations were within the normal range.

The Chvostek sign was positive on many occasions. Serum calcium values reached more normal levels after therapy with AT 10 (hytakerol) and calcium salts, and the patient was discharged on August 19, 1942, after the implantation of pellets of DOCA.

INTERPRETATION. *July 21, 1942.* Sinus arrhythmia at a rate averaging 70; *P–R* interval of 0.15 second; normal *QRS* complexes; upright *T* waves, with long *S–T* intervals. The *Q–T* duration is prolonged and measures 0.42 second (upper limit of normal 0.39 second for this heart rate).

COMMENT. This tracing shows long *Q–T* duration with *T* waves of normal appearance. Prolongation of the *S–T* interval with little shift from the baseline is a distinguishing feature. In this case the electrocardiographic patterns led to the diagnosis of hypocalcemia. The exact cause of the low calcium levels in this patient with Addison's disease was never discovered.

CHAPTER 19

Hypertensive Heart Disease

Essential hypertension or hypertension due to renal disease, to pheochromocytoma or to aortic coarctation may be attended for many years by a normal electrocardiographic pattern, but as the strain increases, either through severity of the hypertension or through its long duration, the left ventricle begins to enlarge. The beginning of such enlargement is generally best shown by increased amplitude of R waves and decreased amplitude of T waves, to the point of inversion, in the precordial leads over the left ventricle, that is, Leads V_4 to V_6 inclusive, especially in Lead V_5. Simultaneously or sometimes more tardily there occur changes in Lead 1 with increased amplitude of the R waves and decrease to inversion of the T's. The pattern

of the full blown case of hypertensive heart disease can be simulated by that caused by other strain on the left ventricle, as from aortic stenosis or aortic regurgitation. See Figures 211, 212, 213, and 214 for examples of the electrocardiogram in cases of systemic hypertension.

Reversal of this pattern to a more normal, or even a completely normal, record is possible in some instances of severe hypertension with enlargement of the heart after correction of the hypertension, partial or complete, by some such procedure as drug therapy (for example, with protoveratrine) (see Fig. 215), lumbodorsal sympathectomy (see Fig. 216) or special diet, in particular the rice diet.

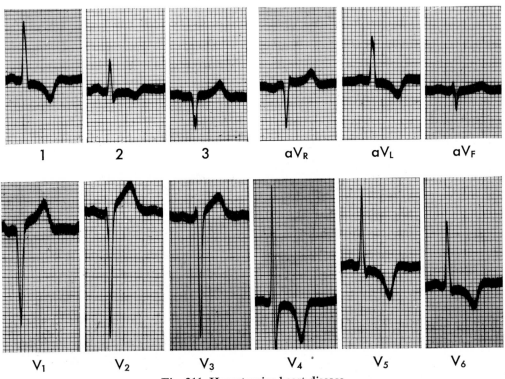

1   2   3   aV$_R$ aV$_L$ aV$_F$

V$_1$ V$_2$ V$_3$ V$_4$ V$_5$ V$_6$

Fig. 211. Hypertensive heart disease.

Hypertensive heart disease in a man of sixty-one with diabetes controlled by diet. He entered the hospital for repair of a right inguinal hernia. For some time there had been known hypertension "up to 210." On admission his blood pressure was 195 mm. of mercury systolic and 115 mm. diastolic. The eyegrounds revealed narrowing and tortuosity of the vessels, but no hemorrhage or exudates. The heart was enlarged with a moderately loud systolic murmur at the apex. There was no edema.

This electrocardiogram was taken the day after admission. An x-ray film of the chest five days later, and four days after right inguinal herniorrhaphy under spinal anesthesia, showed the heart to be prominent in the region of the left ventricle with a tortuous and sclerotic aorta. His blood pressure had stabilized at a level of approximately 180 mm. systolic and 110 mm. diastolic. Two days after the operation he was given daily digitoxin; he was discharged on this maintenance dosage.

INTERPRETATION. Normal rhythm at a rate of 75, with considerable left ventricular preponderance as shown by left axis deviation in the bipolar limb leads, deep S waves in the precordial leads (V$_2$ and V$_3$) over the right ventricle, high R waves over the left ventricle (leads V$_4$, V$_5$ and V$_6$), and inverted T waves in Leads 1, 2, V$_4$, V$_5$ and V$_6$ with upright T waves in Lead aV$_R$. There are small R waves in Leads V$_2$ and V$_3$.

COMMENT: This is a perfectly characteristic picture of advanced hypertensive heart disease, but it is not a pathognomonic pattern, for it can be found also in important grades of aortic stenosis or regurgitation.

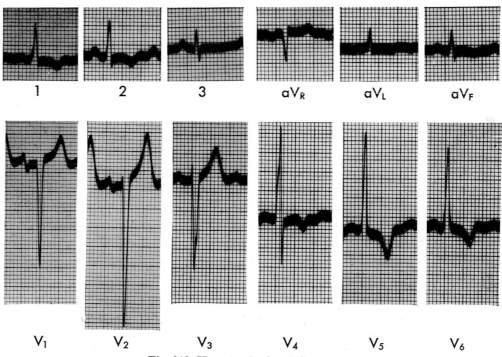

Fig. 212. Hypertensive heart disease.

Hypertensive heart disease in a man aged fifty-five who was referred to our laboratory for an electrocardiogram with the diagnosis of malignant hypertension. He had had no digitalis. He weighed 160 pounds and was 5 feet 6 inches tall. No blood pressure readings were available.

INTERPRETATION. Normal rhythm, rate 100, left ventricular enlargement as indicated by the deep, slightly wide S waves in the precordial leads (V_2 and V_3) over the right ventricle, high R waves in the leads (V_4, V_5 and V_6) over the left ventricle, and inverted T waves in Leads 1, 2, V_4, V_5 and V_6. In contrast to the last case (p. 250), there is no left axis deviation in the classical limb leads.

COMMENT. This record is in full accord with the clinical diagnosis of advanced hypertensive heart disease, but does not reveal, as do the eyegrounds and rapid progress of such a case, its so-called malignant character.

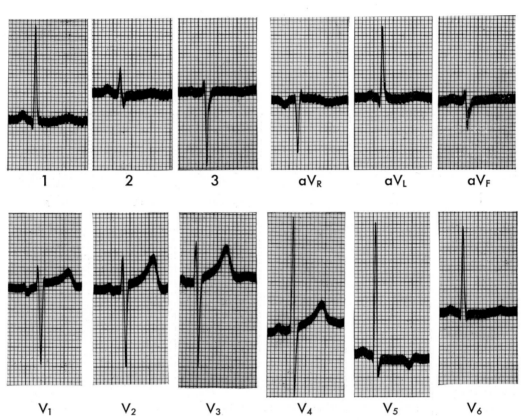

Fig. 213. Hypertensive heart disease.

Essential hypertension of about eight years' duration in an insurance executive aged fifty-two who entered the hospital for consideration of his candidacy for lumbodorsal sympathectomy. His symptoms at this time were limited to paresthesias of the left leg and left hand and to easy fatigability. On physical examination retinal, central nervous system and cardiovascular changes were observed. The heart by roentgenogram showed prominence in the region of the left ventricle and a tortuous aorta. There was no evidence of myocardial or coronary insufficiency, and it was believed that the patient would fit into the group of rather favorable response to surgery, although he was not an ideal case. His blood pressure was 220 mm. of mercury systolic and 120 mm. diastolic on the day of entry; 190 mm. systolic and 120 mm. diastolic on the day before discharge.

The patient was unable to decide upon the operation. He died from a cerebrovascular accident three months later.

INTERPRETATION. Normal rhythm, rate 60, considerable left axis deviation in the frontal plane, as shown by Leads 1 and 3, and high R waves in Leads V_4, V_5 and V_6 over the left ventricle, with upright T waves in Leads 1 and 2 and in all the precordial leads except V_5.

COMMENT. Although the left ventricular enlargement or preponderance is indicated by the high R waves in Leads 1, V_4, V_5 and V_6 and by inversion of the T waves in Lead V_5, there is evidence of less involvement of the left ventricle than in the preceding two cases because of the fairly normal T waves in Leads 1, V_4 and V_6. The evolution of the case indicated much more cerebral vascular strain and damage than cardiac involvement. In fact, death came from cerebral hemorrhage within a few months, doubtless before the heart had become seriously affected. The left axis deviation in this case shown by the classical limb leads was probably chiefly due to a horizontal heart position (in view of upright T waves in Lead 1 and high R in Lead aV_L).

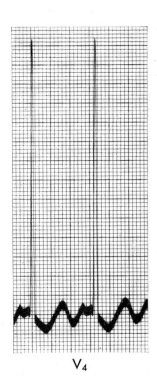

V₄

Fig. 214. Tall *R* in V₄ (hypertensive heart disease).

Unusually tall *R* in V₄ in a male x-ray technician of thirty-two with hypertensive heart disease. Hypertension had first been noted in 1947 (blood pressure 280/140), although he had suffered from severe frontal headaches since 1945. In 1949 he began to have attacks of pulmonary edema, and about mid-January, 1950, he had experienced two such episodes while at bed rest in another hospital; a third severe attack on February 7, 1950, had precipitated his present hospital admission. His blood pressure following this was 210 mm. of mercury systolic and 120 mm. diastolic, with a variation of 10 mm. with respiration.

On February 10 a course of protoveratrine was instituted. This drug was effective in lowering his blood pressure, and he was later taught to give it to himself intramuscularly. The electrocardiographic lead shown here was taken on February 16, 1950, and may show the complicating effect of hyperchloremic alkalosis. In spite of frequent unfavorable reactions to protoveratrine, including nausea, vomiting, sweating, and chilliness of the extremities, his response to it was encouraging, and he was discharged on March 29 on therapy with this drug, with instructions as to the administration of atropine for toxic side effects.

During his hospital stay cardiac catheterization was performed while he was off the medication; he was then given protoveratrine with subsequent follow-up by re-catheterization. A 40 per cent drop in his cardiac output following the therapy was observed; there was, however, no change in peripheral resistance.

It is of interest that this patient, who was hospitalized for further studies and observation on three subsequent occasions during the year 1950, was last seen in the Hypertension Clinic on February 26, 1951, at which time he was doing well on oral protoveratrine every six hours, with only infrequent toxic reactions. His blood pressure on this occasion was 160 to 150 mm. systolic and 90 mm. diastolic.

INTERPRETATION. Precordial Lead V₄, presumably over the left ventricle, shows normal rhythm, rate 90, with extraordinarily high *R* waves (70 mm. = 7 mv.) and markedly diphasic *T* waves with somewhat prolonged systole (0.4 + second).

COMMENT. The high *R* wave here may be due to the combined effect of left ventricular enlargement and nearness to the heart resulting from a thin chest wall. The abnormal *T* waves may be due in part to left ventricular enlargement and to the effect of digitalis, but depletion of potassium may also have played a role.

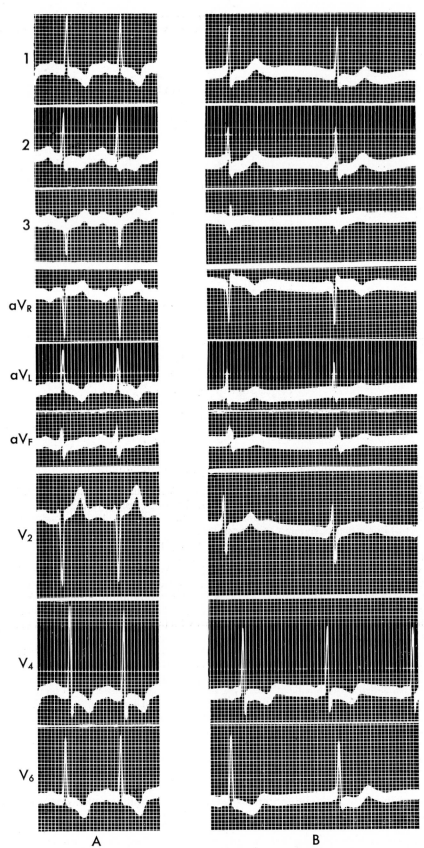

1

2

3

aV_R

aV_L

aV_F

V_2

V_4

V_6

A   B

A, Before, and, *B*, 15 minutes after administration of protoveratrine.

Fig. 215. Hypertensive heart disease. Protoveratrine effect.

(*See facing page for legend.*)

(*Legend continued from opposite page, Figure 215*)

Severe hypertensive cardiovascular disease in an obese and nervous woman of forty-four who entered the hospital as a possible candidate for sympathectomy. Her blood pressure on admission was 240 mm. of mercury systolic and 140 mm. diastolic (right arm), 250/170 (left arm), 200/150 (legs). It was believed that operation might possibly offer relief to the headaches which were her chief and bitter complaint. However, the operation was delayed, pending studies with protoveratrine. Three tenths of a milligram of protoveratrine intravenously caused the blood pressure to fall to an approximately normal level for as long a period as four to five hours. When she received the injections every four hours, she was free from the headaches.

The electrocardiograms shown here were taken (*A*) before (blood pressure, left arm, 194/136, pulse 92) and (*B*) fifteen minutes after 1 to 2 cc. of protoveratrine in saline intravenously (blood pressure, left arm, 90/58, pulse 60). Her response to protoveratrine, though only transient and for a given dose, was thought sufficient to warrant her discharge home on a 1000 calorie diet, sodium restriction, and sedation, to be followed with further protroveratrine studies. These were pursued during three subsequent hospital admissions. However, the use of the drug had to be discontinued finally because it sent her into shock. Without it her pressure could not be controlled, and she died one year and two and a half months after her initial hospital admission.

INTERPRETATION. *A*, Normal rhythm, rate 100, left axis deviation shown by the limb leads, deep *S* waves in Lead V_2, high *R* waves in Lead V_4, and inverted *T* waves in Leads 1, 2, V_4 and V_6.

B, Normal rhythm, rate 50, normal complexes throughout except for slight depression of *S–T* segments in Leads 1, 2, aV_L, aV_F, V_4 and V_6, elevation of *S–T* segments in Lead aV_R, and inversion of *T* waves in Leads V_4 and V_6.

COMMENT. This is an example of the rapid reversibility, at least in part, by an especially effective veratrum alkaloid, of the electrocardiographic pattern of left ventricular strain or enlargement secondary to marked hypertension. Although the exact mechanism of this change has not yet been elucidated, a decrease of left ventricular dilatation with the sharp drop in blood pressure and pulse rate could play an important role.

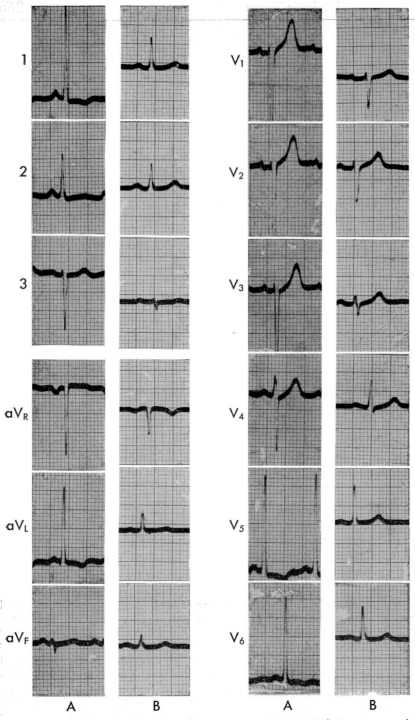

Fig. 216. Hypertensive heart disease. Prelumbodorsal sympathectomy and two years later.*

Prelumbodorsal and postlumbodorsal sympathectomy for hypertension in a woman aged thirty-nine. The electrocardiogram shown in *A* was taken one month preoperatively, on January 20, 1948; at that time her blood pressure was 199 mm. of mercury systolic and 134 mm. diastolic. The electrocardiogram shown in *B* was taken twenty-five months after the second stage operation, on June 15, 1950; at that time her blood pressure was 113 mm. systolic and 77 mm. diastolic.

The dates of operation were February 18 and May 13, 1948. This patient's heart size by x-ray film on February 5, 1948, just before the first operation, was 14.9 cm., with an internal chest diameter of 25.7 cm. On May 12, 1949, one year after the second operation, her heart measured 11.9 cm.

The eyeground changes had been graded "2" when she was seen in 1947. When last determined (May 12, 1949) they were "0" with no evidence of exudates, arteriovenous compression, or hemorrhage.

A

B

January 20, 1948 (one month preop.)
B.P. 199/134

A

B

June 15, 1950 (25 months postop.)
B.P. 113/77

INTERPRETATION. *A*, Normal rhythm, rate 100, striking left axis deviation and left ventricular preponderance as shown by high *R* waves in Leads 1, V_5 and V_6, deep *S* waves in Leads 3, V_2, V_3 and V_4 (still over the right ventricle), and inverted *T* waves in Leads 1, V_5 and V_6.

B, Normal rhythm, rate 70, normal complexes throughout all twelve leads.

COMMENT. This is a clear-cut instance of what is not uncommonly seen, namely, the complete reversibility of hypertensive heart disease by lumbodorsal sympathectomy. Here the normal record is still seen more than two years after operation, along with a normal blood pressure.

* Courtesy of Drs. Dera Kinsey and Reginald Smithwick, Massachusetts Memorial Hospitals, Boston.

CHAPTER 20

Cor Pulmonale

Just as essential hypertension or other causes of systemic hypertension may affect the left ventricle, so also pulmonary hypertension, acute or chronic, due to obstruction of the pulmonary circulation can cause right ventricular enlargement and the electrocardiographic pattern thereof. This may appear either acutely or as a chronic condition.

Acute Cor Pulmonale

When there is massive obstruction of the pulmonary circulation by embolism or thrombosis, there may be a considerable degree of pulmonary hypertension acutely produced, and this may result in turn in acute dilatation of the right heart chambers and myocardial anoxia, with especial hazard to patients with serious coronary heart disease. The pattern is characteristically that of a tendency to right axis deviation in the limb leads, with the appearance of S waves in Lead 1, the appearance or exaggeration of Q waves in Lead 3, and the inversion of the T waves in Lead 3. Sometimes there is lowering or inversion of the T waves in Lead 2 also. Simultaneously there may be a slight increase of the R waves, but more often a decrease

to inversion of the T waves in the precordial leads over the right ventricle, in particular Leads V_2 and V_3, sometimes extending as far over as Lead V_5. Such a pattern may appear acutely and disappear within a few hours or days with subsidence of the right ventricular dilatation. This is particularly true of the limb lead changes; the precordial lead changes may lag behind those of the limb leads. See Figure 217.

Chronic Cor Pulmonale

Chronic enlargement of the right ventricle (see Fig. 218) may follow the acute cor pulmonale or more often may slowly develop under the strain of chronic pulmonary hypertension secondary to such conditions as silicosis, pulmonary endarteritis obliterans (see Fig. 219) and kyphoscoliosis (see Fig. 220). The pattern is that of enlargement of the right ventricle: right axis deviation shown in the limb leads and increased amplitude of R waves with decreased amplitude of the T waves in the precordial leads over the right ventricle, especially V_2 and V_3, and increased S waves in the precordial leads over the left ventricle, V_4 to V_6.

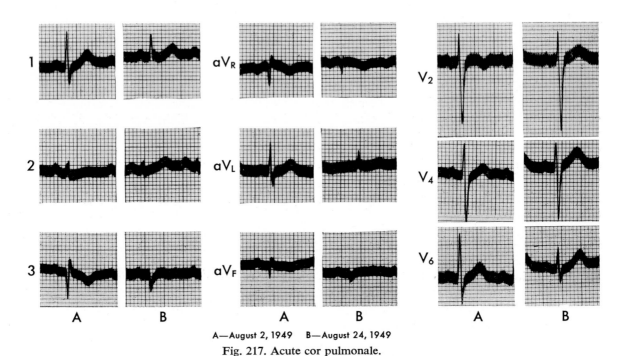

A—August 2, 1949   B—August 24, 1949

Fig. 217. Acute cor pulmonale.

Cor pulmonale, acute, in a man of fifty-six, one month after partial removal of a left acoustic neuroma (June 30, 1949). The patient had fever with an irregular temperature from 100° to 104° F. for some time after this operation, with the appearance on July 17 of a cough (later productive of blood-streaked sputum) and coarse rales over the chest. These persisted, and an x-ray film on July 27 revealed a broad streak of increased density at the left lung base, which at the time was thought to represent atelectasis in association with pneumonitis or possibly an old scar. X-ray findings failed to establish definitely the presence of acute pneumonia, although the left lobe was thought to be somewhat suspicious. On August 1 the x-ray appearance of the chest was considered suggestive of pleuritis, possibly owing to an infarct in the base of the right upper lobe. The patient was also having occasional pleuritic discomfort in the right lower chest. It was observed on August 2 that, prior to the appearance of these signs and symptoms, he had experienced "soreness" of his left calf: at this time the legs appeared to be normal except that the left leg was 1½ inches longer than the right. A review of these findings pointed to the presence of a pulmonary infarct due to an embolus from the left leg.

The electrocardiogram shown in *A* was taken on August 2. On the following day bilateral common femoral vein interruption and ligation were performed and a large white venous thrombus was removed from the left leg. The electrocardiogram in *B* was taken three weeks later, on August 24. Although his clinical course had been complicated after this procedure by a pneumonitis secondary to resolving infarcts, this tracing shows definite change and improvement over the first record. On August 25 digitalization was begun, and the patient left the hospital improved on September 16.

INTERPRETATION. *A, August 2, 1949.* Normal rhythm, rate 100, prominent *S* waves in Lead 1 and *Q* waves in Leads 3 and aV$_F$, and inverted *T* waves in Leads 3, aV$_F$, and V$_2$.

B, August 24, 1949. Normal rhythm, rate 105, no *S* waves in Lead 1, much smaller *Q* waves in Leads 3 and aV$_F$, higher *T* waves in Lead 2, flat *T* waves in Lead 3, and upright *T* waves in Lead V$_2$.

COMMENT. This change in the electrocardiographic complexes, especially in Leads 1, 3 and V$_2$ (which lies over the right ventricle), is characteristic of the subsidence of dilatation of the right ventricle which constitutes the basis of the entity called acute cor pulmonale.

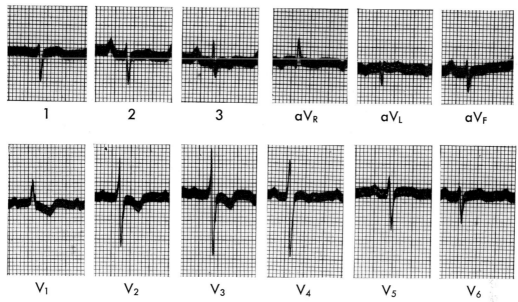

Fig. 218. Chronic cor pulmonale.

Cor pulmonale, chronic, in a man of thirty-nine who had been admitted to the hospital in January, 1950, because of dyspnea and cough with hemoptysis for the past six months. His history included thrombophlebitis ten years before, followed in 1946 by a pulmonary embolus with subsequent right common and left superficial vein ligations. In 1947 superficial saphenous stripping operations had been performed.

Upon physical examination he was of ruddy complexion, possibly slightly cyanotic. His blood pressure was 122 mm. of mercury systolic and 80 mm. diastolic. The neck veins were not distended. Lymphadenopathy was evident with enlarged nodes in both axillae and in the epitrochlear and inguinal regions. There were fine rales at both lung bases. The heart was enlarged. A Grade 1 systolic murmur was audible at the cardiac base and apex. The liver was felt 3 to 4 cm. below the costal margin. There was evidence of many healed varicose ulcers on both legs, and varicosities were present as well on the right upper arm and down the anterior axillary line to, and including, the trunk.

X-ray film of the chest demonstrated general enlargement of the heart; in the oblique view there was apparent increase in the size of the right ventricle and the undivided portion of the pulmonary artery. The right leaf of the diaphragm was somewhat irregular laterally, suggesting atelectasis or scarring in the adjacent lung. In the lower lung fields the pulmonary vessels were fewer than would be expected. The pulmonary artery to the left lower lobe appeared sharply cut off at its lower end. These findings were consistent with pulmonary embolism without infarction and thrombosis of the major pulmonary arteries, or with multiple pulmonary emboli to the small pulmonary arteries.

A photoelectric hemoglobin determination registered 14.9 gm. His vital capacity was 4.3 liters. Venous pressure (antecubital) was 86 mm. An exercise test with measurement of the oxygen consumption was believed to be consistent with a fixed flaw through the pulmonary arterial system. Cardiac catheterization was recommended, but not carried out at this time. The electrocardiogram shown here was taken the day after admission.

Biopsy of an axillary node and a subcutaneous nodule from the thigh demonstrated no malignancy. Two days after his discharge on January 16 the patient was again admitted with a diagnosis of bacteremia due to undetermined organism, migrating thrombophlebitis, and chronic cor pulmonale secondary to multiple pulmonary emboli. He was discharged on February 11 on a daily ration of 0.15 mg. of digitoxin and 50 mg. of Dicumarol, with prothrombin determinations to be done twice weekly at a neighborhood hospital. However, the anticoagulant therapy did not prevent further thrombophlebitis and embolism, and vena cava ligation was advised on the occasion of his last visit to the Out Patient Clinic, December 8, 1950.

INTERPRETATION. Normal rhythm, rate 90, marked right axis deviation (shown by limb leads), prominent R waves and inverted T waves in precordial leads V_1 to V_4 inclusive, and prominent S waves in Leads 1 and 2 and precordial leads V_2 to V_6 inclusive.

COMMENT. This record is typical of enlargement of the right ventricle with normal rhythm. Such a combination, rare with mitral stenosis (which almost always shows atrial fibrillation with this high degree of right ventricular enlargement), is found with certain congenital defects and with the cor pulmonale. Since there is no evidence of congenital heart disease by physical signs, roentgenogram or history, and since there has been definite pulmonary embolism (doubtless massive or multiple) from leg vein thrombosis in the past, the diagnosis is clearly that of chronic cor pulmonale. Pulmonary embolism is one of the rarer causes of chronic cor pulmonale. Usually there is complete recovery, including electrocardiographic, after pulmonary embolism, or there is, in the minority of cases, rapid death. In the establishment of such a diagnosis the electrocardiogram is of the greatest help.

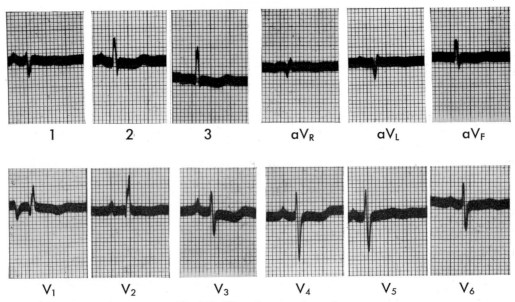

Fig. 219. Chronic cor pulmonale.

Cor pulmonale on a basis of extensive pulmonary endarterial thrombosis of unknown cause in a woman amateur golf champion (seven times) aged forty-six. About one year before her first hospital admission (July 27, 1949) there had begun without apparent cause the gradual onset of fatigue, dyspnea, edema of face and legs, swelling of the abdomen, and slight cyanosis. Treatment consisted of three months of bed rest, injections of 2 cc. of salyrgan twice weekly, ammonium chloride, a low sodium diet, adrenal cortical extract, and injections of vitamin B, with some digitalis (probably none for the past month). Improvement on this regimen had been only temporary. The symptoms had recurred, and she had failed to respond to mercurial injections. In June she had been seen at our Cardiac Rounds, where the possibility of an atrial septal defect was considered likely, in view of the right ventricular hypertrophy by electrocardiogram, as shown here, and the x-ray finding of a large pulmonary artery.

Physical examination on July 30 revealed a slightly cyanotic woman in no acute distress, but appearing chronically ill. The pulse was regular at a rate of 100. Her blood pressure was 110 mm. of mercury systolic and 80 mm. diastolic. There was no finger clubbing. The superficial and deep veins of the neck were distended, and there was a deep systolic jugular pulse. The chest was clear, although the diaphragm was high. The heart was enlarged to the left anterior axillary line, with a diffuse apical impulse. There was a Grade 4, harsh systolic murmur heard best at the lower end of the left sternal border and at the apex, without transmission to the neck or back and only poorly transmitted to the left axilla and to the base of the heart. A thrill was also present. The pulmonary second sound was greatly accentuated and louder than the aortic second sound. There were no diastolic murmurs. She had marked ascites, and the liver dullness extended 3 to 4 cm. below the costal margin. There was moderate edema of the legs, but no calf tenderness. The possibility of an interventricular septal defect with secondary pulmonary arteriosclerosis causing right ventricular hypertrophy and right heart failure with functional tricuspid regurgitation was entertained at this time on the basis of the aforementioned physical findings.

X-ray examination of the chest on July 30 revealed the heart shadow to be enlarged, with a cardiothoracic ratio of 16.5:28 cm. and increased size apparently in the region of both ventricles. The main pulmonary artery shadow and the hilar vessels were more than usually prominent, and the peripheral vessels in the lungs somewhat less prominent than usual. These findings increased the likelihood of diffuse pulmonary disease and cor pulmonale.

An abdominal paracentesis, productive of 3900 cc. of rather cloudy, straw-colored fluid, was performed on August 2. By August 18 fluid had begun to reaccumulate, and on the 28th, 2500 cc. of clear, straw-colored fluid were removed by a second abdominal paracentesis. The day after this, digitalis had to be stopped because of toxic symptoms. Two days later she was discharged with her condition unaltered. She died at home within forty-eight hours of leaving the hospital.

Postmortem examination showed pulmonary thrombosis, old and recent, cor pulmonale without valvular disease, ascites, bilateral hydrothorax, severe chronic passive congestion of the liver, and peripheral edema.

INTERPRETATION. Normal rhythm, rate 75, with right axis deviation by limb leads and prominent R waves in precordial leads V_1, V_2 and V_3, deep S waves in Leads V_4, V_5 and V_6 (over the left ventricle?), and flat to diphasic to slightly inverted T waves in all leads.

COMMENT. This record shows evidence of right ventricular enlargement, this time the result of one of the rare causes of the chronic cor pulmonale, namely, multiple pulmonary emboli and thrombi, recent and old, with recanalization. Associated with the multiple clots found throughout the pulmonary circulation there were numerous atheromatous plaques in the secondary and tertiary pulmonary arterial branches, doubtless secondary to the pulmonary hypertension. The hydrothorax and edema may have played a role in flattening the T waves and lowering the voltage of the complexes in general.

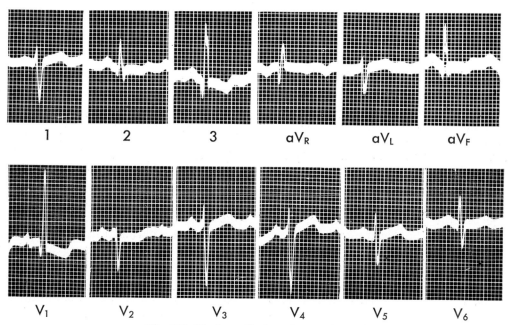

Fig. 220. Kyphoscoliosis and cor pulmonale.

Cor pulmonale, secondary to thoracic deformity, in a kyphoscoliotic man of forty-four who entered the hospital in 1950 with the complaint of increasing dyspnea and shortness of breath. Seventeen years before, from 1933 to 1936, this patient had been in a sanatorium for treatment of tuberculosis, which he had apparently contracted from a friend. Despite bilateral pneumothorax he was again hospitalized in 1940, at which time a three-stage thoracoplasty was performed. Since 1941 his sputum has been negative for tubercle bacilli, although he was again admitted to the sanatorium for a brief period in 1945.

The electrocardiogram shown here was taken on March 8, 1950. A left-sided thoracoplasty and the deformity of kyphoscoliosis were apparent upon physical examination, with good chest expansion. The left lung field was resonant, but showed moist rales, squeaks and wheezes. Examination of the heart revealed normal rhythm at a rate of 96, no cardiac enlargement to percussion, and sounds of good quality. There was a harsh, rasping Grade 3 apical systolic bruit. One-plus pitting edema of the legs was evident. The blood pressure was 120 mm. of mercury systolic and 90 mm. diastolic. The neck veins were pulsating 4 cm. above the clavicles, and the liver edge was somewhat tender 5 cm. below the costal margin. An x-ray film of the chest revealed enlargement of the right ventricle with left thoracoplasty, tuberculous scars in the lungs, and possibly bronchiectasis on the right.

Mercurial diuresis and digitalis therapy were of benefit in treating the congestive failure, and on March 17 cardiac catheterization was carried out with results as follows: (1) rather marked pulmonary and right ventricular hypertension, 100 mm. of mercury systolic and 40 mm. diastolic, (2) low, fixed cardiac output, 2.8 liters per minute, (3) arterial oxygen unsaturation of 89 per cent. Later, pulmonary function tests were performed. The patient was discharged March 22 on a regimen including daily digitoxin and ammonium chloride.

INTERPRETATION. Normal rhythm, rate 100, well-marked right axis deviation in the limb leads with prominent R waves in precordial Lead V_1 and S waves in Leads V_5 and V_6, and inverted T waves in Leads 3, aV_F and V_1, with low diphasic T waves in Leads 2 and V_2.

COMMENT. This electrocardiogram clearly belongs to the pattern of right ventricular enlargement, for which there is an evident explanation clinically in the presence of thoracic deformity (kyphoscoliosis) secondary to thoracoplasty and of extensive pulmonary disease with fibrous scarring. This is thus another type of chronic cor pulmonale.

CHAPTER 21

Coronary Heart Disease

The electrocardiographic method has its greatest usefulness in the diagnosis and treatment of coronary heart disease, especially in myocardial infarction. The diagnostic significance of the electrocardiographic alterations covers a wide range; at one extreme they are pathognomonic, while at the other they merge into the range of normal variation. Inasmuch as coronary heart disease is frequently associated with some other type of heart disease, most often hypertensive, the electrocardiogram in such cases may be influenced by more than one factor. Under these circumstances and in the presence of certain arrhythmias and conduction defects, the interpretation of the curves becomes more difficult and the information obtained from them may be less valuable.

Myocardial Infarction

From the standpoint of its effects on the electrocardiogram, an acute myocardial infarct may be regarded as comprising three zones, namely, a central "dead zone," an outer "ischemic zone" and an intermediate "injury zone." In the dead zone the tissue is either electrically inert or dead and no longer contributes to the electrical forces of the heart. This causes a change in the pathway taken by both the depolarization and the repolarization processes, which are declared in the electrocardiogram by alterations in QRS and T respectively. The loss of any considerable amount of muscle tissue results in a shift in the "center of gravity" of the muscle mass which produces electrical forces, and a consequent shift in orientation of the mean spatial vector representing the electrical field of the heart.

The ischemic zone is usually much larger than the central dead zone and often eccentrically located. Here the muscle cells are not sufficiently damaged to influence significantly the depolarization process; hence QRS is not affected, but repolarization is retarded and this produces alterations in the T waves. With

recovery the T waves revert toward their initial form.

Between the dead and ischemic zones are muscle cells which are living but severely injured, and which give rise to a "current of injury." This injury current is constant throughout the cardiac cycle except for a short period following depolarization; at this time the injured cells, having been depolarized along with the others, produce no current. Thus the effect of the injury current on the electrocardiogram is to displace the baseline except for a short period following QRS when the baseline ($RS-T$) rises or falls to its true zero position. This is a passive phenomenon, but the illusion is created that the $RS-T$ shift is a deviation from, rather than to, the zero position, and it is customary so to regard it. Injury currents are ephemeral and disappear after a few hours, days or weeks.

In addition, there may appear alterations in rate, either sinus bradycardia or tachycardia, various arrhythmias, and conduction defects. It is important to remember that secondary changes in T waves are associated with conduction defects.

The diagnosis of infarction is possible on the basis of the electrocardiographic changes alone if they are typical. In the absence of typical QRS changes, however, the evidence is only presumptive and must be considered along with the other clinical findings before a definite diagnosis can be made. The electrocardiogram also furnishes information regarding the size and location of the infarct, the evolutionary changes during healing, and the extent of the residual damage. This information is not precise, but properly used is very valuable.

The discussion which follows is organized on the basis of the location of the infarct in the different regions of the heart. In most instances the infarct involves the epicardial portion or the entire thickness of the heart wall. Occasionally it may be intramural, producing only slight electrocardiographic changes. More rarely it may be subendocardial; this makes diagnosis difficult because the electrocardiographic changes are not pathognomonic of infarction.

Anterior Infarction

Anterior myocardial infarction is very common and often includes involvement of the septal, lateral, or posterior wall. Examples of anterior wall infarction are shown in many of the following figures.

Anteroseptal Infarction

Significant changes in anteroseptal myocardial infarction are illustrated in Figures 221–224 and may be summarized as follows. In the limb leads the alterations, characteristically, are limited to the RS–T segments and T waves; QRS changes are minor or absent. In the acute stage there may be slight elevation of RS–T in Lead aV_L and Lead 1, with lowering or inversion of T; reciprocal changes are seen in Lead 3 and Lead aV_F. The RS–T segment changes usually disappear within a short time. The T wave changes either disappear or tend to do so.

In the precordial leads the characteristic QRS changes are observed in one or more of Leads V_1 through V_4. They consist in a disappearance of the R wave or the appearance of a Q wave. The RS–T segments are elevated in the leads showing QRS changes and sometimes in one or more additional leads. The T waves are reduced in amplitude or become inverted in the leads showing QRS and RS–T segment changes and in other leads as well. The QRS changes may remain as permanent alterations or may disappear. The RS–T segment changes nearly always disappear, and the T wave abnormalities tend to disappear in leads not showing QRS abnormalities and to remain in leads showing QRS changes.

Lateral Infarction

Infarction may be limited to a portion of the left lateral wall of the heart, but more commonly is only part of a more extensive involvement. In lateral or low lateral infarction the alterations in the limb leads may be insignificant. Sometimes, however, abnormal Q waves appear in Leads 1 or 2 and are accompanied by characteristic changes in RS–T and T. In the precordial leads abnormal Q or RS waves do not appear in Leads V_1 through V_4, but do appear in Leads V_5 or V_6, or both; the RS–T segment and T wave changes may be more widespread.

High lateral infarction may be missed if only the standard six precordial leads are taken; it is necessary to obtain leads from over the upper left side of the chest wall. In high lateral infarction abnormal Q waves are not seen in precordial Leads V_1 through V_6, but do appear in one or more leads obtained in the left axillary region. Abnormal Q or QS waves may or may not appear in Lead 1 or aV_L, or both. RS–T segment and T wave changes may be more widespread than the QRS changes.

Anterolateral Infarction

Anterolateral myocardial infarction involves the anterior wall of the left ventricle, the apex, and a portion of the left lateral wall of the heart as well. It is usually a more extensive process than anteroseptal infarction, and the electrocardiographic changes are more widespread. In the limb leads abnormal Q or QS waves appear in Lead 1, the RS–T segments become elevated and the T waves inverted; similar changes may occur in Leads 2 and aV_L. Changes reciprocal to those occurring in Lead 1 are seen in Leads 3, aV_R, and sometimes in aV_F. In the precordial leads there appear, in addition to the changes characteristic of anteroseptal infarction, abnormal Q or QS waves in V_5 or V_6, or both. These QRS alterations are accompanied by elevation of the RS–T segments and inversion of the T waves. Typical examples are shown in Figures 225, 226 and 227.

Posterior Infarction

Infarction of the posterior and diaphragmatic wall of the heart usually produces characteristic changes in the limb leads and lower esophageal leads, but not in the precordial leads. In the limb leads, Q or QS waves appear in Leads 3 and aV_F and sometimes in Lead 2. Elevation of the RS–T segments and inversion of the T waves accompany the QRS changes. In Leads 1 and aV_L reciprocal RS–T segments and T waves are seen. In the lower esophageal leads, Q or QS complexes appear, accompanied by elevation of the RS–T segments and inversion of the T waves. In the precordial leads, significant QRS changes are absent. In the early stages there may be marked depression of the RS–T segments in one or more leads on the right side of the chest, and this may be followed by an increase in amplitude of the T waves (Fig. 228). These RS–T segment changes are transitory and may last for a few hours or a day or two at the most. In precordial leads on the left side, particularly V_5 and V_6, lowering or inversion of the T waves may appear, which indicates that the area of injury has extended to the left lateral wall. Typical electrocardiograms illustrating posterior wall infarction are shown in Figures 228 to 232, inclusive.

Posterolateral Infarction

If the infarction involves the lateral as well as the posterior wall, characteristic electrocardiographic changes are seen in precordial leads V_5 or V_6 in addition to those already described for posterior wall infarction. These changes consist in the appearance of abnormal Q waves associated with elevation of the $RS-T$ segments and inversion of the T waves. The $RS-T$ segment and T wave changes frequently involve leads in which QRS alterations do not appear. In precordial leads on the right side the T waves may become abnormally tall. Typical electrocardiographic changes in posterolateral infarction are shown in Figures 233 and 234.

Anteroposterior Infarction

The electrocardiographic alterations in anteroposterior infarction are essentially a combination of the changes observed in anterior and posterior wall infarction. If, however, the area involved is much greater in one wall than in the other, the electrocardiographic alterations associated with the more largely infarcted area may predominate. Infarction of the anterior and posterior walls may occur simultaneously or at different times. In the latter case serial electrocardiograms are helpful in establishing the diagnosis. Typical electrocardiographic changes are shown in Figures 235 and 236.

Subendocardial Infarction

Thus far we have described electrocardiographic alterations associated with infarction involving the epicardial portion of the heart wall, or its entire thickness. It now remains to describe briefly the findings in subendocardial infarction. This diagnosis is made when the clinical findings are characteristic of infarction and the electrocardiographic findings are confined to alteration in the $RS-T$ segments and T waves. In both limb and precordial leads depression of the $RS-T$ segments is associated with lowering or inversion of the T waves. A probable example of the electrocardiographic

alterations in subendocardial infarction is shown in Figure 237.

Infarction and Bundle Branch Block

When infarction occurs in a patient with bundle branch block, or when bundle branch block is a complication of myocardial infarction, the electrocardiographic alterations are a mixture of those seen in both disorders. It is important to remember that in these instances alterations in the $RS-T$ segments and in the T waves may be secondary to the conduction difficulty. The changes are best observed in those instances when infarction occurs in a patient with pre-existing bundle branch block, or when there is alternating bundle branch block and normal rhythm.

The electrocardiographic alterations of infarction complicating right bundle branch block are more readily interpreted than those complicating left bundle branch block. Infarction of the posterior wall of the heart in the presence of right bundle branch block is sometimes declared by the appearance of abnormal Q waves in Leads 3 and aV_F, associated with elevation of the $RS-T$ segments and inversion of the T waves in these leads. Infarction of the anterior wall of the heart in the presence of right bundle branch block is usually declared by the disappearance of the R wave in precordial Leads V_1 or V_2, associated with elevation of the $RS-T$ segments and inversion of the T waves.

Infarction of the posterior wall of the heart in the presence of left bundle branch block may produce no significant QRS changes, but concordant T waves may become discordant. A diagnosis of infarction cannot be based upon such a change, however, unless demonstrated by serial electrocardiograms and supported by clinical evidence of infarction. Infarction of the anterior wall of the heart in the presence of left bundle branch block may likewise produce no significant QRS changes, and serial electrocardiograms may be necessary for the detection of $RS-T$ segment and T waves changes. Some examples of bundle branch block with infarction are shown in Figures 238 through 241.

Ventricular Aneurysm

It has already been pointed out that, as a rule, the $RS-T$ segment changes following infarction are short-lived. Exceptionally, however, displacement of the $RS-T$ segment remains as a permanent residuum, and in such instances a ventricular aneurysm may be suspected. A typical example is shown in Figure 242.

Atypical Myocardial Infarction and Infarction with Other Complications

It is generally agreed that a definite diagnosis of myocardial infarction cannot be made on the basis of the electrocardiographic findings unless typical QRS changes are present. However, in many instances the QRS alterations are either absent or slight and the electrocardiographic evidence for infarction may be valuable even though QRS changes are not present. In some of these instances a more thorough exploration may disclose abnormal QRS complexes in one or more chest or esophageal leads. When QRS changes are absent it is safe to assume that the infarcted area is not large, and frequently the T wave changes disappear and the electrocardiogram once again becomes normal or nearly so.

In some instances the QRS changes following myocardial infarction are not typical of infarction in any of the specific locations described earlier. Furthermore, when myocardial infarction is complicated by severe congestive failure, anoxia or other disorders, localization of the area of infarction may be difficult or impossible. Examples of such difficulties are shown in Figures 243, 244 and 245.

Coronary Heart Disease without Infarction

Coronary heart disease or coronary insufficiency without myocardial infarction may produce electrocardiographic alterations which are helpful in diagnosis. Many illustrations have already been given, including such disturbances as partial or complete atrioventricular block, intraventricular block, low voltage of the QRS complexes, and alterations of the $RS–T$ segments and T waves. (See also Figs. 246–248.) The evidence is usually presumptive, and a definite diagnosis of coronary heart disease cannot be made on these electrocardiographic findings alone. In some instances a patient at rest may have a normal electrocardiogram, but if the heart is placed under stress or a work load, electrocardiographic changes may appear. These alterations are sometimes observed if records are obtained in the morning under basal conditions and again at the end of a day's activities. They may also appear as seemingly spontaneous changes when the patient is examined at different times during the day or on different occa-

sions. In addition, such changes may be seen following paroxysmal tachycardia or when the patient is subjected to generalized induced anoxemia (Fig. 249) or to strenuous physical activity.

The Anoxia Test

This is carried out as follows. After a control period a patient is given 10 per cent oxygen to breathe for a period of twenty minutes. Electrocardiograms are obtained before and at 5-minute intervals throughout the test. Levy* considers the test positive if it has to be stopped because of anginal pain or if the following electrocardiographic changes appear:

1. The arithmetic sum of the $RS–T$ deviations in all four leads (1, 2, 3, and 4) totals 3 mm. or more
2. There is partial or complete reversal of the direction of T in Lead 1, accompanied by an $RS–T$ deviation of 1 mm. or more in this lead
3. There is complete reversal of the direction of T in Lead 4, regardless of $RS–T$ deviation
4. There is partial reversal of the direction of T in Lead 4, accompanied by an $RS–T$ deviation of 1 mm. or more in this lead.

The Electrocardiographic Work Test

Master** has described a standardized procedure based on the so-called "two-step test" which consists of climbing up and down two 9-inch steps, the number of ascents depending upon the subject's sex, age and weight.‡ An electrocardiogram is obtained (three bipolar limb leads and CF_4) before the exercise is begun, after its completion and three and eight minutes later. An $RS–T$ segment depression greater than 0.5 mm. (using the $P–Q$ interval as the control level) indicates a "positive test." A change from an upright to a flat or inverted T wave is also abnormal. If the test is negative, a "double step-test" consisting of twice the standard number of steps should be made at a later time.

* Levy, R. L., Patterson, J. E., Clark, T. W., and Bruenn, H. G.: The Anoxemia Test as an Index of the Coronary Reserve. J.A.M.A., *117:* 2113, 1941.

** Master, A. M.: The Electrocardiogram after Exercise: A Standardized Heart Function Test. U. S. Nav. M. Bull., *40:* 346, 1942.

‡ Master, A. M., Friedman, R., and Dack, S.: The Electrocardiogram after Standard Exercise as a Functional Test of the Heart. Am. Heart J., *24:* 777, 1942.

In our tests we have used a single step of variable height with conveniently placed bars to be used as hand holds. The subject steps up and down once every two or three seconds, the rate depending on the degree of cardiac reserve. The exercise is continued until the rate of work is no longer maintained. Electrocardiograms are taken before, at the completion of exercise and five minutes later.

Lastly, it should be pointed out that the electrocardiogram may be normal in the presence of serious coronary heart disease. The electrocardiogram in Figure 251 is an example of this.

(Legend continued from facing page, Figure 221)

INTERPRETATION. *A*, Electrocardiogram obtained five days after the onset of symptoms. There is no definite abnormality in the limb leads. In the precordial leads QS complexes are seen in V_1 and V_2 and the R wave is unusually, if not abnormally, low in V_3.

B, Electrocardiogram obtained one day later, showing a significant alteration of the T waves in the limb leads. In Lead 1 the T waves are abnormally low, and in Lead 3 they have become slightly taller. In the precordial leads the R wave in V_3 is barely perceptible; the change may be the result of a slightly different location of the electrode. In Leads V_1 through V_5 the T waves have become diphasic with a tendency toward slight late inversion of T.

C, The T waves are now frankly inverted in Lead 1, and in the precordial leads the tendency toward late inversion of T is still more apparent.

COMMENT. These serial electrocardiographic changes substantiate the diagnosis of myocardial infarction probably involving the anteroseptal region. If an earlier record had been taken showing R waves in Leads V_1 or V_2, or both, their disappearance in later records, together with RS–T segment and T wave changes, would be unequivocal evidence of infarction.

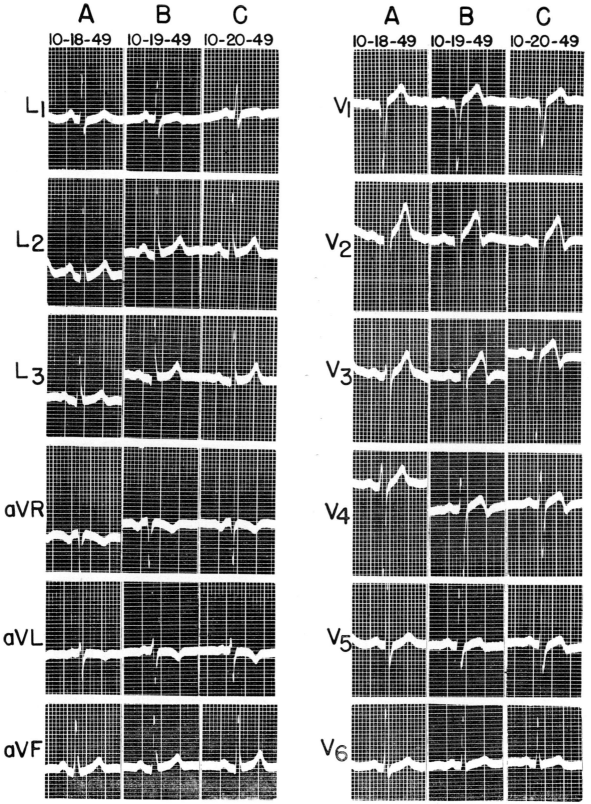

Fig. 221. Anteroseptal myocardial infarction.

The electrocardiograms shown here were obtained on a physician forty-one years of age who suffered substernal pain with radiation to the left arm while performing an operation. As soon as was practicable he went home, where he rested for several days. His clinical course was characteristic of myocardial infarction involving a small area.

(*Legend continued on opposite page*)

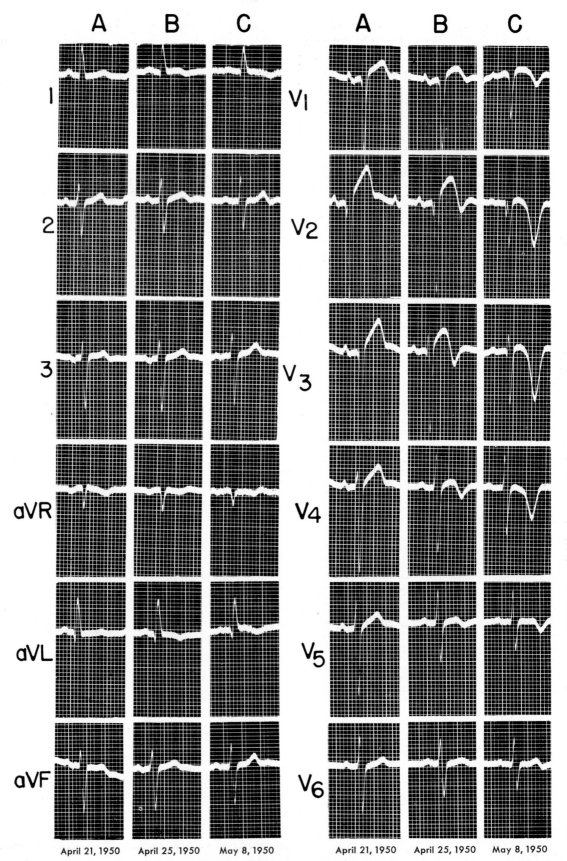

Fig. 222. Anteroseptal myocardial infarction.

(See facing page for legend.)

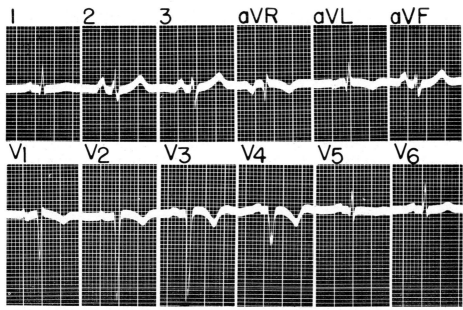

Fig. 223. Anteroseptal myocardial infarction.

The electrocardiogram shown here was obtained from a man of average build, fifty-eight years of age, who had suffered a typical attack of acute myocardial infarction five months previously. Since that time he had had easily provoked angina pectoris. The heart was not enlarged, the blood pressure was normal, and there were no congestive phenomena. Therapy did not include digitalis.

INTERPRETATION. The P waves and P–R interval are normal. In the limb leads there is low voltage of QRS and slight slurring near the baseline. Small Q waves are seen in Leads 1 and aV_L. The T waves in Lead 1 are low but upright, and are inverted in Lead aV_L. In the precordial leads a Qr complex is seen in Lead V_1 with QS complexes in Leads V_2 to V_4. A broad Q of small amplitude is seen in V_5. The T waves are inverted in Leads V_1 through V_4 and nearly flat in V_5.

COMMENT. These changes are typical of *healed myocardial infarction* involving mainly the anteroseptal area. The processes originally may have extended into the left lateral wall, and the Q wave and relatively small R wave in V_5 may represent residual changes due to damage in this region.

(Legend continued from opposite page, Figure 222)

These electrocardiograms were obtained from a tailor sixty-six years of age who had suffered, six days prior to hospital admission, a typical attack of myocardial infarction. This had been followed by recurrent episodes of angina pectoris, complicated by right shoulder and arm pain which was later diagnosed as gout. He had not received digitalis.

INTERPRETATION. *A*, Record obtained three hours after entry to the hospital. The P waves and the P–R intervals are normal. The QRS complexes in the limb leads show moderate left axis deviation, and the duration of QRS is about 0.1 second. In Lead 1 a tiny Q wave is seen, and in Lead aV_L the duration of Q is about 0.03 second. There is no abnormality of the RS–T segments, and the T waves in Lead 1 are rather low but upright. In the precordial leads QS complexes are seen in Leads V_1 to V_3, and the R waves are low in Lead V_4. The RS–T segments are abnormally elevated in Leads V_1 to V_3, and the T waves are unusually tall.

B, Electrocardiogram taken four days later, showing significant changes in the limb leads. There is slight elevation of the RS–T segment in Lead 1, and the T waves in this lead and in Lead aV_L are now inverted. In the precordial leads an abnormal Q wave is seen in Lead V_3. The RS–T segments are abnormally elevated in Leads V_1 to V_3, and the T waves are diphasic or inverted in Leads V_1 to V_5.

C, Record obtained a little over three weeks after the initial episode, two weeks after hospital admission. There has been a further change. The RS–T segment has returned to the baseline in Lead 1, and the T wave in this lead is more deeply inverted than before. In Lead 3 the T wave is taller than formerly. In the precordial leads there has been no significant change in QRS, but the RS–T segments have returned to the baseline or nearly so, and T waves are now deeply inverted in Leads V_1 to V_5 and are diphasic in Lead V_6.

COMMENT. These changes are typical of myocardial infarction involving the anteroseptal region of the heart. The changes in the limb leads are relatively minor. In the precordial leads the changes are pathognomonic of infarction; the significant QRS changes are confined to Leads V_1 to V_3, but the RS–T segment and T wave changes involve all six precordial leads.

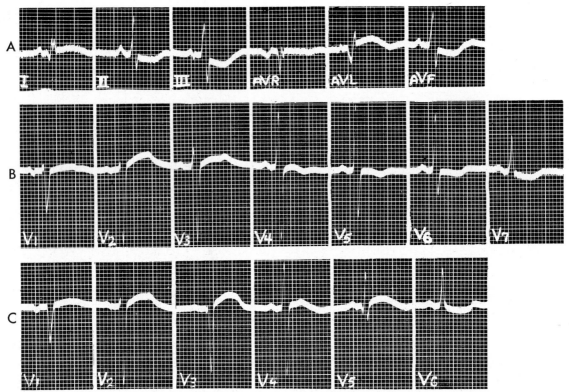

Fig. 224. Anteroseptal myocardial infarction.

This electrocardiogram was obtained from a retired shop worker of average build, sixty-eight years of age, one week after his second myocardial infarct. Just a year prior to this episode he had suffered myocardial infarction from which he had recovered without subsequent angina pectoris or dyspnea. Therapy did not include digitalization.

INTERPRETATION. *A*, In the limb leads the *P* waves and *P–R* intervals are normal. There is slight slurring of the *QRS* complexes, and abnormally prominent *Q* waves are seen in Leads 1 and aV_L. There is elevation of the *RS–T* segments in Leads 1 and aV_L and depression of these segments in Leads 2, 3 and aV_F.

B, In precordial leads V_1 through V_7 the *R* waves are unusually, if not abnormally, low in V_2 and the *T* waves tend to be low or inverted in Leads V_3 through V_7.

C, Precordial leads corresponding to V_1 through V_6, but obtained by placing the electrode approximately one interspace higher, show a *QS* complex in strip 3. A *Q* wave is seen in the strip (5) corresponding to V_5, but one interspace higher.

COMMENT. This tracing illustrates the value of supplementary chest leads. The standard precordial leads do not show *QRS* changes typical of anterior wall infarction, but moving the electrodes one interspace higher discloses an area above the V position which yielded a *QS* complex indicative of infarction involving the anteroseptal region.

(*Legend continued from facing page, Figure 225*)

INTERPRETATION. *A*, Electrocardiogram taken two and a half days after the onset of symptoms. In the limb leads the *P* waves and *P–R* interval are normal. The *QRS* complexes are abnormally low in voltage; prominent *Q* waves are seen in Lead 1, and a *QS* complex is seen in Lead aV_L. The *RS–T* segments are abnormally elevated in Leads 1, 2 and aV_L with reciprocal changes in Leads 3 and aV_R. The *T* waves tend to be low or diphasic in all leads. In the precordial leads an *rS* complex is seen in V_1, a *QS* complex in V_2 through V_4, and *Q* waves, in association with low voltage of *QRS*, are seen in Leads V_5 and V_6. The *RS–T* segments are abnormally elevated in Leads V_2 through V_5, and the *T* waves are rather low in all leads.

B, Obtained twelve days later. Significant changes have occurred. In the limb leads the *T* waves are deeply inverted in Leads 1 and aV_L and slightly inverted in Lead 2. In the precordial leads the *QRS* complexes are not changed significantly, but the *RS–T* segments have returned to, or nearly to, the baseline, and the *T* waves are now upright in Lead V_1 and diphasic or inverted in the remaining five leads.

C, Obtained about two weeks after *B*. A slight further change has occurred. The *T* waves have become more deeply inverted in Leads 1 and aV_L and are taller in Lead 3. Slight further changes are also noted in the *T* waves and in the precordial leads.

COMMENT. These changes are typical of infarction involving the anterior wall of the heart. Abnormal *QRS* complexes are seen in the limb leads and in precordial leads V_2 through V_6. *RS–T* segment and *T* wave changes have corresponded to the widespread *QRS* alterations. The involvement is more extensive than that seen in anteroseptal infarction and probably involves the lateral wall as well.

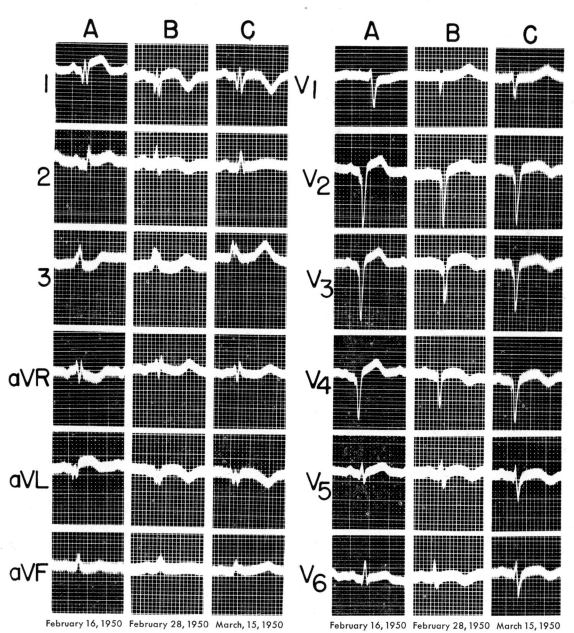

February 16, 1950   February 28, 1950   March, 15, 1950   February 16, 1950   February 28, 1950   March 15, 1950

Fig. 225. Anterolateral myocardial infarction.

These electrocardiograms were obtained from a purchasing agent forty-eight years of age who had experienced *acute* myocardial infarction a day or two before tracing *A* was taken. For the past four weeks he had had mild angina pectoris on effort. Tracings *B* and *C* were obtained respectively about ten days and one month later. Therapy did not include digitalization.

(*Legend continued on opposite page*)

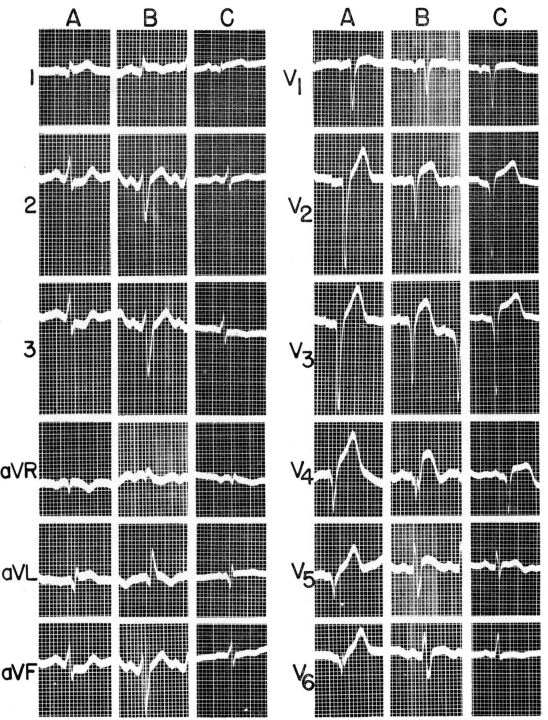

February 14, 1950   February 17, 1950   February 21, 1950   February 14, 1950   February 17, 1950   February 21, 1950

Fig. 226. Anterolateral myocardial infarction.

(*See facing page for legend.*)

(Legend continued from opposite page, Figure 226)

These electrocardiograms were obtained from a fifty year old taxicab driver. The first record was taken shortly after his hospital admission in acute distress, which was attributed to myocardial infarction with pericarditis secondary thereto. At the time of the second tracing, obtained three days later, he had no complaints of pain beyond a vague ache in the left shoulder. However, on the following day his blood pressure fell to 80 mm. of mercury systolic and 60 mm. diastolic, with a pulse rate of 118, although he was comfortable at this time. The third record was taken two weeks after entry, when he was progressing favorably. Therapy did not include digitalization.

INTERPRETATION. *A,* Tracing obtained within a few hours of the onset of symptoms. In the limb leads the *P* waves and the *P–R* intervals are normal. The *QRS* complexes show rather low voltage, and *Q* waves of abnormally long duration are observed in Leads 1 and aV_L. The *RS–T* segments are elevated in Leads 1 and aV_L and abnormally depressed in Leads 2, 3 and aV_F. In the precordial leads *QS* deflections are seen in all leads. The *RS–T* segments are abnormally elevated in Leads V_2 through V_6 and the *T* waves are unusually, if not abnormally, tall.

B, Record obtained three days later, showing significant changes in both limb and precordial leads. The electrical axis of *QRS* in the limb leads has shifted markedly to the left, and the *S* waves in Leads 2, 3 and aV_F have become much more prominent. The *RS–T* segment is still upwardly displaced in Lead 1, and the *T* wave in Lead 1 is now inverted. The downward displacements of the *RS–T* segments in Leads 2, 3 and aV_F have disappeared, and the *T* waves in these leads are tall and upright. In the precordial leads the voltage of all the waves is lower in V_1 through V_4, and *RS* complexes have appeared in Leads V_5 and V_6. There is an extreme degree of upward displacement of the *RS–T* segment in Lead V_4, and there is late inversion of the *T* wave in this lead.

C, Electrocardiogram obtained one week later, showing still further changes. There is low voltage of all complexes in the limb leads. The *Q* waves are abnormally prolonged in Leads 1 and aV_L. The *RS–T* segments are slightly elevated, and the *T* waves, which formerly were inverted, are now upright. The *T* waves in Leads V_3 and aV_F, which were formerly upright, are now inverted. In the precordial leads there has not been any great change in the *QRS* complexes except in Lead V_6, where the chief *QRS* deflection consists of an *R* wave. The *RS–T* segments are abnormally elevated in Leads V_2 through V_4, and the *T* waves in Leads V_4 through V_6 are diphasic or inverted.

COMMENT. These changes are typical of acute myocardial infarction involving the anterior and lateral wall of the left ventricle. Even allowing for considerable differences in technique, the acute injury has resulted in profound and progressive changes in both the depolarization and repolarization processes, as indicated by the changing patterns. The presence of the *RS–T* segment displacements suggests that an injury current or perhaps a newly developed cardiac aneurysm was still present at the time the last record was obtained.

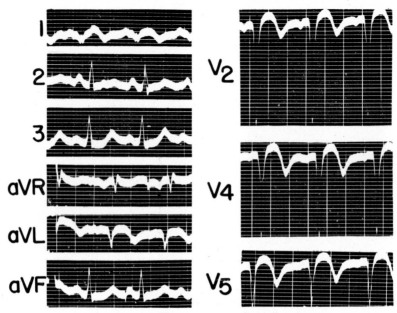

Fig. 227. Anterolateral myocardial infarction.

This electrocardiogram was obtained from a man of stocky build, thirty-six years of age, during convalescence following acute myocardial infarction.

INTERPRETATION. The *P* waves and *P–R* intervals are normal. In Leads 1 and aV$_L$, *QS* complexes are seen, and there is rather low voltage of *QRS* in the other limb leads. The *RS–T* segments are slightly elevated in Lead 1 and slightly depressed in Lead 3, and the *T* waves in Lead 1 are deeply inverted. The precordial leads are all similar and consist of *QS* complexes followed by elevation of *RS–T* and inversion of the *T* waves.

COMMENT. These changes are characteristic of extensive infarction involving the anterior and lateral walls of the left ventricle.

(Legend continued from facing page, Figure 228)

These electrocardiograms were obtained from a taxicab driver forty-six years of age who had suffered acute myocardial infarction. The first two records were taken, respectively, shortly after hospital admission and about one week thereafter. The third tracing was obtained three weeks after admission and two days after the recurrence of severe pain which required Demerol and persisted into the next day. Digitalization was begun two days after the first electrocardiogram was taken.

INTERPRETATION. *A,* Electrocardiogram obtained within a few hours of the onset of symptoms. In the limb leads the *P* waves and *P–R* intervals are normal; the latter measure 0.18 second. The *QRS* complexes are normal in amplitude, but the duration of *QRS* is approximately 0.12 second, and prominent *Q* waves are seen in Leads 3 and aV$_F$. The *RS–T* segments are displaced to a striking degree; the displacement is downward in Leads 1 and aV$_L$ and upward in Leads 2, 3 and aV$_F$. In the precordial leads there is marked downward displacement of the *RS–T* segments in V$_1$ through V$_3$ and the *T* waves are of low amplitude and diphasic.

B, Electrocardiogram obtained six days later. In the limb leads the *QRS* complexes show a moderate degree of left axis deviation, and prominent *Q* waves are seen in Leads 2, 3 and aV$_F$. The *RS–T* segments have returned nearly to the baseline, and the *T* waves are now inverted in Leads 2, 3 and aV$_F$. Striking changes have occurred in the precordial leads. In Lead V$_1$ r*Sr*^{1} complexes are seen, and in Leads V$_5$ and V$_6$ there are small *Q* waves. The *RS–T* segments have returned nearly to the baseline, and the *T* waves are abnormally tall in V$_2$ and V$_3$, abnormally low in V$_5$ and V$_6$.

C, Electrocardiogram obtained two weeks later. The duration of the *P–R* interval is now 0.13 second; the duration of *QRS* is normal. Prominent *Q* waves are seen in Leads 2, 3 and aV$_F$. The *RS–T* segments show no significant deviation; the *T* waves are inverted in Leads 2, 3 and aV$_F$. In the precordial leads small *Q* waves are still present in Leads V$_5$ and V$_6$, and the *T* waves are low and diphasic in V$_4$ and V$_5$, slightly inverted in V$_6$.

COMMENT. These changes are typical of acute myocardial infarction involving mainly the posterior wall of the heart. In order that *RS–T* segment changes, such as those observed here in Leads V$_1$ through V$_3$, may be captured electrocardiographically, it is necessary to obtain a record soon after the onset of infarction. The changes in precordial leads V$_4$ through V$_6$ indicate that the area of injury extends at least around to the left lateral wall.

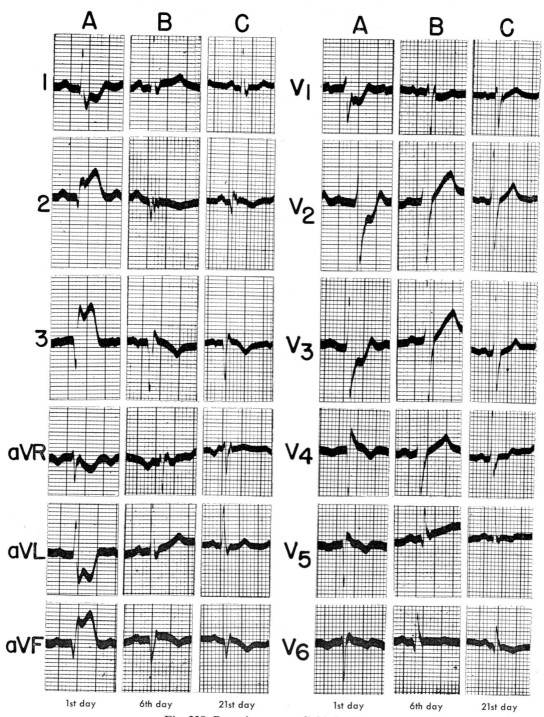

Fig. 228. Posterior myocardial infarction.

(See opposite page for legend.)

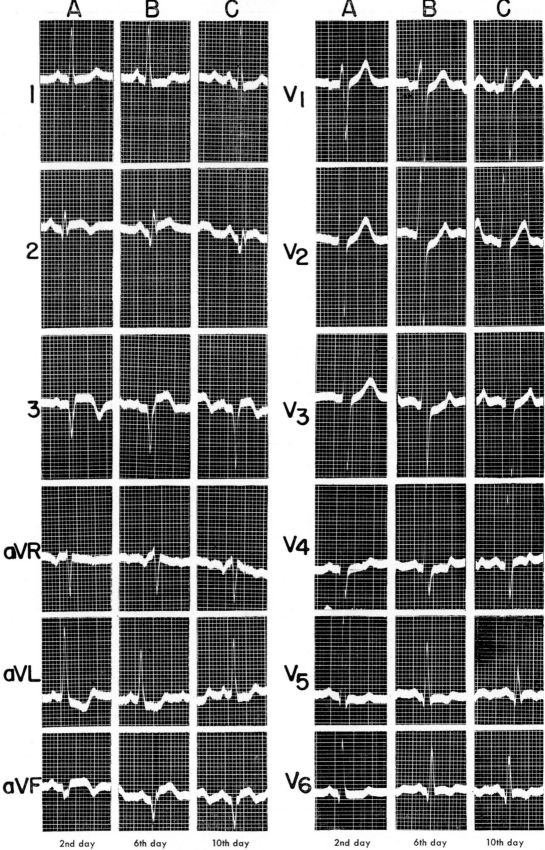

2nd day   6th day   10th day   2nd day   6th day   10th day

Fig. 229. Posterior myocardial infarction.

(See facing page for legend.)

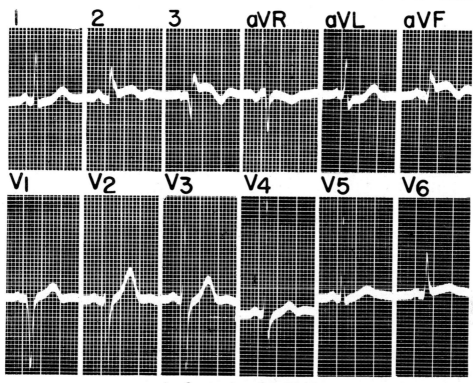

A—September 25, 1949

Fig. 230. Posterior myocardial infarction.

(See page 278 for legend.)

(Legend continued from opposite page, Figure 229)

These electrocardiograms were obtained from a man sixty years old who had had an acute myocardial infarct. Severe substernal pain had persisted intermittently over the two days prior to his hospital entry, following which the record shown in *A* was taken. At that time he was comfortable, but on the third hospital day, despite subjective improvement, his blood pressure dropped from 175 mm. of mercury systolic and 90 mm. diastolic to 120/70, the heart sounds were weaker than they had been on admission, and a tachycardia of about 112 persisted. The records shown in *B* and *C* were taken on the fifth and ninth hospital days, respectively. He was receiving no digitalis therapy at this time.

INTERPRETATION. *A*, Record obtained two days after the onset of symptoms. In the limb leads the *P* waves are normal and the *P–R* interval is 0.16 second. The *QRS* complexes show moderate left axis deviation; *QS* complexes are seen in Leads 3 and aV_F. The *RS–T* segments are upwardly displaced in Leads 2, 3 and aV_F. In the precordial leads the *T* waves are unusually tall in V_1 through V_3 and abnormally low in V_4 through V_6.

B, Electrocardiogram obtained four days later, showing significant changes when compared with the original record: the *Q* waves have become more prominent in Lead 2, the displacement of the *RS–T* segments is greater in Leads 2 and aV_F, and the *T* waves have become upright in these leads. In the precordial leads there is slight downward displacement of the *RS–T* segments in Leads V_1 through V_3 which was not present formerly.

C, Electrocardiogram obtained four days after the record in *B*. In the limb leads the *RS–T* segments have returned toward the baseline, and diphasic *T* waves are seen in most leads. In the precordial leads the *RS–T* segments are now normal; the *T* waves are diphasic in V_4, slightly diphasic or inverted in V_5 and V_6.

COMMENT. These changes are typical of acute myocardial infarction involving mainly the posterior and diaphragmatic walls of the left ventricle, although the area of injury extends into the lateral wall. The changes shown in these three records indicate that the evolutionary course of the healing process following acute infarction was interrupted by an extension of the injury. This is indicated in record *B* by the development of more prominent *Q* waves in Lead 2 and the more marked displacement of the *RS–T* segments in both the limb and precordial leads.

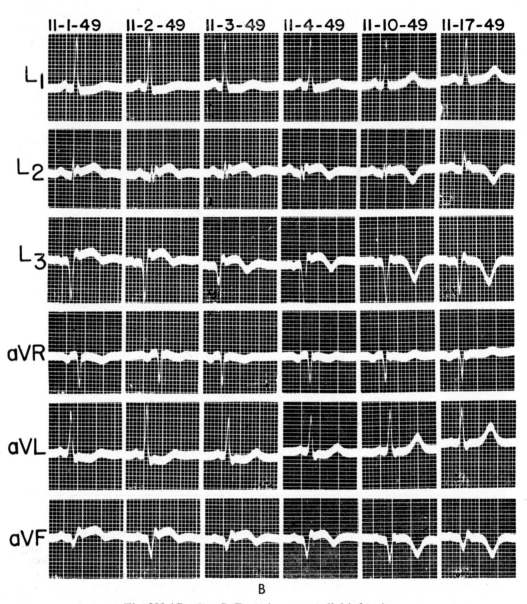

II-1-49   II-2-49   II-3-49   II-4-49   II-10-49   II-17-49

L₁

L₂

L₃

aVR

aVL

aVF

B

Fig. 230 (*Continued*). Posterior myocardial infarction.

These electrocardiograms were obtained from a man of stocky build, forty-four years of age, with hypertension and acute myocardial infarction. The symptoms of infarction developed one day prior to the date when the first record (*A*) was taken.

INTERPRETATION. *A* (September 25, 1949), This tracing shows normal *P* waves and *P–R* intervals. In the limb leads abnormally prominent *Q* waves are seen in Leads 3 and aV_F. The *RS–T* segments are upwardly displaced in Leads 2, 3 and aV_F and downwardly displaced in Leads 1 and aV_L. The *T* waves are inverted in Lead 3 and are diphasic in Leads 2 and aV_F. In the precordial leads *QS* complexes are seen in V_1 and *rS* complexes in V_2. The *T* waves are rather low in amplitude in V_4, abnormally low in V_5 and V_6.

B, Typical evolutionary changes in pattern. The principal alterations are seen in the limb leads. In the precordial leads there are changes in the *T* waves, particularly in V_4 through V_6.

COMMENT. These alterations are typical of acute myocardial infarction involving principally the posterior and diaphragmatic walls of the left ventricle. The absence of *R* in V_1 and the disappearance of *R* in V_2 suggest that the septum si also involved.

(*See facing page for Figure 230 B.*)

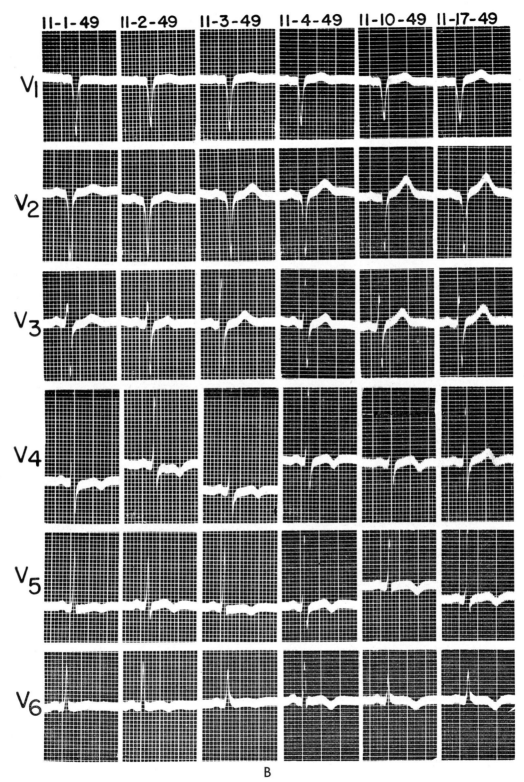

B

Fig. 230 (*Continued*). Posterior myocardial infarction.

(*See opposite page for legend.*)

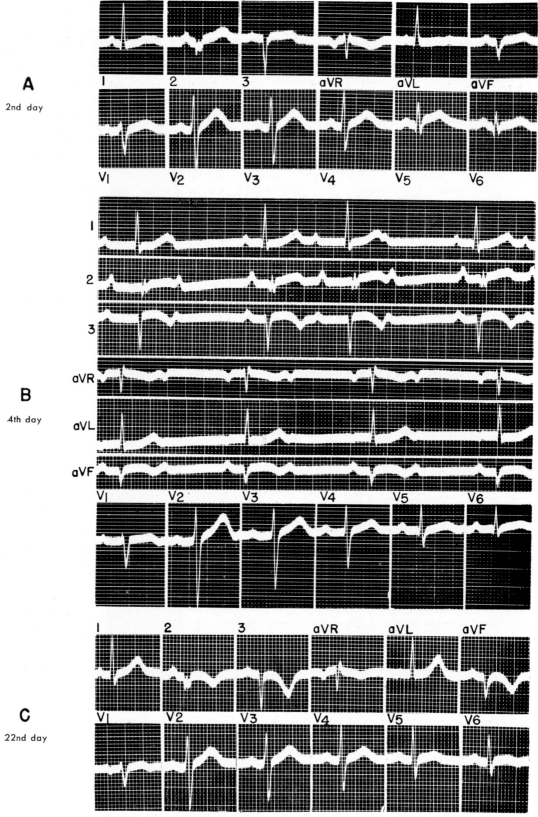

Fig. 231. Posterior myocardial infarction.

(*See facing page for legend.*)

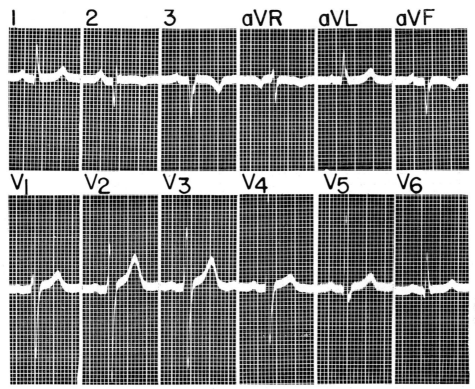

Fig. 232. Posterior myocardial infarction.

This electrocardiogram was obtained from a man forty-nine years of age with hypertension, healed myocardial infarction and angina pectoris. The blood pressure was 210 mm. of mercury systolic and 125 mm. diastolic. The heart was full-sized but not definitely enlarged. No murmurs were heard, and there were no congestive phenomena. Therapy did not include digitalization.

INTERPRETATION. Here the abnormal findings are confined to the limb leads. The Q waves in Lead 2 and QS waves in Leads 3 and aV$_F$, associated with inversion of the T waves in these three leads, are typical of the final evolutionary pattern in myocardial infarction involving the posterior and diaphragmatic walls of the heart. There is also widening of the S waves in precordial Leads V$_2$ to V$_5$ inclusive.

(Legend continued from opposite page, Figure 231)

These electrocardiograms were obtained from a salesman forty-seven years old who had had acute myocardial infarction. The day before the tracing shown in A he had experienced the classic symptoms of coronary occlusion; an electrocardiogram at that time had demonstrated S–T and T wave alteration, but no change in the QRS. Tracings B and C were obtained respectively three days and three weeks after the onset of his attack. The therapy did not include digitalization.

INTERPRETATION. A, Record obtained the day after the onset of symptoms. In the limb leads the P waves and P–R intervals are normal. The QRS complexes show moderate left axis deviation, and QS waves are seen in Leads 2, 3 and aV$_F$. There is slight elevation of the RS–T segments in Leads 2 and 3 and slight depression in Lead 1. The T waves tend to be low in amplitude in all leads. In the precordial leads the QRS complexes show no definite abnormality except for the possibility that their amplitude is smaller than it should be in Leads V$_5$ and V$_6$.

B, Record taken two days later. In the limb leads there is seen to be partial heart block with dropped beats. QS complexes are still evident in Leads 3 and aV$_F$, and small Q waves are present in Lead 2. There has been little change in the RS–T segments, but the T waves are now typically inverted in Lead 3 and slightly inverted in aV$_F$. There has been no significant change in the precordial leads.

C, Obtained fifteen days later. Atrioventricular conduction is normal. In the limb leads there are QS complexes in Leads 2 and aV$_F$ and also in Lead 3 (if an embryonic R wave is disregarded). The RS–T segments have returned to the baselines; the T waves are typically inverted in Leads 2, 3 and aV$_F$ and abnormally tall in Leads 1 and aV$_L$. The precordial leads show little change, although the T waves in the V$_6$ position have become slightly inverted.

COMMENT. These changes following acute infarction again typify involvement of the posterior and diaphragmatic walls of the heart. Atrioventricular block of this type is not infrequently present as a temporary complication in these cases.

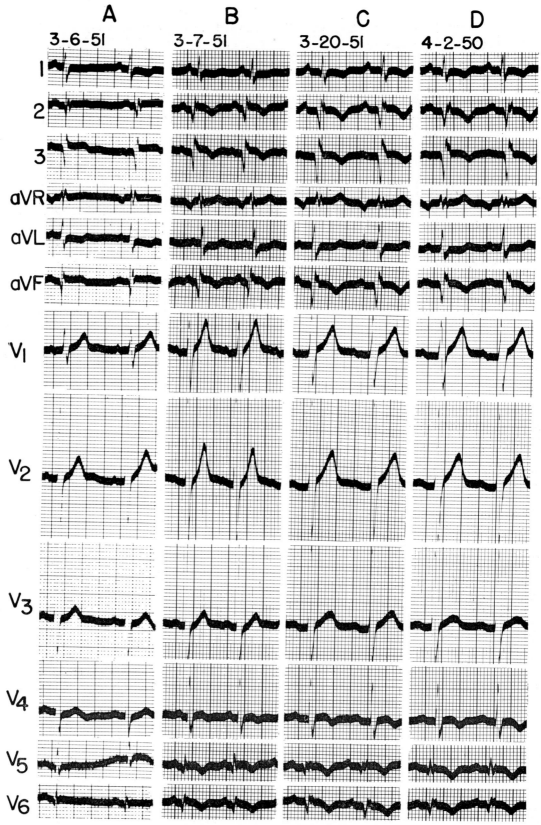

Fig. 233. Posterolateral myocardial infarction.

(*See facing page for legend.*)

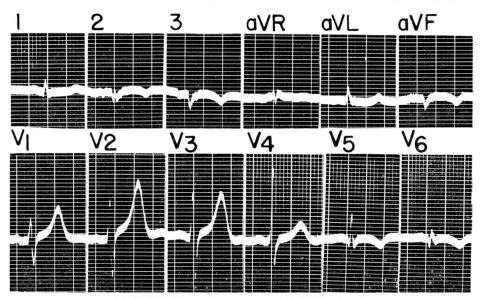

Fig. 234. Posterolateral myocardial infarction.

This electrocardiogram was obtained from a man of average build, fifty-three years of age, with healed myocardial infarction. The heart was not enlarged, the blood pressure was normal, and there were no congestive phenomena. Therapy did not include digitalization.

INTERPRETATION. In the limb leads there is low voltage of all the waves. The P waves are barely perceptible, but the P–R intervals are normal. There is extremely low voltage of the QRS complexes, and QS waves are seen in Leads 2, 3 and aV_F with inversion of the T waves in these leads. In the precordial leads there is low voltage of the QRS complex in V_5 and extremely low voltage of QRS in V_6; in both these leads Q waves are seen. The T waves are abnormally tall in V_1 through V_3 and inverted in V_5 and V_6.

COMMENT. These changes are consistent with the diagnosis of healed myocardial infarction involving the posterior and lateral walls of the left ventricle.

(*Legend continued from opposite page, Figure 233*)

These electrocardiograms were obtained from a man of stocky build, thirty years of age, who was suffering from acute myocardial infarction.

INTERPRETATION. *A*, Record showing normal P waves and P–R intervals. In the limb leads the QRS complexes are of low voltage, and prominent Q waves are seen in Leads 2, 3 and aV_F. There is slight elevation of the RS–T segments in Leads 3 and aV_F, and the T waves are low or diphasic in all leads. In the precordial leads the QRS complexes are abnormally low in voltage in Leads V_5 and V_6 and the T waves are low in these leads.

B, Electrocardiogram taken one day later, showing progressive changes in both limb and precordial leads. In the limb leads the T waves are slightly inverted in Lead 1 and deeply inverted in Leads 2, 3 and aV_F. In the precordial leads the Q waves have become abnormally prominent in Leads V_5 and V_6; associated with this is slight elevation of the RS–T segments and inversion of the T waves. In Leads V_1 and V_2 the T waves have become more upright.

C and *D* show still further changes. In the limb leads the voltage of QRS has increased, and the Q waves in Leads 2, 3 and aV_F have become prominent. The RS–T segments have returned to, or nearly to, the baseline, and the T waves are deeply inverted in Leads 2, 3 and aV_F, slightly inverted in Lead 1. In the precordial leads the voltage of QRS is abnormally low in Leads V_5 and V_6, the Q waves are prominent, and the T waves are deeply inverted.

COMMENT. These changes are characteristic of infarction involving not only the posterior and diaphragmatic walls of the heart, but the left lateral wall as well.

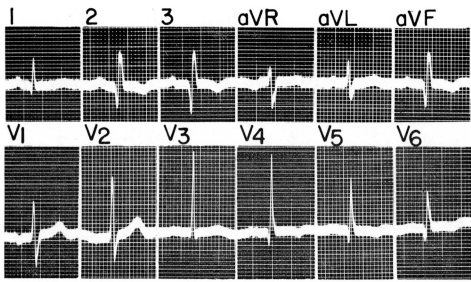

Fig. 235. Anteroposterior myocardial infarction.

This electrocardiogram was obtained from a physician seventy-eight years of age who had suffered myocardial infarction twenty-two years before the electrocardiogram shown here was taken. There had been no further episodes, and he had continued to lead an active but careful life. At the time this record was obtained he was working three days a week as a consultant. He was smoking twenty cigarettes a day and was considerably limited in walking by intermittent claudication. Therapy did not include digitalization.

INTERPRETATION. The P waves are normal, and the P–R intervals measure approximately 0.2 second. In the limb leads abnormal Q waves are seen in Leads 2, 3 and aV_F, and the Q wave in Lead 1 is probably abnormal as well. The T waves are abnormally low in amplitude in Lead 1 and are inverted in Leads 2, 3 and aV_F. In the precordial leads abnormal Q waves are seen in Leads V_4 through V_6; the T waves are abnormally low in V_3 and are inverted in V_4 through V_6.

COMMENT. These changes are consistent with the diagnosis and indicate that the infarction, while primarily involving the posterior and diaphragmatic walls of the heart, also extends laterally and anteriorly as indicated by the abnormal Q waves in Lead 1 and in precordial Leads V_4 through V_6.

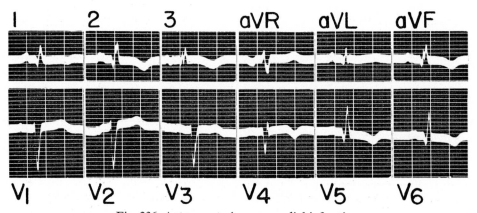

Fig. 236. Anteroposterior myocardial infarction.

This electrocardiogram was obtained from a man of average build, twenty-nine years of age, with healed myocardial infarction. The heart was slightly enlarged. No murmurs were heard, and the blood pressure was normal. There was evidence of slight congestion of the lungs. Therapy did not include digitalization.

INTERPRETATION. The P waves and P–R intervals are normal. In the limb leads there is low voltage of the QRS complexes, and prominent Q waves are seen in Leads 1, 2 and aV_F. The RS–T segments are normal. The T waves are slightly inverted in Lead 1, deeply inverted in Leads 2, 3 and aV_F. In the precordial leads small R waves may be seen in V_1 and V_2. In V_3 a QS complex is present, and in Leads V_4 through V_6 there are abnormal Q waves. The RS–T segments are normal, but the T waves are abnormally low in V_3 and inverted in V_4 through V_6.

COMMENT. These changes are consistent with a diagnosis of healed myocardial infarction involving both the anterior and posterior walls of the heart.

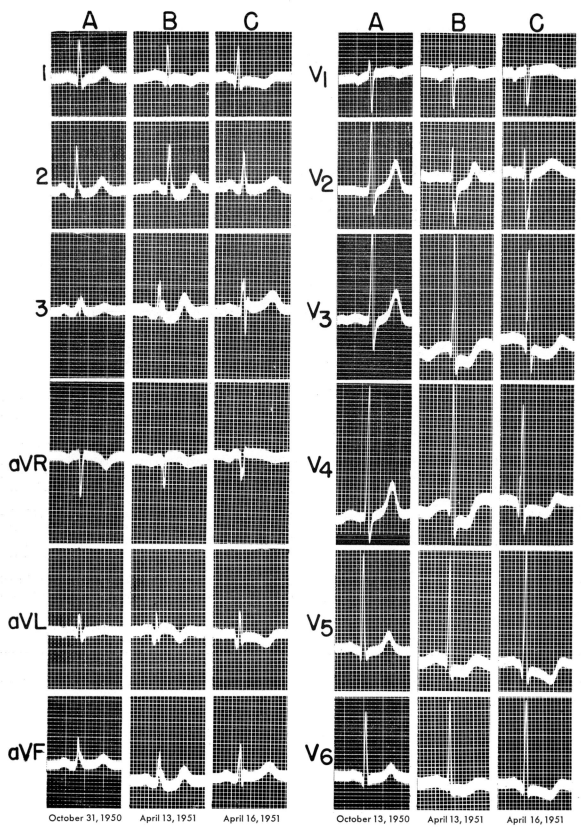

October 31, 1950   April 13, 1951   April 16, 1951   October 13, 1950   April 13, 1951   April 16,1951

Fig. 237. Subendocardial infarction.

(*See text, page 264.*)

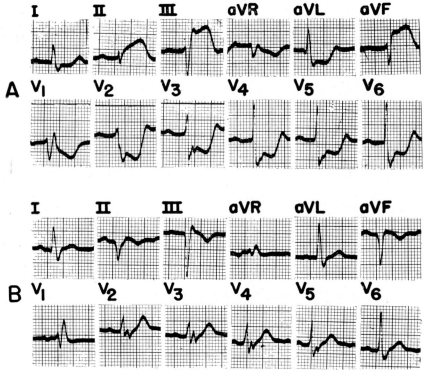

Fig. 238. Posterior myocardial infarction and right bundle branch block.

Electrocardiograms obtained from a man seventy-four years of age who had suffered an acute myocardial infarct on the day that tracing *A* was taken. *B* was obtained three weeks later. His history included rheumatic fever at the age of thirty-three, but there had been no known coronary or other cardiovascular involvement.

INTERPRETATION. *A*, Record obtained a few hours after the onset of symptoms. The *P* waves are normal, and the *P–R* interval is 0.24 second, which indicates first stage of atrioventricular block. There is right bundle branch block. In the limb leads the *RS–T* segments are markedly elevated in Leads 2, 3 and aV_F and depressed in Leads 1 and aV_L. The *T* waves are upright or diphasic in all leads except aV_F. In the precordial leads an *rSR'* complex is seen in Lead V_1. The *RS–T* segments are markedly depressed in all leads, and the *T* waves are diphasic in character.

B, Record obtained three weeks later. The *P–R* interval is normal, but bundle branch block is still present. Significant changes have occurred in the *QRS* complexes: *QS* waves are seen in Leads 2 and aV_F, and a prominent *Q* wave has appeared in Lead 3. The *RS–T* segments are no longer displaced. The *T* waves are upright in Leads 1 and aV_L and inverted in Leads 2, 3 and aV_F. In the precordial leads only minor changes have occurred in the *QRS* complexes. The *T* waves are flat in V_1, but tall and upright in V_2 through V_6.

COMMENT. These records illustrate the changes which occur in acute posterior myocardial infarction complicated by right bundle branch block. Except for the initial displacement of the *RS–T* segments, the significant changes occurred in the limb leads.

(*Legend continued from facing page, Figure 239*)

This electrocardiogram was obtained from a salesman fifty-nine years of age with hypertensive and coronary heart disease and myocardial infarction. It was thought at this time that the infarct was of recent origin, inasmuch as three weeks prior to this examination he had experienced a brief fainting attack; although no chest pain had accompanied this, he thought he might have had slight shortness of breath on walking up stairs that day. When he was seen again two weeks later, the electrocardiogram was unchanged, however, and it was believed that his infarct might have occurred three years before, coincident with a transitory episode of aphasia and left hemiplegia.

INTERPRETATION. The *P* waves and *P–R* intervals are normal. The *QRS* complexes reveal that there is intermittent right bundle branch block. The influence of the infarction on this electrocardiogram is best observed by consideration of the normal cycles. In the limb leads *Q* waves are seen in Leads 1 and aV_L, and the *T* waves in these leads are low and diphasic. In the precordial leads an *rS* complex followed by an upright *T* wave is seen in Lead V_1. In Leads V_2 and V_3 the *R* wave is absent. The *RS–T* segments are slightly elevated and the *T* waves upright. In Leads V_4 through V_6 the *T* waves are low or diphasic.

COMMENT. This is a typical example of the electrocardiographic findings in anteroseptal infarction complicated by intermittent right bundle branch block.

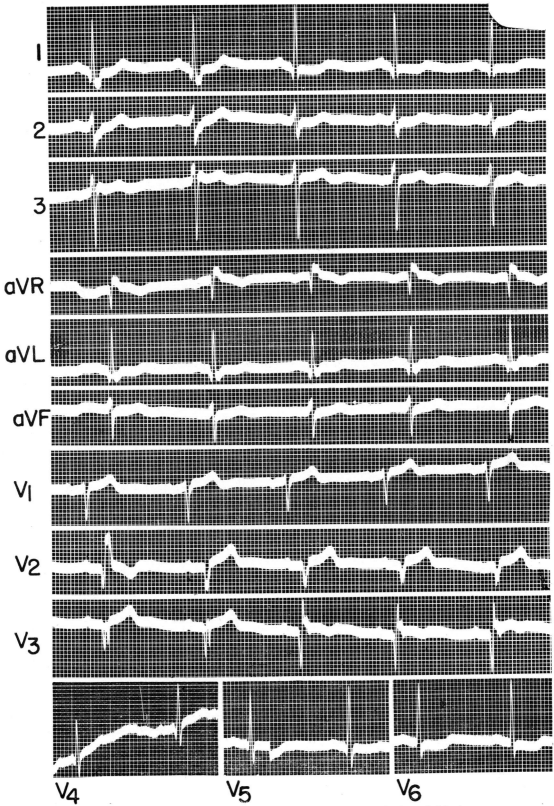

Fig. 239. Anterior myocardial infarction and right bundle branch block.

(See opposite page for legend.)

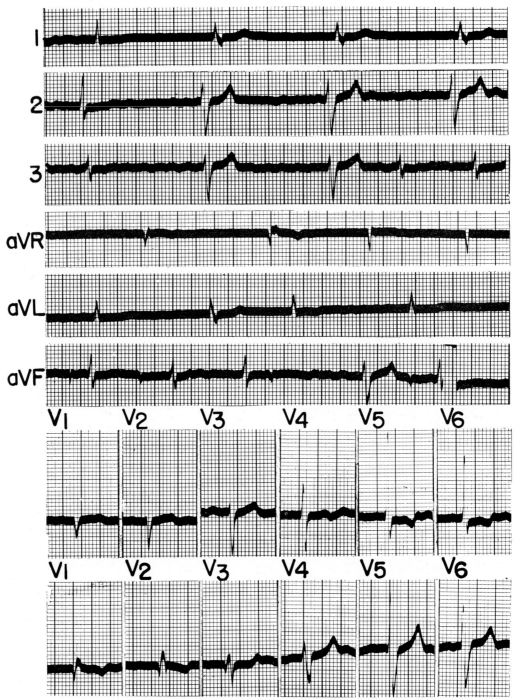

Fig. 240. Anterior myocardial infarction and right bundle branch block.

This electrocardiogram was obtained from a Negro man seventy-two years of age with healed myocardial infarction and intermittent right bundle branch block. Atrial fibrillation is also present.

INTERPRETATION. The influence of the bundle branch block on the *RS–T* segments and *T* waves may be seen in the limb leads by comparing the first two cycles in each lead (except in aV_F, where the last two cycles should be compared). In the precordial leads the influence of the bundle branch block may be seen by comparing the upper with the lower set of leads.

An analysis of the *QRS* complexes in cycles where normal conduction is present reveals low voltage of *QRS* in the unipolar limb leads, absent *R* waves in Leads V$_1$ and V$_2$, and abnormally small *R* waves in V$_3$. The *T* waves are nearly isoelectric in Leads 1 and aV$_L$ and are inverted or diphasic in Leads V$_4$ through V$_6$.

COMMENT. These findings are consistent with a diagnosis of healed myocardial infarction involving the anteroseptal region of the heart and complicated by atrial fibrillation and right bundle branch block.

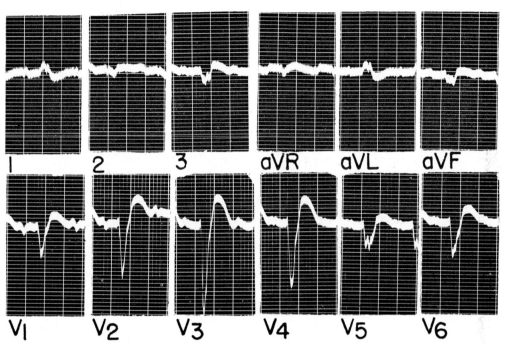

Fig. 241. Anterior myocardial infarction and left bundle branch block.

This electrocardiogram was taken on a woman sixty-seven years of age who had suffered myocardial infarction six weeks previously. At the time this record was obtained the heart was considerably enlarged, the sounds were of poor quality, and a Grade 1 systolic murmur was heard at the apex. Her blood pressure was 110 mm. of mercury systolic and 60 mm. diastolic, and there was moderate congestive failure. Therapy included digitalization.

INTERPRETATION. There is extremely low voltage of all complexes in the limb leads. The *P* waves are poorly made out, but the *P–R* intervals measure approximately 0.19 second. There is left bundle branch block. In Leads 1 and aV_L there is sagging of the *RS–T* segments, and in Leads 3 and aV_F there is slight elevation. In the precordial leads embryonic *R* waves are seen in V_1 through V_6; the chief *QRS* deflection is downward, the *RS–T* segments are elevated, and the *T* waves are low in amplitude in all leads.

COMMENT. From a consideration of the limb leads a diagnosis can be made of left bundle branch block. The extremely low voltage of all the waves is consistent with severe myocardial damage and congestive failure, but there is little to support the diagnosis of myocardial infarction. In the precordial leads, however, the marked upward displacement of the *RS–T* segments and the downward direction of the chief *QRS* deflection in V_5 and V_6 indicate extensive infarction involving the anterior wall of the heart with or without cardiac aneurysm.

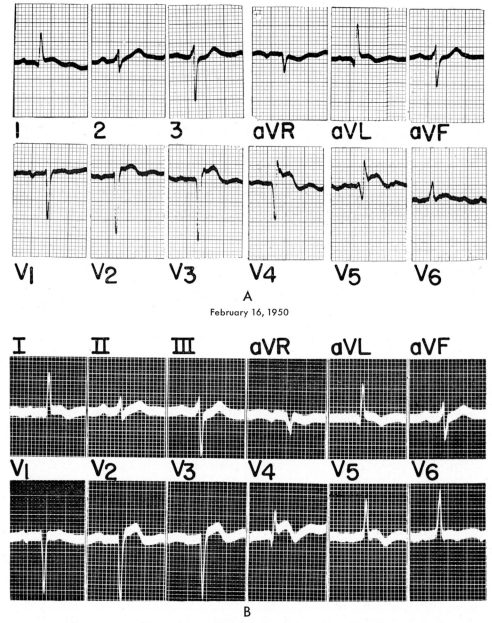

A

February 16, 1950

B

February 19, 1951

Fig. 242. Ventricular aneurysm.

These electrocardiograms were obtained from a woman sixty-seven years of age who suffered an acute myocardial infarct in August, 1948. Except for phlebitis that fall and acute pulmonary edema one year later, her course had been uneventful. Examination on February 16, 1950, showed the heart to be enlarged. The sounds were of poor quality, and gallop rhythm was present. Her blood pressure was normal, and there were no congestive phenomena. Fluoroscopic examination revealed a bulging of the left ventricle which was thought to be an aneurysm.

INTERPRETATION. *A*, Electrocardiogram taken on February 16, 1950. The *P* waves and *P–R* intervals are normal. In the limb leads the *QRS* complexes show well marked left axis deviation, and *Q* waves are seen in Leads 1 and aV_L. There is elevation of the *RS–T* segments in Leads 1 and aV_L, and the *T* waves are low and diphasic in these leads. The *RS–T* segment in Lead 3 is slightly depressed; the *T* waves are tall and upright in Leads 3 and aV_F. In the precordial leads small *R* waves are seen in V_1 and V_2, but not in V_3; in V_4 and V_5 the *Q* waves are abnormally prominent. The *RS–T* segments are elevated in Leads V_2 through V_5, and the *T* waves are low and diphasic in these leads.

B, Record obtained one year later. During this interval the cardiac status has remained relatively the same. In the limb leads only minor changes have taken place. The displacement of the *RS–T* segments in Leads 1 and aV_L is less than before, and the *T* waves are more deeply inverted. In the precordial leads the displacement of the *RS–T* segments is less, and the *Q* wave in V_4 is less prominent; in V_5 a *Q* wave is no longer seen.

COMMENT. These electrocardiograms have changed but little in configuration from those that were taken during the more acute process and are characteristic of the presence of an aneurysm of the left ventricle, associated with a large healed anterior myocardial infarct of the left ventricle.

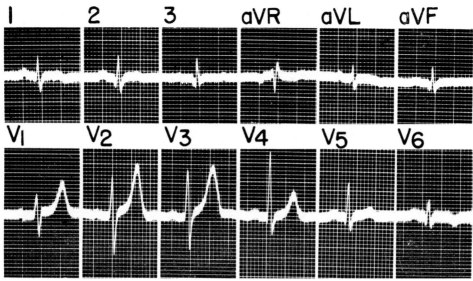

Fig. 243. Posterolateral myocardial infarction.

This electrocardiogram was obtained from a fifty-two year old superintendent of an electric company who had had angina pectoris for a period of one year prior to acute myocardial infarction. Upon hospital admission his blood pressure was 125 mm. of mercury systolic and 86 mm. diastolic, and his sedimentation rate was elevated.

INTERPRETATION. This record was obtained three weeks after the onset of symptoms. The P waves and P–R intervals are normal. In the limb leads there is low voltage of the QRS complexes, and small Q waves are seen in Leads 2, 3 and aV_F. The RS–T segments are normal, but the T waves are low or slightly inverted in all leads. In the precordial leads there is no definite abnormality of the QRS complexes. However, the T waves are abnormally tall in Leads V_1 rough V_3, abnormally low in V_5, and slightly inverted in V_6.

COMMENT. These findings are consistent with a diagnosis of acute posterolateral myocardial infarction occurring three weeks previously, even though there are no pronounced QRS changes.

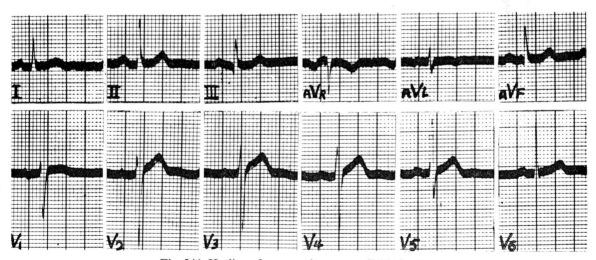

Fig. 244. Healing after posterior myocardial infarction.

The electrocardiogram shown here was obtained from a man fifty-six years of age with healed myocardial infarction.

INTERPRETATION. The P waves and the P–R intervals are normal. Small Q waves are seen in Leads 3 and aV_L. The T waves are rather low in Lead 1 and are inverted in aV_L. In all other respects the electrocardiogram is within the usual normal range.

COMMENT. This patient had a small myocardial infarct in 1941, at which time the T waves in Lead 1 were inverted. In 1948 he had a second attack involving the posterior wall of the heart. Upon this occasion prominent Q waves and inverted T waves appeared in Leads 2 and 3. The electrocardiogram shown here was obtained a year after the second episode and demonstrated remarkably little indication of previous damage. He died suddenly in a third attack a year after this record was taken.

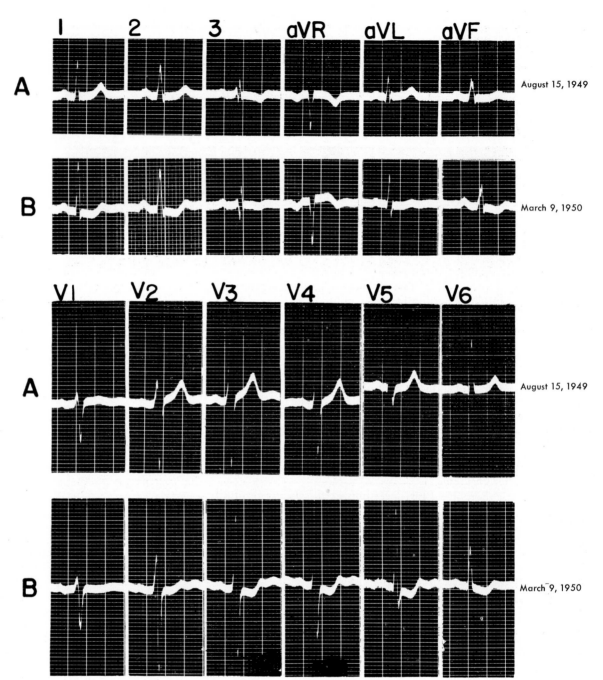

Fig. 245. Myocardial anoxia due to coronary insufficiency in a patient with a healed infarct.

These electrocardiograms were obtained from a man of average build, forty-seven years of age, with healed myocardial infarction. Prior to the attack he had always been well and strong, but subsequently his exercise tolerance was considerably reduced and he suffered from angina pectoris. Therapy did not include digitalization.

INTERPRETATION. *A*, Record obtained one year and nine months after the attack; no significant abnormality seen.

B, Record taken seven months later; during this interval no new symptoms had arisen. In the limb leads there is well marked sagging of the *RS–T* segment in Leads 1, 2 and aV$_F$, and the *T* waves are abnormally low in these leads. In the precordial leads there is sagging of the *RS–T* segments in Leads V$_2$ through V$_6$, and the *T* waves are abnormally low in these leads.

COMMENT. These *RS–T* and *T* wave changes can be the result of temporary anoxia from effort or other cause or of so-called left ventricular strain, which is prone to occur in patients with coronary or hypertensive heart disease.

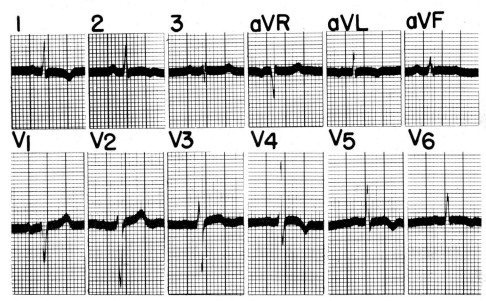

Fig. 246. Coronary heart disease without infarction.

The electrocardiogram shown here was obtained from a Negro man seventy years of age with coronary heart disease and congestive failure. He was unusually well and strong until three years previously, when he gradually became limited by shortness of breath and "spells of pressure in the chest." At no time did the symptomatology suggest acute myocardial infarction. The heart was moderately enlarged, and a faint systolic murmur was heard over the mitral area. The blood pressure was 126 mm. of mercury systolic and 70 mm. diastolic. There was evidence of fluid in the pleural cavities, and there was moderate edema over the shins.

INTERPRETATION. *P* waves and *P–R* intervals are normal. In the limb leads there is deep inversion of the *T* waves in Leads 1 and slight inversion in Leads 2 and aV_L. In the precordial leads the *T* waves are abnormally low in V_3 and inverted in V_4 through V_6.

COMMENT. Coronary insufficiency may be associated with inversion of the *T* waves in the electrocardiogram, as this case illustrates.

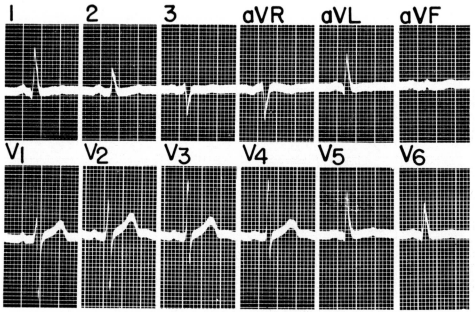

Fig. 247. Probable coronary heart disease.

The electrocardiogram shown here was obtained from a man of stocky build, forty-one years of age. He had no complaints, but desired a check-up because hypertension had been discovered incidentally four months before. The heart was full-sized, but not definitely enlarged. The sounds were of good quality, and no murmurs were heard. His blood pressure was 142 mm. of mercury systolic and 92 mm. diastolic. There were no congestive phenomena. He was not receiving digitalis.

INTERPRETATION. P waves and P–R intervals are normal. In the limb leads there is slight slurring of the QRS complexes and a tendency toward left axis deviation. Small Q waves are seen in Leads 1 and aV_L. The T waves are abnormally low in all limb leads and in Leads V_5 and V_6. Also, in the precordial leads, minute Q waves are seen in V_5 and V_6.

COMMENT. T wave changes in this electrocardiogram are consistent with the diagnosis of coronary disease. No conclusions can be drawn about the significance of minute Q waves, since these may well represent septal depolarization.

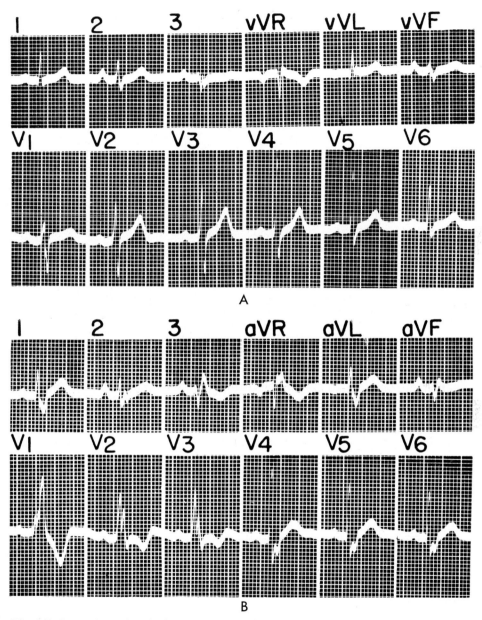

Fig. 248. Intermittent bundle branch block as the only evidence of coronary heart disease.

These electrocardiograms were taken on a man of stocky build, sixty-one years of age, with coronary heart disease and angina pectoris and intermittent right bundle branch block.

INTERPRETATION. The electrocardiogram in *A* (September 27, 1950) demonstrates no definite abnormality, but the one in *B* (October 19, 1950), obtained three weeks later, shows right bundle branch block.

COMMENT. The only electrocardiographic evidence of coronary heart disease and insufficiency in this case was a conduction defect.

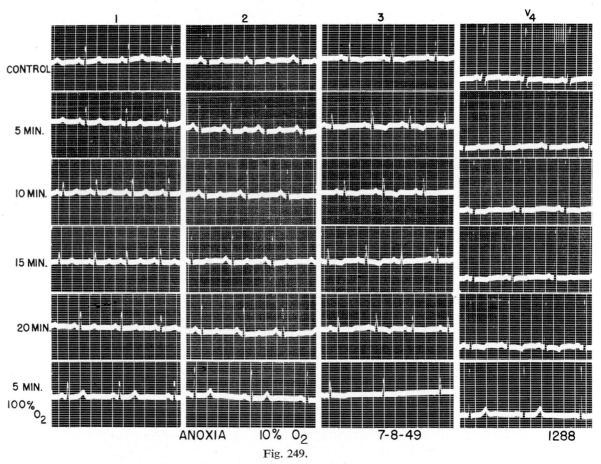

Fig. 249.

The electrocardiogram shown here was obtained from a man twenty-five years of age who had complained of pain in the chest at frequent intervals for over a year. The heart was not enlarged, the sounds were of fairly good quality, and no murmurs were heard. The blood pressure was 140 mm. of mercury systolic and 100 mm. diastolic. X-ray examination revealed a full-sized heart, with slight prominence in the region of the left ventricle; marked calcification was visible in the aortic arch. There were no congestive phenomena. Therapy did not include digitalization.

INTERPRETATION. Serial tracings were obtained while the patient breathed 10 per cent oxygen. In the control record the T waves are unusually, if not abnormally, low in Leads 2 and V_4.

Four electrocardiograms taken at five minute intervals while the patient breathed 10 per cent oxygen reveal progressive lowering of the T waves in all the leads. In addition, there is slight downward displacement of the RS–T segments in Leads 1 and 2. The last record was obtained after the patient had breathed 100 per cent oxygen for five minutes. The T waves have now become normal, or nearly normal, in appearance.

COMMENT. These electrocardiographic changes were interpreted as positive evidence of coronary insufficiency and helped in making the diagnosis in this case.

(*Legend continued from facing page, Figure 250*)

These electrocardiograms were obtained before and immediately after exercise from a man fifty-nine years of age with coronary heart disease and angina pectoris of three years' duration. The heart was not enlarged. A soft blowing systolic murmur was heard at the mitral area. Blood pressure was 130 mm. of mercury systolic and 68 mm. diastolic. There were no congestive phenomena.

INTERPRETATION. *A*, The P waves are normal and the P–R interval is about 0.2 second. In the limb leads there is slurring of the QRS complexes, but their amplitude, axis and duration are normal. There is sagging of the RS–T segments in Leads 2 and 3, and the T waves are low and diphasic in these leads. In the precordial leads there is sagging of the RS–T segments in Leads V_5 and V_6, and the T waves in these leads are low.

B, Electrocardiogram obtained after the patient had exercised for three minutes. The exercise consisted of stepping up 20 inches once every $2\frac{1}{2}$ seconds. The heart rate has increased, and the P waves are more prominent in Leads 2 and 3. The RS–T segments are depressed in Lead 1 and severely depressed in Leads 2, 3, V_5 and V_6.

COMMENT. The slurring of the QRS complexes, the sagging of the RS–T segments and the abnormally low T waves in *A* are consistent with the diagnosis of coronary heart disease. The greater abnormality of the RS–T segments and T waves following the slight amount of exercise confirms the fact that coronary insufficiency is the cause and suggests that even this degree of exercise is too much for the patient to undertake.

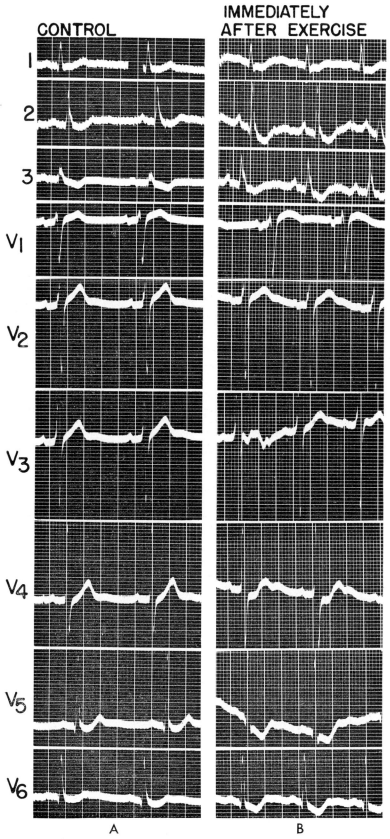

CONTROL

IMMEDIATELY
AFTER EXERCISE

1
2
3
V1
V2
V3
V4
V5
V6

A

B

Fig. 250. Coronary insufficiency revealed by the exercise test.

(*See opposite page for legend.*)

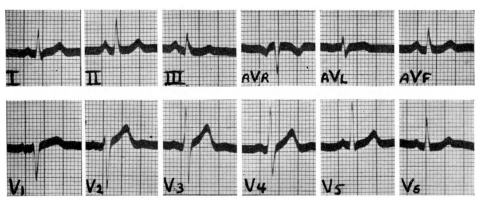

Fig. 251. Normal electrocardiogram in coronary heart disease.

This electrocardiogram was obtained from a man fifty-six years of age with coronary heart disease and easily provoked angina pectoris of seventeen months' duration. The heart was slightly enlarged in the region of the left ventricle, and a Grade 1 systolic murmur was heard at the mitral area. The blood pressure was 132 mm. of mercury systolic and 78 mm. diastolic. Recent treatment included digitalization.

INTERPRETATION. The electrocardiogram shows no definite abnormality.

COMMENT. This electrocardiogram is shown to emphasize the fact that normal records may be obtained from patients with a severe degree of coronary insufficiency.

CHAPTER 22

Miscellaneous

In this category remain all other diseases, noninfectious in nature, that have not been discussed in previous chapters. Some are manifested by disorders of body chemistry, as in nephritis and diabetes, others by changes in the blood, as in the leukemias, polycythemia and anemia, and others by pathologic changes in the tissues, as in amyloid disease, collagen disease, avitaminosis, sarcoidosis, trauma and the neoplasms (benign and malignant). In the majority of cases of all these diseases the electrocardiogram remains normal, but now and then nonspecific abnormalities of rate, rhythm, conduction or of individual complexes (*P* waves, *QRS* waves, *S–T* segments, and *T* waves) are found.

Disorders in Potassium Balance

In recent years the clinical importance of disturbances in potassium balance has become increasingly apparent, and at the same time the usefulness of the electrocardiogram in the detection of these disturbances has become well established. Deviations in content and distribution of the potassium ion in the body which produce values in serum concentration above or below the normal range of 3.5 to 5 milliequivalents per liter (hyperpotassemia or hyperkalemia and hypopotassemia or hypokalemia, respectively) effect changes in contractile power of skeletal and cardiac muscle, with muscle weakness increasing in proportion to the degree of electrolyte imbalance. Clinical syndromes result in which weakness of the muscles of the extremities progresses to paralysis. Respirations become labored as a consequence of involvement of the respiratory muscles, with eventual paralysis of respiration if the underlying fault is not corrected. Decrease in intensity of heart sounds, cardiac dilatation and congestive failure may result from involvement of heart muscle. Changes in heart rate and rhythm also occur and are discussed in greater detail later. Hypotension may be present, possibly as a result of several factors, including heart muscle weakness,

dehydration, and imbalance of other electrolytes, especially sodium. These clinical states may rapidly progress to a fatal issue, and since treatment is often effective, the ability to recognize the electrocardiographic patterns associated with significant degrees of potassium imbalance is assuming considerable importance.

The clinical syndromes associated with hyperkalemia and hypokalemia are similar enough to make their differentiation difficult without the use of laboratory aids; their effective treatment is almost impossible without the valuable information given by the electrocardiogram and blood chemistry determinations. Both methods should be used in evaluating therapeutic results. Occasionally the electrocardiogram is a more reliable indicator of impending disaster than the serum potassium levels. This is especially true in hyperkalemia, in which the complication of cardiac standstill may be the terminal event.

Hyperpotassemia (Hyperkalemia)

Following are some of the disorders in which high levels of serum potassium may be expected: (1) renal disease, in which urinary excretion of the electrolyte is reduced, especially when potassium salts are given therapeutically—hyperkalemia in its most dramatic forms usually occurs in association with oliguria; (2) hemolytic crises, burns, starvation and other pathologic states characterized by tissue breakdown and consequent release of large quantities of potassium; (3) Addison's disease, in which adrenal cortical insufficiency leads to loss of sodium and retention of potassium.

In the progression of hyperpotassemia toward critical levels a certain evolution of electrocardiographic pattern has been recorded by many observers. This was summarized recently by Merrill and his co-workers* as follows:

* Merrill, J. P., Levine, H. D., Somerville, W., and Smith, S., III: Clinical Recognition and Treatment of Acute Potassium Intoxication. Ann. Int. Med., *33:* 797, 1950.

(1) the development of tall, narrow, pointed T waves; (2) depression of the S–T segment which tends to become a direct line from the nadir of the S to the apex of the T wave; (3) auriculoventricular block; (4) decreased amplitude and increased duration of the P waves, and eventually auricular standstill; (5) intraventricular block of progressively increasing grade associated with a decreased height of the R waves and an increased depth of the S waves; (6) prolongation of the Q–T interval; (7) a ventricular arrhythmia variously regarded as due to auricular fibrillation or sinus arrhythmia and occasionally due to ventricular ectopic beats; (8) sinus bradycardia; (9) disintegration of the ventricular complexes culminating in a baseline having the appearance of a continuous sine wave; and (10) ventricular standstill. Although there is some overlap in their time relationships, a certain degree of intraventricular block, for example, developing simultaneously with auriculoventricular block, this is the general sequence of the changes noted.

The relationship of this series of changes to serum potassium concentrations is not an absolutely quantitative one. It can be stated, however, that this is the sequence most likely to occur in response to rising serum concentrations of potassium above the normal. It should be observed that prolongation of the Q–T interval does not occur until a relatively late stage in the development of these definitive patterns has been reached, and it is usually seen in association with intraventricular block. This is an important point to remember in deciding whether the potassium imbalance lies in the direction of too much or too little.

In hypopotassemia, prolongation of the Q–T duration is nearly always present and usually is not accompanied by intraventricular block. When it is so accompanied, certain characteristics of the QRS complexes and the absence of atrial standstill may be of assistance in establishing the proper diagnosis.

Hypopotassemia

Low levels of serum potassium are encountered in diabetic acidosis as a result of increased urinary excretion and migration of the electrolyte from extracellular fluid into body cells. Potassium loss by diuresis, vomiting and diarrhea, or by suction from the gastrointestinal tract, may be sufficient to produce the clinical states described earlier. Hypokalemia may complicate the nephrotic state, especially when ammonium chloride is given as a diuretic. The resulting acidosis and diuresis combine to increase urinary excretion of potassium, while altered respiratory exchange, decreasing from

muscle failure, leads to retention of carbon dioxide and enhances the acidosis.

Excessive amounts of adrenal cortical hormone stimulate urinary excretion of potassium; thus hypokalemia may complicate Cushing's disease and the therapeutic use of cortisone and ACTH—it has been reported following treatment of Addison's disease with desoxycorticosterone acetate. In familial periodic paralysis the essential defect appears to be low serum potassium. The development of hypokalemia in many of the disorders listed here may be accelerated by the additional factor of low potassium intake as a sequel of anorexia.

The progression of electrocardiographic patterns described in association with increasingly high serum levels of potassium has already been outlined. Falling levels of potassium below the normal might be expected to produce an equally clear-cut sequence of distinctive patterns in the electrocardiogram. Several characteristics of the electrocardiogram in hypokalemia are of diagnostic value, but no systematic arrangement of these changes to indicate successive degrees of decreasing serum potassium levels has been possible. The work of Bellet and associates* suggests that the etiologic factor is of some specific importance in producing certain changes. In their series U waves were observed less frequently in diabetic acidosis and were a prominent feature in the alkalosis of vomiting. It seems possible that imbalance of electrolytes other than potassium or that factors as yet unknown may influence the electrocardiogram in hypokalemia and distort the quantitative relationship of serum potassium levels to electrocardiographic changes in that disorder. At present it can be said only that prolongation of the Q–T duration bears some rough relationship to the degree of hypopotassemia: difficulties in measuring this interval with accuracy in many instances makes any precise definition of the relationship impossible.

Bellet and associates* have described five electrocardiographic patterns in hypopotassemia. These are summarized as follows: (1) depression of the S–T segment accompanied by lengthening of the Q–T duration; (2) T wave inversion accompanied by prolongation of Q–T duration, with or without U waves; (3)

* Bellet, S., Steiger, W. A., Nadler, C. S., and Gazes, P. C.: Electrocardiographic Patterns in Hypopotassaemia: Observations on 79 Patients. Am. J. M. Sc., *219:* 542, 1950.

upright T waves with prolonged Q–T duration. In many instances the T wave occupies the whole Q–T time; that is, there is no isoelectric period between QRS and T. (4) Very low T waves with large U waves. It may be difficult to measure the Q–T duration in this pattern. (5) T waves normal in amplitude and length followed by large, isolated U waves. Other workers* have described changes in P waves, premature beats and atrioventricular block. It is not necessary to remember this classification in detail, but it serves as a good summary of the important changes to be found in hypokalemic states. It is evident that the important changes to look for are prolongation of the Q–T duration, S–T segment depression, alterations in amplitude, contour, direction and duration of T waves, and prominent U waves. U waves are best seen in the chest leads.

There is another abnormality of the electrocardiogram which we have observed in two cases (Figs. 253, 254). This consists in slurring of the final portion of the QRS complex, just before its junction with the S–T segment; the early part of QRS is little affected. In the first strip in Figure 254 the slurring is so pronounced that the exact point of junction with the S–T segment is difficult to define; this led to a mistaken diagnosis of bundle branch block in this case, although the diagnosis of hypokalemia was made on the appearance of the T waves. This conduction abnormality has not yet been established as indicative of hypokalemia.

Anemia

Electrocardiographic changes described in

* Darrow, D. C., and Pratt, E. L.: Fluid Therapy. J.A.M.A., *143*: 432, 1950.

association with anemia are nonspecific, and include S–T segment depressions and low to inverted T waves. Because severe anemia may produce functional alteration in heart muscle, with dilatation and even congestive failure, one might expect to see an electrocardiographic abnormality produced by severe anemia. However, this is not always the case. The electrocardiogram may be normal under those circumstances.

Amyloidosis

Some pathologic processes characterized by deposit of "foreign" substances in tissue also involve the heart. Hemochromatosis and amyloidosis are examples of such disorders, in which the deposit of ferrous compounds and amyloid respectively are associated with changes in structure and function of heart muscle. Involvement in this fashion may lead to cardiac dilatation and failure, and possibly to interference with the atrioventricular and intraventricular conduction mechanisms. Amyloidosis secondary to chronic infection (tuberculosis, osteomyelitis) most often involves the liver, spleen and kidneys, while so-called "primary" amyloidosis involves the heart, smooth muscle of the upper gastrointestinal tract, and striped muscle of the larynx and tongue in varying degrees. The electrocardiographic pattern is not specific, but often suggests extensive damage to the myocardium.

It is of considerable importance to note that the Congo red test in primary amyloidosis is usually within normal limits, presumably because the substance deposited is different from that encountered in secondary amyloidosis and does not take up the dye.

A—December 15, 1949—3:30 P.M.

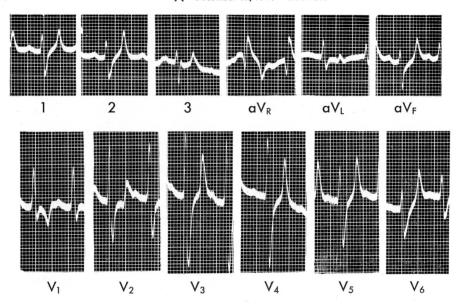

B—December 15, 1949—11 P.M.

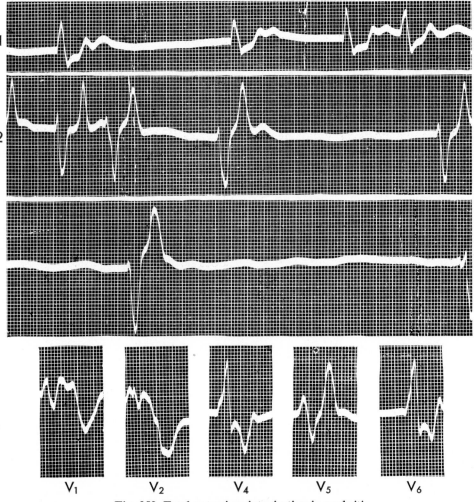

Fig. 252. Fatal potassium intoxication in nephritis.

(See facing page for legend.)

(Legend continued from opposite page, Figure 252)

Hyperpotassemia in nephritis in a four year old boy who was admitted to the hospital on December 9, 1949, with the symptom of dribbling of urine in the daytime for a period of one year. Physical examination revealed little except retarded growth and questionable icterus of the skin. There was no edema. The blood pressure was 110 mm. of mercury systolic and 70 mm. diastolic. Repeated urine examinations showed consistent acid reaction, low specific gravity (1.010 at the highest), 2-plus albumin, and gross pyuria. Urine cultures were positive for Streptococcus beta-hemolyticus.

The first clinical impression was pyelonephritis or possibly polycystic disease of the kidneys, and the patient was placed on a diet high in carbohydrates and fat, and low in protein. Blood chemical studies on December 12, 1949, showed the nonprotein nitrogen to be 100 mg. per cent; sodium, 127.4 milliequivalents per liter; chlorides, 96 milliequivalents per liter; carbon dioxide, 17 milliequivalents per liter; potassium, 3.9 milliequivalents per liter. On December 15 the patient became drowsy and by late afternoon was stuporous. His respirations were sighing in nature. He was given an intravenous solution of 5 per cent dextrose in water and put in an oxygen tent, but died at midnight. Postmortem examination revealed hydronephrosis with dilatation of the ureters, hypertrophy of the bladder, and chronic bilateral pyelonephritis.

INTERPRETATION. *A* (December 15, 1949—3:30 P.M.), Sinus rhythm at a rate averaging 120 with *P–R* interval of 0.20, prolonged for this age. (The *P–R* interval of 0.30 second in Lead aV$_L$ is apparent only. Actually, what looks like a *P* wave is a small sharp *T*.) The *QRS* complexes are wide, measuring up to 0.14 second, with slurred and depressed *S–T* segments. The *T* waves are high with narrow bases.

B (December 15, 1949—11:30 P. M.), Grossly irregular rhythm proceeding almost to standstill in Lead 3. No atrial activity is evident. The *QRS* complexes are wide. The *T* waves are large and of varying width.

COMMENT. This patient had hydronephrosis with chronic pyelonephritis, acidosis, nitrogen retention, and hyperpotassemia. While potassium values were normal up to December 12, three days before death, the first electrocardiogram taken on the day of death suggested a high value of serum potassium. The final serum potassium level, at the time of the last tracing, was 9.1 milliequivalents per liter. In this patient with grave renal disease, the final progression of hyperpotassemia was rapid, accentuated by potassium retention from failing renal function and possibly by increased potassium intake in the form of orange juice during his hospital stay. No potassium salts were given therapeutically.

These electrocardiograms demonstrate a typical progression of pattern in potassium intoxication. Tracing *A* shows an atrioventricular conduction defect, narrow pointed *T* waves and wide *QRS* complexes, with slurred and depressed *S–T* intervals. The final tracing, *B*, taken forty-five minutes before death, showed the terminal state of potassium intoxication with deformed complexes of ventricular origin, high *T* waves, and no atrial activity.

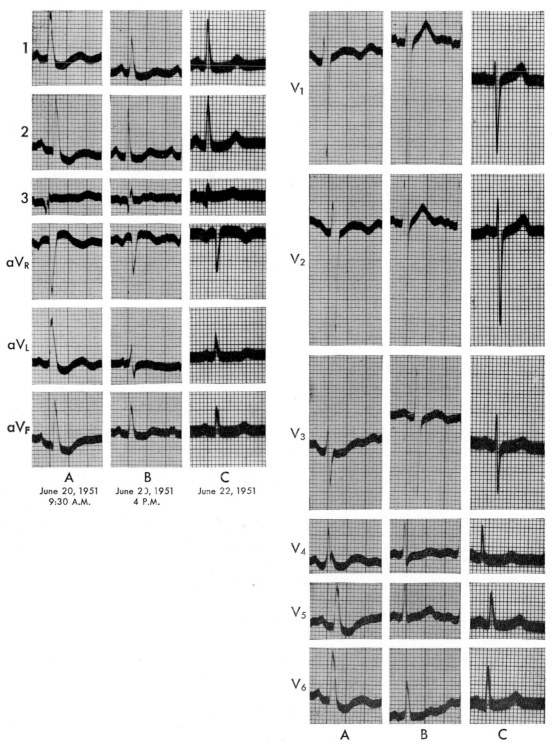

Fig. 253. Hypopotassemia in the nephrotic syndrome.

(*See facing page for legend.*)

(*Legend continued from opposite page, Figure 253*)

Hypopotassemia in the nephrotic syndrome in a fifty-one year old housewife who exhibited the first signs of fluid retention after 1939, seven years after an attack of scarlet fever. Treatment was begun with confirmation of the diagnosis in 1944. This produced temporary relief, but in 1945 she was again hospitalized because of increasing fluid retention. After treatment with a low sodium diet, mercurial diuretics, concentrated human serum albumin, and gum acacia, her fluid retention was reasonably well controlled. For the year preceding her most recent hospital admission on June 19, 1951, she had continued the program of salt restriction, ammonium chloride, 6 to 9 gm. daily, and weekly injections of mercurial diuretics. During the month preceding this admission she had become weak, anorexia had developed, and she had eaten very little. However, the ammonium chloride had been continued.

On admission to the hospital she showed almost total paralysis of the extremity and neck muscles; this paralysis had developed within a period of twenty-four hours. Blood chemistry values on admission were as follows: sodium, 143.6 milliequivalents per liter; chloride, 120 milliequivalents per liter; potassium, 2.5 milliequivalents per liter; carbon dioxide, 10.6 milliequivalents per liter; calcium, 8.9 mg. per cent; nonprotein nitrogen, 47 mg. per cent. After eight hours of treatment with intravenous potassium chloride and sodium lactate, her serum potassium on June 20 dropped to 1.6 milliequivalents per liter. Respiratory paralysis developed, and she was placed in a respirator. Intravenous administration of potassium chloride was increased at that time. Eight hours later she had recovered the use of her arms and legs, and was breathing without difficulty. On June 22 the blood chemistry values were as follows: sodium, 135.6 milliequivalents per liter; chloride, 101 milliequivalents per liter; carbon dioxide, 25.5 milliequivalents per liter; potassium, 4 milliequivalents per liter. This patient has never shown evidence of significant nitrogen retention. Her blood pressure has averaged 150 mm. of mercury systolic and 90 mm. diastolic.

INTERPRETATION. *A* (June 20, 1951—9:30 A.M.), Sinus rhythm at a rate of 85, with P–R interval of 0.16 second. The T waves in Leads 2 and aV_F and in all the chest leads are low in amplitude. S–T segment depression is marked in Leads 1, 2, aV_L, aV_F, V_5 and V_6. The Q–T duration is difficult to measure with precision, but probably averages 0.44 second (upper limit of normal for this heart rate = 0.37 second). Prominent U waves are seen in the chest leads. The QRS complexes are somewhat widened, but the longest interval is 0.1 second; the final portion of the QRS complex is slurred.

B (June 20, 1951—4 P.M.), Sinus rhythm at a rate of 100. The T waves in all leads are low. The Q–T duration is 0.36 second (upper limit of normal for this heart rate = 0.35 second). Small U waves are seen in the chest leads.

C (June 22, 1951), Sinus rhythm at a rate of 75, with P–R interval of 0.12 second; T waves of normal amplitude in the classical leads, rather low in the chest leads V_3 through V_6. The Q–T duration averages 0.39 second (upper limit of normal for this heart rate = 0.39).

COMMENT. The rapid development of a critical state of hypopotassemia in this patient can be attributed to several factors. The acidosis produced by ammonium chloride and the presence of a tubular renal lesion predisposed to loss of potassium, while anorexia cut down the oral intake of this ion. Acidosis was enhanced by carbon dioxide retention resulting from respiratory failure.

This sequence of electrocardiograms illustrates the classical electrocardiographic changes encountered in low potassium states. The characteristic features include S–T segment depression, diminution in amplitude and increase in duration of T waves, and the presence of U waves. The last tracing shows a return to a more normal pattern. Although the Q–T duration looks longer in this tracing, the heart rate is slower, and the Q–T time is just within normal limits. However, low calcium (7.3 mg. per cent on June 21) may have been responsible for prolongation of the Q–T time to the upper limit of normal, without significant S–T or T deviation: the long S–T segment suggests this.

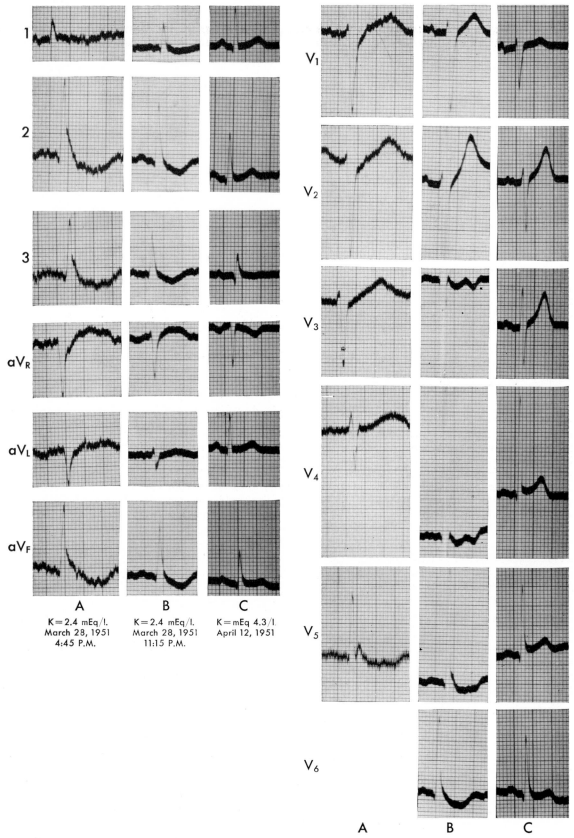

Fig. 254. Hypopotassemia in diabetic acidosis.

(*See facing page for legend.*)

(*Legend continued from opposite page, Figure 254*)

Hypopotassemia in diabetes in a fifty year old unemployed diabetic man who was admitted to the hosptial on March 28, 1951, in diabetic coma. He responded well to therapy and was discharged on April 20. On admission the degree of dehydration was extreme. At the end of six hours of treatment the acidosis improved and hydration was satisfactory. However, the potassium level at that time was only 1.5 milliequivalents per liter.

INTERPRETATION. *A* (March 28, 1951—4:45 P.M.), Sinus rhythm at a rate of 60, with *P–R* interval of 0.18 second. The *T* waves show a broad base occupying most of the *Q–T* duration. *S–T* segments are difficult to define because of slurring heart rate = 0.42 second).

B (March 28, 1951—11:15 P.M.), Sinus rhythm at a rate of 85, with *P–R* interval of 0.18 second. The *T* waves are low to inverted in the standard leads, upright in V_1, V_2, low and diphasic in V_3 through V_6. The *QRS* complexes show slight terminal slurring, especially in Leads V_5 and V_6. The *Q–T* duration measures 0.44 second (upper limit of normal for this heart rate = 0.36 second).

C (April 12, 1951), Normal electrocardiogram, with *QRS* and *T* waves normal in duration, amplitude and direction.

COMMENT. This sequence of tracings demonstrates the development of hypopotassemia in diabetic acidosis. Low serum potassium levels result from massive diuresis, low potassium intake, and shift of potassium into the cells in response to glucose and insulin therapy. The interesting characteristics of these electrocardiograms include (1) long *Q–T* duration with *T* waves occupying most of the *Q–T* period, and (2) slurring of the terminal portion of the *QRS* (mentioned in the introduction to this section), especially marked in tracings *A* and *B*. This slurring led to an erroneous diagnosis of bundle branch block at first. The return of the patterns to normal with replacement of potassium is of special interest. It is also of interest to observe that tracing *A*, taken four hours after the onset of therapy, shows the abnormal characteristics to a greater degree than does tracing *B*, which was taken ten hours after the beginning of therapy. Although the serum potassium levels were the same at both times, it is probable that the tissue cell level of potassium had risen.

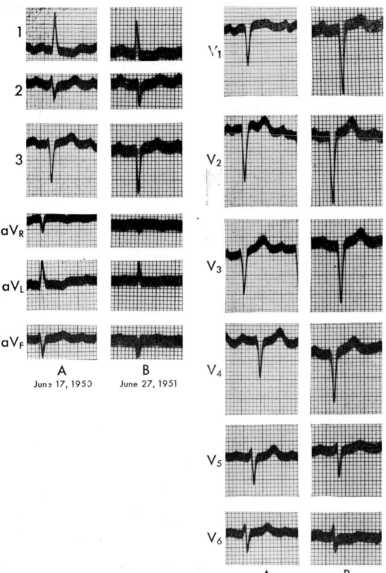

A June 17, 1950 **B** June 27, 1951

Fig. 255. Pernicious anemia.

Pernicious anemia in a sixty-three year old housewife who entered the hospital on June 16, 1950, with a history of anorexia, weight loss and vague abdominal discomfort. On admission she looked extremely pale and ill. Her blood pressure was 160 mm. of mercury systolic and 50 mm. diastolic. The heart was enlarged to percussion. A definite diastolic gallop rhythm was heard at the apex. Examination of the blood revealed the hemoglobin to be 4 gm., white blood cell count 4000 per cu. mm., and the differential count normal. The smear showed considerable variation in size of red cells with many macrocytes. Nucleated red cells were present. The chest film showed diffuse cardiac enlargement with a transverse cardiac diameter of 15 cm., in comparison with an internal diameter of the thorax measuring 25 cm.

Because of the cardiac findings the patient was digitalized on the third hospital day. On the basis of the blood smear, a diagnosis of pernicious anemia was made and treatment was started. On liver therapy the level of hemoglobin gradually increased. A check-up one year later showed a hemoglobin of 13.7 gm. There were no murmurs or gallop present.

INTERPRETATION. *A* (June 17, 1950). Sinus rhythm at a rate of 100; *P–R* interval equal to 0.2 second (slightly prolonged for this heart rate); low *T* waves in Lead 1 with sagging *S–T* segments; upright *T* waves in the chest leads V_1 through V_6, and inverted *T* waves in aV_L.

B (June 27, 1951). Comparison with the first tracing shows little change in standard leads or precordial leads, except for slightly increased amplitude of the *QRS* complexes.

COMMENT. With rise in the hemoglobin level following treatment of pernicious anemia, the patient's functional cardiac status improved considerably, and the heart size decreased. It is interesting to observe that practically no change took place in the electrocardiogram after recovery of normal function (tracing *B*). It was at first thought that these changes could have been due to anemia; it is possible that they are on the basis of chronic coronary artery disease.

(We are indebted to Dr. John T. Quinby of Boston for permission to use this case history.)

(Legend continued from facing page, Figure 256)

COMMENT. In this case of proved amyloidosis involving the heart, minor abnormalities of *T* waves and *QRS* complexes are present in the first tracing. In the second tracing, atrioventricular and bundle branch block are the important abnormalities. This pattern can be explained by involvement of myocardium, coronary vessels and possibly the conduction system by the destructive process of amyloidosis. What part, if any, was played by atherosclerosis in the production of heart block was not determined at autopsy. In any case, cardiac enlargement and congestive failure may be attributed to amyloidosis of the myocardium with involvement of the valves as a possible added factor.

In this patient the apparent predominance of elevation of the systemic venous pressure over that in the pulmonary vessels may be explained as a possible result of three factors: (1) generalized involvement of all the myocardium; (2) predominant deformity of the tricuspid valve; (3) rigidity of the heart muscle infiltrated with amyloid. This has produced a syndrome indistinguishable clinically from constrictive pericarditis. Rigidity of muscle wall is thought to interfere with diastolic filling. This is the basic underlying fault in constrictive pericarditis.

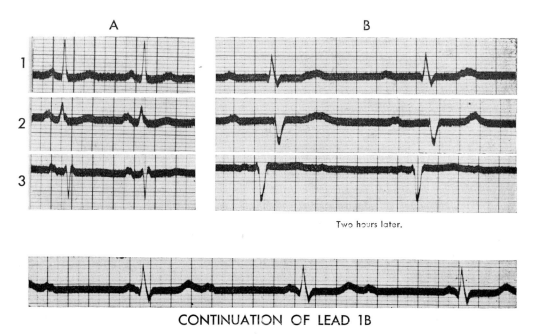

A	B
1	1
2	2
3	3

Two hours later.

CONTINUATION OF LEAD 1B

Fig. 256. Amyloidosis.

Primary amyloidosis in a fifty-nine year old man who began to notice fatigue, eructation and hoarseness two years before admission to the hospital. One year before admission a gastrointestinal series showed sluggish peristalsis and an ulcer of the first portion of the duodenum. Nine months before admission another gastrointestinal series showed a constant projection on the lesser curvature of the stomach in the prepyloric region. Examination of the larynx revealed thickening of the vocal cords. A biopsy was reported as showing "inflammatory tissue." At this time the patient began to notice dyspnea on effort. Two months before admission 2:1 block was reported in the electrocardiogram.

On admission to the hospital (August 9, 1945) physical examination revealed the pulse regular at 48, blood pressure 100 mm. of mercury systolic and 60 mm. diastolic. There was marked distention of the veins over the face, neck, arms, chest and abdomen. The heart was enlarged, with the apex lying 2 cm. to the left of the midclavicular line. Heart sounds were distant, with the pulmonary second sound greater than the aortic second sound. A systolic murmur was heard, Grade 1 in intensity in the aortic area and Grade 2 at the cardiac apex. A mid-diastolic rumble without presystolic accentuation was also heard at the apex. The lungs were clear. The liver was enlarged, extending 2 cm. below the costal margin in the midclavicular line. The spleen was not felt, and no masses were palpable. Pitting edema was present over the extremities. The voice was hoarse.

X-ray examination of the chest revealed well marked enlargement of the heart shadow with poor ventricular pulsations. No pericardial calcification was seen. Vascular shadows in the lungs were increased, and a small amount of pleural fluid was present bilaterally. Repeated gastrointestinal series revealed obstruction in the region of the pylorus or duodenum, but structural details could not be made out.

Examination of the urine showed nothing remarkable, and examination of the blood revealed only hypochromic anemia of slight degree.

The patient responded well to routine therapy of congestive heart failure. During the fourth hospital week several irregular masses were seen below the vocal cords by direct examination with the laryngoscope. One of these was biopsied and reported as amyloidosis of the larynx.

With this evidence it was felt that a diagnosis of primary amyloidosis could explain involvement of the stomach and duodenum as well as the cardiac findings of enlargement, congestive failure and atrioventricular block. Two negative Congo red tests were not considered conclusive evidence against the diagnosis.

The patient was discharged somewhat improved on October 5, 1945, to the care of his physician.*

The clinical course began a downward trend shortly after discharge, and the patient died a month later after operation for relief of pyloric obstruction. On postmortem examination, extensive amyloidosis of the heart, tongue, epiglottis, larynx, stomach and intestines was found. The serous surfaces of the pericardium, pleura and peritoneum were heavily involved. Amyloidosis in the myocardium was extensive, as expected, and, in addition, all heart valves, especially the tricuspid, were deformed. Little involvement of the parenchymatous organs was evident.

INTERPRETATION. A (August 9, 1945). This tracing, taken the day after admission, shows normal sinus rhythm at a rate of 80 with P–R interval of 0.13 second. The T waves in Leads 1 and 2 are upright. The T in Lead 3 is flat. The QRS complexes are slurred and rather broad, measuring 0.1 second in Lead 3.

B (August 9, 1945). Two hours later. This tracing, taken because of a sudden drop in heart rate, shows 2:1 atrioventricular block with P–R interval of conducted complexes varying from 0.12 second to 0.40 second. Alteration in QRS complexes, with duration increased to 0.12 second and appearance of S waves in Lead 1, suggests right bundle branch block. The T waves are upright in Leads 1 and 2, low in Lead 3. *(Legend continued on opposite page)*

* We are indebted to Dr. Frank T. Fulton of Providence, Rhode Island, who referred the patient to one of us (PDW) and later provided information about the autopsy findings.

PART VIII

Electrocardiograms for Practice in Interpretation

Fig. 257.

INTERPRETATION. Normal rhythm, rate 75, considerable left axis deviation with deep S waves in Leads V_1, V_2 and V_3, high R waves in Leads 1, V_4, V_5 and V_6, and inverted T waves in Leads 1, aV_L, V_4, V_5 and V_6.

CLINICAL FINDINGS. J.G., an unemployed man of fifty-nine years, entered the hospital for study after three episodes of precordial pain with radiation down both arms, coming on after effort and disappearing with rest. The day of admission he had an attack of this pain, which he described as "pinching" in character, which lasted for five minutes without radiation. It was accompanied by a feeling of weakness and coldness (but no sweating) and nausea without vomiting; it was followed by loss of consciousness for two or three minutes. When he regained consciousness, the pain was gone. For ten years he had had known hypertension, and for the past eight years the intermittent "pinching" pain over the precordium, following exertion, radiating down both arms, and relieved by rest. Seven months before the present episode a perforated peptic ulcer had been found upon operation, with relief of epigastric pain which he had experienced over the previous ten years; this pain had recurred, however, two months before the present hospital entry.

On physical examination his blood pressure was found to be 190 mm. of mercury systolic and 90 mm. diastolic. The heart was enlarged. Grades 1 and 2 systolic murmurs were heard at the aortic area and apex respectively; there was a questionable Grade 1 diastolic murmur at the aortic area and along the left sternal border. A gastrointestinal series demonstrated an ulcer crater in the duodenum. The white blood cell count was 7800 per cu. mm. A Hinton test was reported negative. X-ray examination of the chest showed clear lung fields and a greatly enlarged heart, with a cardiothoracic ratio of 17.5:28.5. The aorta was tortuous. The electrocardiogram presented here was taken the day after admission and showed no change from an emergency recording made the day he came into the hospital. He was not taking digitalis.

COMMENT. This record is absolutely characteristic of marked left ventricular enlargement, more commonly seen in hypertensive heart disease than in any other condition. There happens to be in this case, in addition to chronic hypertension, clinical evidence of coronary insufficiency, but the electrocardiogram does not show any indication thereof.

Fig. 258.

INTERPRETATION. Normal rhythm, rate 95, high R and inverted T waves in Leads 1, 2, V_4, V_5 and V_6 and deep S waves in Leads V_1, V_2 and V_3 indicative of left ventricular enlargement.

CLINICAL FINDINGS. S.R., a housewife of fifty-six years, came in for examination in October, 1949, because of recurring episodes of fainting over the past year. At the age of eight she had had rheumatic fever, with a heart murmur from that time. During the past year she had experienced four attacks of syncope characterized by a feeling of tightness in her chest and light-headedness, culminating in unconsciousness which lasted for several minutes and was followed by light-headedness and blurring of speech. Between attacks she had been well, without substernal oppression or other difficulty.

Upon physical examination there was found to be a harsh, Grade 4, aortic systolic murmur heard as far as the apex and axilla. There was a systolic thrill in the aortic area. The heart rhythm was regular at a rate of 85. The liver was slightly enlarged, and the spleen was palpable. There was no jaundice. The blood pressure was 125 mm. of mercury systolic and 85 mm. diastolic. By orthodiagram the heart measured 12 cm., with an internal thoracic diameter of 22 cm.; the left ventricle was moderately enlarged.

The electrocardiogram shown here was taken on April 13, 1950, at the time of a check-up examination. In the interim nasal congestion had developed, with a loose cough, daily raising of bloody sputum, and an occasional night sweat. There had been no jaundice and no fainting, but slight effort would produce dyspnea and substernal constriction, and the patient had tended to wheeze at night. She had lost 5 pounds. Physical examination, fluoroscopy and electrocardiogram revealed the same findings as before. There was no congestion of the veins, lungs or liver. She had been taking digitoxin daily. Studies to determine the cause of the hemoptysis were undertaken promptly, and bronchoscopy a few days later revealed left bronchial stenosis of unknown cause.

COMMENT. This record reveals a characteristic pattern of left ventricular hypertrophy which could be due to any factor causing great strain on the left ventricle; the most common causes of such strain are hypertension and aortic valve disease. In this case a high degree of aortic stenosis was responsible for this particular pattern and probably also for the syncopal attacks.

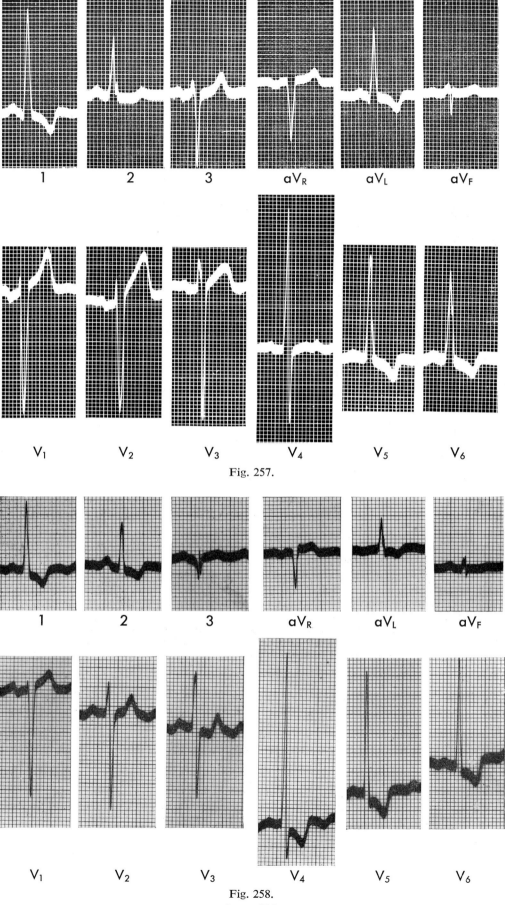

Fig. 257.

Fig. 258.

Fig. 259.

INTERPRETATION. Normal rhythm, rate 65 to 75, with prominent Q waves in Leads 2, 3, aV_F and V_6, depressed $S-T$ segments in Leads 1 and aV_L and elevated $S-T$ segments and inverted T waves in Leads 2, 3, aV_F, V_5 and V_6.

CLINICAL FINDINGS. R.H., a fifty year old tailor, entered the hospital May 27, 1949, after twenty-four hours of severe chest discomfort, initiated by a crushing substernal pain which was felt across the upper anterior chest, but did not radiate. The pain lasted about two hours. The following day, while he was working at his desk, there was a recurrence of crushing pain which extended to his jaw. This time the pain lasted about six hours, until he was given Demerol with relief. He had noted three "dizzy spells" during the second attack. On the day of admission the pain occurred repeatedly; its duration varied, and he suffered some discomfort between the attacks. A fever had developed. The past history included varicose veins of the right leg, with ligation of the long saphenous in 1941, and intermittent claudication from 1942, increasing until March, 1949, when he stopped smoking. Three or four years before the present episode he had had, while lifting a desk, an attack of shortness of breath with wheezing and chest discomfort. This lasted about one and a half hours, but had not recurred.

On physical examination he was found to be slightly obese and rather pale. There was no venous distention and no edema. Respirations were rapid and shallow, and there was slight orthopnea. The blood pressure was 96 mm. of mercury systolic and 60 mm. diastolic. The heart appeared to be enlarged to percussion, with sounds of poor quality, including a split first sound. No murmurs were heard. The rate was slow at 56, with a slightly irregular rhythm. The sedimentation rate on admission was 34 mm. in one hour, photoelectric hemoglobin 13.6 gm., and white blood cell count 16,900 per cu. mm.

The electrocardiogram shown here was taken on May 28. A course of Dicumarol was instituted, and recovery was uneventful. He was discharged home improved on June 26.

COMMENT. This record is characteristic, in fact pathognomonic, of acute posterolateral infarction of the left ventricle.

Fig. 260.

INTERPRETATION. Normal rhythm, rate 85, with prominent Q waves in Leads 1, aV_L, V_4 and V_5, small R_1, absent R in V_4, elevated $S-T$ segments in Leads 1 and V_5, sagging $S-T$ segments in Leads 2, 3 and V_6, and low T waves in the limb leads, with inversion in V_5 and V_6.

CLINICAL FINDINGS. C.M., a fifty-four year old restaurant owner, had been hospitalized after extensive anterior myocardial infarction in November, 1943. This was complicated on the thirteenth hospital day by embolism to the left femoral artery, for which an embolectomy was performed. He was checked thereafter first at monthly, then at bimonthly intervals. Dyspnea and occasional chest pain persisted, but he improved slowly on a regimen of daily digitalis and ammonium chloride. Two years after his myocardial infarction he was doing well except for mild angina pectoris, for which he used nitroglycerin when necessary. On the third anniversary of his hospital admission he reported that walking in the cold weather regularly produced substernal discomfort. Four years after the myocardial infarction pulsus alternans developed, and he appeared to be on the edge of congestive failure, but continued to get along without too much trouble.

Physical examination in March, 1949, revealed a regular pulse rate of 80, a blood pressure of 130 mm. of mercury systolic and 80 mm. diastolic. There was no engorgement of the neck veins. The heart sounds were good. There was a Grade 3 apical systolic murmur and a slight apical protodiastolic gallop. By fluoroscopy the heart was found to be enlarged; the lungs were clear.

On April 29, 1949, at the time the electrocardiogram shown here was taken, there had been no significant change in his cardiac status.

COMMENT. This record is entirely in keeping with chronic myocardial infarction involving the anterior wall of the left ventricle. Evidently the scar and continued coronary insufficiency, as indicated by the persistent angina pectoris, have had a deleterious effect on the myocardial reserve, as shown by the findings of pulsus alternans and apical protodiastolic gallop rhythm.

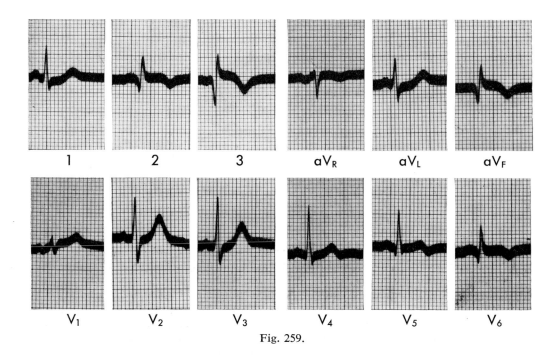

Fig. 259.

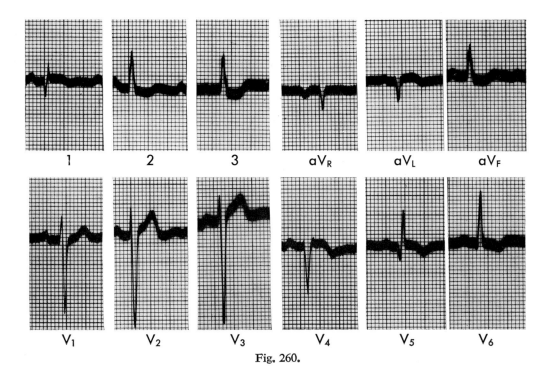

Fig. 260.

Fig. 261.

INTERPRETATION. Normal rhythm, rate 100, right axis deviation with upright T waves in all leads except aV_R. The precordial leads are all normal.

CLINICAL FINDINGS. A.S., an active young woman of eighteen, came in for an opinion as to the significance of a precordial systolic murmur which had been discovered at the age of twelve years after two episodes of faintness. She had been well and athletic as a child, but at the age of eleven had had several rather severe sore throats. One of the heart specialists who saw her when she was twelve considered that she might have a patent ductus arteriosus; two other consultants disagreed with this diagnosis. She had been well thereafter, but somewhat restricted as to her activity because of the questionable significance of the heart murmur.

On physical examination she was found to be tall and of slender build. She looked well and had a good color. There was no cyanosis or finger clubbing. There were no abnormal pulsations in the neck, and no palpable thrills. The heart sounds were of good quality. The pulmonary second sound was slightly accentuated. In the upright position, varying but not completely disappearing with respiration, was a slight, Grade 1 systolic murmur, heard in the precordial area as far as the apex and along the left border of the heart. The murmur was unchanged in the recumbent position and after exercise; there was a slight third sound. No diastolic murmurs were heard. The heart action was regular at 80. The blood pressure was 125 mm. of mercury systolic and 80 mm. diastolic. By fluoroscopy the heart was normal in size and vertically placed in the chest. Its transverse diameter was 9.5 cm., with an internal thoracic diameter of 21 cm. There was no fullness of the left atrium in the oblique view, and the pulmonary root shadows were normal.

COMMENT. Both physical examination and electrocardiography indicate the probability, though not certainty, of a normal heart, despite the slight murmur (probably physiologic) which has been heard for years. Her build with vertical heart readily accounts for the considerable right axis deviation in the limb leads; the precordial leads are well within normal limits, showing no evidence of right ventricular enlargement.

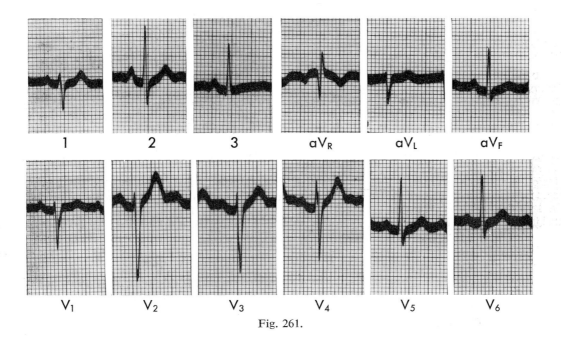

1   2   3   aV_R   aV_L   aV_F

V₁   V₂   V₃   V₄   V₅   V₆

Fig. 261.

Fig. 262.

INTERPRETATION. Regular tachycardia at an extreme rate of 230, probably paroxysmal atrial tachycardia, possibly atrial flutter with 1:1 rhythm. The record is not otherwise remarkable, although there are prominent S waves in Leads V_4 and V_6, as well as in Lead V_2.

CLINICAL FINDINGS. L.S., a forty-three year old department head of a printing company, was admitted to the hospital on January 28, 1949. At the time of an office examination a few hours before, he had appeared extremely ill, vomiting and in a state of semicollapse, with a heart rate of over 200 per minute. The electrocardiogram shown here was taken at this time. The patient was given 0.1 gm. of quinidine lactate intramuscularly, with reversion to normal rhythm about two hours later. Because he appeared to be much sicker than could be accounted for by the tachycardia alone, and because of an old history of hypertension and possibly old coronary thrombosis, it was thought that he might be having another coronary attack. The characteristic pain was not present, however.

Physical examination after entry to the hospital revealed a thready pulse at a rate of 100. There were hypertensive changes in the fundi, and the blood pressure was 160 mm. of mercury systolic and 120 mm. diastolic.

On the following day an electrocardiogram, which proved quite different from one taken two years before, demonstrated inverted T waves in Leads 1, aV_L, V_4 and V_6. A white blood cell count on this date was 9000 per cu. mm. A further electrocardiogram on January 31 showed more normal T waves. The patient was discharged home on February 1. One week later, upon the occasion of a second office visit, his blood pressure was 120 mm. systolic and 70 mm. diastolic.

COMMENT. There is no proof of heart disease in this record, simply evidence of an irritability which could, of course, be superimposed on chronic heart disease not apparent in this electrocardiogram. The later inversion of the T waves with normal rhythm can be ascribed to "myocardial fatigue" (secondary to the excessive tachycardia) whether or not heart disease was present.

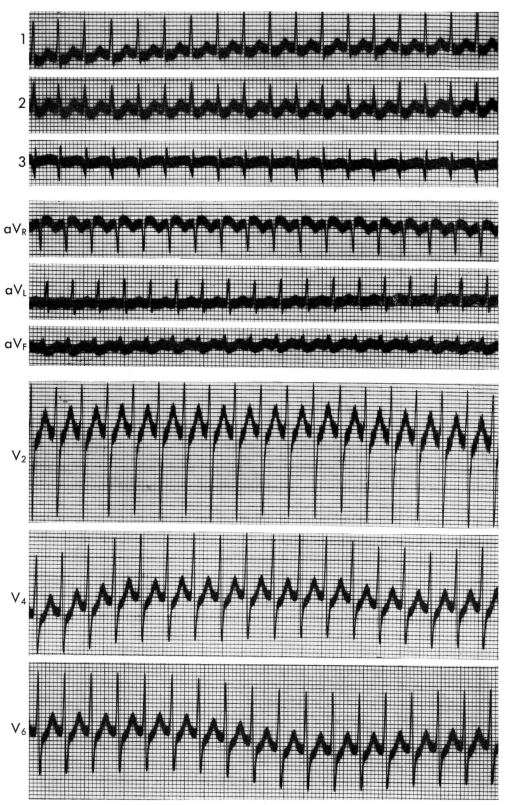

Fig. 262.

Fig. 263.

INTERPRETATION. Sinus rhythm at an average rate of 100; *P–R* interval of 0.16 second. The *T* waves in all leads are diphasic in character, possibly combined with ill defined *U* waves. The *Q–T* duration is difficult to measure exactly, but is obviously prolonged, occupying most of diastole. The *S–T* segments show slight depression, especially in the chest leads.

CLINICAL FINDINGS. L.S., a thirty-six year old housewife, was first admitted to the hospital in December, 1949, with paralysis of the legs and arms for a period of four days. At that time a diagnosis of alkali-losing nephritis with associated hypokalemia was made. She was thought to have a predominantly tubular lesion with good glomerular function, in view of the fact that her nonprotein nitrogen remained at normal levels with a low urine concentration and a high output. Urinalysis consistently revealed albumin, with little in the way of formed elements in the sediment. After correction of her electrolyte balance she did well until May 3, 1950, when she was again admitted to the hospital with a two-day history of malaise, occasional vomiting, and polyuria.

Physical examination at the time of this second hospital admission showed a moderately sick woman, with a pulse rate of 80 and a blood pressure of 120 mm. of mercury systolic and 85 mm. diastolic. Except for a chronic post-thrombotic syndrome in the right leg, her examination, including the deep tendon reflexes, was essentially negative. Blood chemistry values on admission were as follows: sodium, 144 milliequivalents per liter; chlorides, 109 milliequivalents per liter; carbon dioxide 13.3 milliequivalents per liter; potassium, 1.7 milliequivalents per liter; nonprotein nitrogen, 24 mg. per cent. The electrocardiogram shown here was taken on May 5, 1950.

After treatment with oral solutions containing the necessary electrolytes, she responded satisfactorily.

COMMENT. This tracing with obviously prolonged *Q–T* durations and depressed *S–T* segments is suggestive of hypopotassemia. Chemical determination of the serum level (potassium, 1.7 milliequivalents per liter) confirmed the diagnosis. A careful review of this patient's interval therapy before her last hospital admission showed that the potassium intake had been low. This factor, combined with potassium loss through the kidneys, produced the syndrome of hypopotassemia.

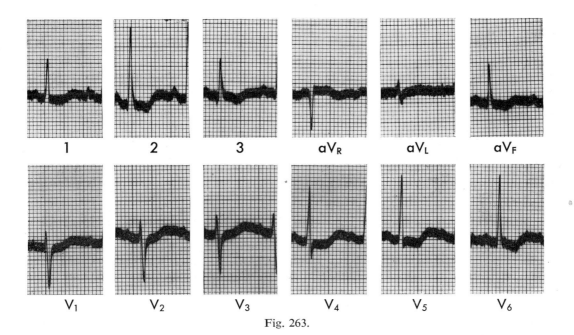

1   2   3   aV_R   aV_L   aV_F

V₁   V₂   V₃   V₄   V₅   V₆

Fig. 263.

Fig. 264.

INTERPRETATION. Partial atrioventricular block varying from the grade of 2:1 to that of 3:2. Atrial rate 80; ventricular rate varies from 40 to 54. Prominent Q waves in Leads 2, 3 and aV_F. Slight elevation of $S-T$ segments in Leads 2 and 3. Late cove-plane inversion of T_3.

CLINICAL FINDINGS. W.R., a forty-seven year old salesman, was admitted to the hospital on January 24 by way of the Out Patient Dispensary, where he had presented himself with the complaint of heavy substernal pain which had come on that morning and had lasted for several hours. The pain was accompanied by radiation to the neck and was associated with weakness, sweating and a feeling of nausea. His past history was noncontributory, and the family history was negative for heart disease. He was given 10 mg. of morphine sulfate intramuscularly with some relief of the discomfort, and an additional dose of 8 mg. two hours later with further relief.

On physical examination after admission his heart rate was found to be regular at 80, the sounds were of fair quality, and there were no murmurs. P_2 was greater than A_2. There was no gallop or rub. Pulsations in the feet were good. The blood pressure was 110 mm. of mercury systolic and 70 mm. diastolic. There was no evidence of congestive failure. His condition continued to be fairly good, despite persistent substernal oppression, unaffected by inhalation of oxygen or by an injection of Demerol.

On January 25 the white blood cell count was 15,600 per cu. mm., photoelectric hemoglobin 14.6, and the prothrombin time 18 seconds. Courses of Dicumarol and of quinidine sulfate were instituted and continued until just before his discharge on February 17. An x-ray film taken three days before he went home showed clear lungs and no enlargement of the heart.

Two days after admission the patient complained of a slight cough and a feeling of palpitation at the upper end of the sternum. The sense of pressure on the chest had disappeared. His blood pressure was 100 mm. systolic and 70 mm. diastolic. On the third day a definite cardiac arrhythmia was present, which is apparent in the electrocardiogram shown here. This tracing revealed further changes in $S-T$ displacement and considerable change in the QRS complexes from the record taken on entry.

COMMENT. Transient heart block is an occasional complication of acute posterior myocardial infarction, which was present in this case. It is due to the fact that the blood supply to the bundle of His is derived largely from either the right coronary artery or the circumflex branch of the left; thrombosis of either of those vessels usually results in a posterior myocardial infarct.

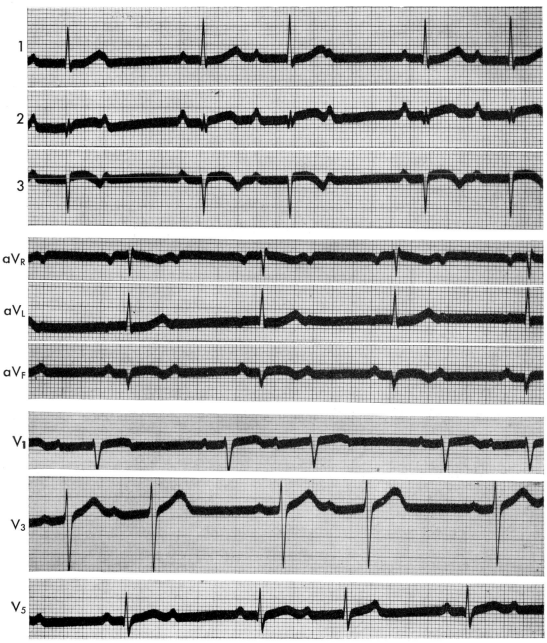

Fig. 264.

Fig. 265.

INTERPRETATION. Regular rhythm, ventricular rate 85 to 90, with ectopic atrial tachycardia (rate 190) and 2:1 atrioventricular block. The P waves are inverted in Lead 1. The blocked P waves are poorly seen in the limb leads, superimposed as they are on the T waves, but they are well made out in the special atrial lead taken in the third intercostal space just to the right of the sternum. The QRS waves are slightly widened (0.11 second).

CLINICAL FINDINGS. M.M., a forty-year old Polish pants-maker, entered the hospital on June 30, 1950, for treatment of congestive heart failure. Eighteen years before, he had undergone a subtotal thyroidectomy, which relieved palpitation and tachycardia of long standing. Eleven years later, with the recurrence of these symptoms and subsequent treatment (quinidine at first and then, more successfully, digitalis), he had been found upon several occasions to have a rapid atrial tachycardia. Upon slowing of the ventricular rate the murmurs of mitral stenosis and regurgitation and slight aortic regurgitation had become apparent. Two and one half months prior to the present illness and after the grippe, he had had a persistent tachycardia, in spite of 0.2 mg. of digitoxin twice daily, and for the past three weeks he had been nauseated, dyspneic and orthopneic, and had had ankle edema. He neither smoked nor used alcohol.

Physical examination on July 1 revealed an obese man, somewhat dyspneic at rest. The neck veins were pulsating just above the clavicles in the upright position. There was slight prominence of the eyes, with lid-lag but no periorbital edema. A well-healed thyroidectomy scar was present; the skin was warm and moist, and there was no tremor. There was some increase in the anteroposterior diameter of the chest, which was clear. The heart was considerably enlarged to the left; the rate was regular at 160. There was a Grade 2 apical systolic murmur. A_2 equaled P_2 and was not accentuated. There was 2 plus edema of the lower legs.

The electrocardiogram shown here was taken on July 5. On this day a total of 3.2 gm. of quinidine had been administered between 10 A.M. and 6 P.M. This tracing was recorded at 5 P.M. after 2.4 gm. By 8 P.M. the ventricular rate had fallen to 80 (atrial tachycardia with 2:1 block electrocardiographically); there were no toxic symptoms. It was concluded that it might be satisfactory to continue with 3 or 4 gm. of quinidine daily and resumption of digitalis and maintenance of other measures for the control of his congestive failure. At the time of discharge on July 12 the presence of masked thyrotoxicosis was still unproved, the possibility existing, but the evidence being against it.

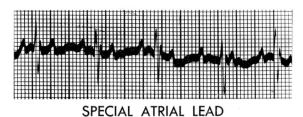

SPECIAL ATRIAL LEAD

COMMENT. Such a record as this of ectopic atrial tachycardia with 2:1 block is not unusual, except that as a rule the abnormal P waves are better seen. The value of the special atrial lead is well illustrated here.

Fig. 266.

INTERPRETATION. Normal rhythm, rate 105 to 110, with low voltage of QRS and T waves throughout except for Leads V_1 and V_2.

CLINICAL FINDINGS. R.B., a nurse aged forty-nine, entered the hospital on June 1, 1950. In 1944 she had undergone a radical mastectomy for carcinoma of the right breast, with subsequent hospitalizations in 1945 for x-ray treatment of recurrent skin nodules in the right supraclavicular region, in 1948 for sterilization by x-ray radiation to the pelvis after pleural effusion due to metastases, and in 1949 for further x-ray therapy of skin nodules. About one month before the present admission she had begun to notice slight dyspnea on exertion and, one week before, a feeling of constriction across the upper abdomen. For the past two days she had had no appetite and had vomited frequently.

On physical examination she was in no acute distress. The chest was dull to percussion, with diminished breath sounds and tactile fremitus in the left chest rising to the sixth interspace. There was no mediastinal shift. The abdomen was not distended, but there was slight, diffuse tenderness, most noticeable over the liver, which appeared to be considerably enlarged. Peristalsis was normal.

An x-ray film showed left pleural effusion and slight effusion on the right, with ascites and a large liver, and obvious increase in the cardiac outline as compared with a chest film taken three months earlier. Paracentesis of the left chest the day after entry yielded 500 cc. of straw-colored fluid, but was stopped at the onset of pulse irregularity and cyanosis. She was very ill for the next few days, and a cardiac consultation was requested on June 8. The electrocardiogram shown here was taken on this same day. Pericardial tamponade appeared to be most likely, and 75 cc. of nonclotting mulberry-colored hemorrhagic fluid were removed from the pericardium.

X-ray therapy was begun again on June 10, followed on June 11 by open thoracotomy, pericardiotomy and punch thoracotomy, with the removal of approximately 300 cc. of bloody fluid. Dyspnea, cyanosis and paradoxical pulse continued. On June 13 she was digitalized and continued on digitoxin until June 27. On June 17 a thoracentesis was done, but no fluid was removed. By July 1 she had improved, and was discharged, somewhat relieved, one week later.

COMMENT. This record is consistent with, in fact, per se suggestive of, pericarditis with effusion (or extensive myocardial disease) without distinction as to etiology. Here the pericardial and pleural lesions responsible for the effusions were the result of metastatic malignancy. Low voltage is common with pericardial effusion, and also with pericardial fibrosis and subjacent myocardial involvement.

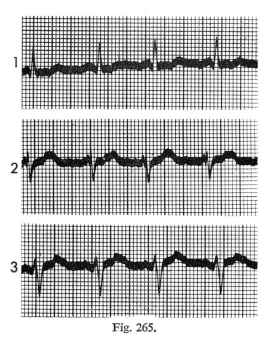

Fig. 265.

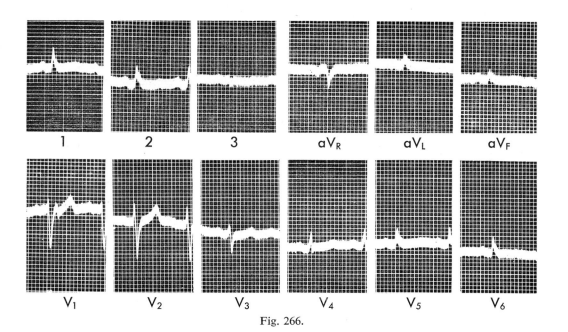

Fig. 266.

Fig. 267.

INTERPRETATION. Normal rhythm, rate 105, extremely high R waves with inverted T waves in Leads 3, aV_F, and V_1 to V_4 inclusive, and prominent S waves in Leads 1, aV_L and V_5 to V_8 inclusive.

CLINICAL FINDINGS. K.DiB., a seven year old girl, was admitted to the hospital on February 4, 1950, for evaluation of a heart murmur. She had had a single episode of cyanosis five days after birth, with elevated temperature and labored respiration. Her mother's pregnancy had been uneventful, and the delivery was full-term. In 1943 the patient had been examined for the complaints of a heart murmur and an imperforate nasolacrimal duct. X-ray film of the chest at that time revealed the heart to be somewhat enlarged to the left, with prominence of the right ventricle. The patient had always been smaller than her playmates and had not played so vigorously as they. She tended to become cyanotic occasionally when cold or when swimming.

Physical examination revealed a well developed, rather small child with strabismus. The front upper incisor teeth were pegged and notched. The blood pressure was 90 mm. of mercury systolic and 60 mm. diastolic in the right arm, 95 mm. systolic and 65 mm. diastolic in the left arm. Upon examination of the heart a Grade 4 systolic murmur was heard over the precordium, most loudly in the third left interspace; it was transmitted to the left axilla and minimally to the neck. There were no diastolic murmurs. A precordial thrill was maximal at the third interspace to the left of the sternum. The liver was palpable 1 to 2 cm. below the costal margin. The spleen descended to the costal margin with inspiration.

X-ray film of the chest a few weeks before was interpreted as showing a greatly enlarged heart, with the left heart border at the left chest wall. It was thought that the left atrium might also be enlarged. It was not possible to identify certainly the aorta or the pulmonary arteries. These findings were considered to be consistent with congenital heart disease of undetermined type. The electrocardiogram taken on February 7 is shown here.

Cardiac catheterization was performed on February 6, and the finding of a significant discrepancy of pressures between the right ventricle and the pulmonary artery was thought to indicate considerable pulmonary stenosis. No other anomalies were defined by the procedure. The patient was discharged on February 8. She was believed to be a suitable candidate for angiocardiography and possibly for pulmonary valvulotomy.

COMMENT. This record demonstrates to an extreme degree the pattern of right ventricular enlargement, greater than in any other record that we can remember. It is confirmatory, though probably not pathognomonic, of a high degree of congenital pulmonary stenosis.

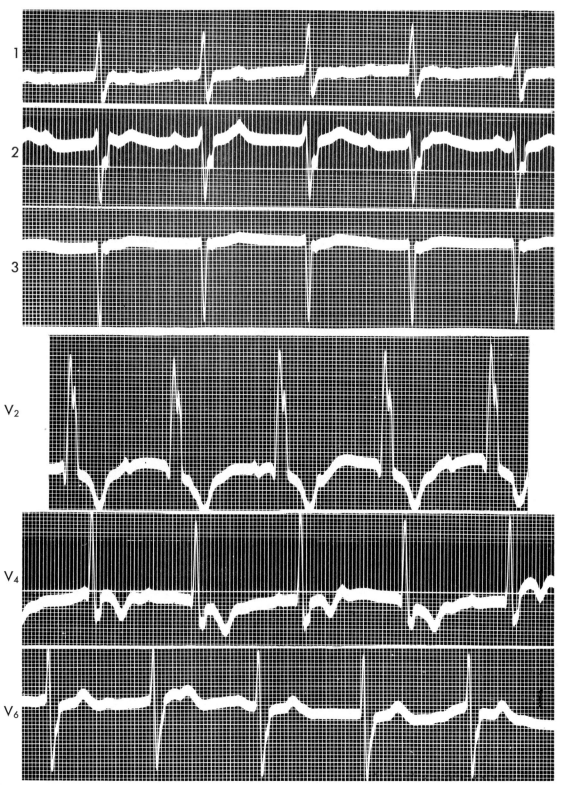

Fig. 268.

Fig. 269.

INTERPRETATION. Normal rhythm and rate in all these records: *A*, control before an exercise test; *B*, immediately after exercise; *C*, control after resting two hours. The tracings in *A* and *C* are essentially normal in all leads except for rather prominent *S* waves over the right side of the precordium (V_1 to V_3 inclusive) and rather high *R* waves over the left side (V_4 to V_6 inclusive).

In *B* there is little or no change in the limb leads from records *A* and *C*, but in the precordial leads there is a striking elevation of the *S–T* segment, most marked in Lead V_4.

CLINICAL FINDINGS. N.McL., a woman of forty-nine and assistant manager of a New York clothing store, entered the hospital on July 3, 1950, for evaluation of brief episodes of chest pain which she had noted since 1943, increasingly over the past several weeks. Examination at the time of their first occurrence had revealed a normal electrocardiogram and no objective findings. Her symptoms were described as a sudden substernal choking, at which time "everything was closing up and I couldn't breathe," accompanied by pain in her left arm. These episodes were sufficiently troublesome for her to stop work for a while in January of 1950, with good results until a few weeks prior to the present admission, when they recurred rather suddenly, coming on while she was at work, upon walking, and during attendance at a ball game. She saw her physician on the morning of July 3, after three severe attacks, and an electrocardiogram at this time demonstrated depression of the *RS–T* segments in Leads 2, 3 and aV_F, which was not present in the tracing taken in 1943. One episode occurring in the doctor's office was relieved by 0.03 mg. of nitroglycerin. However, their brief duration of one to three minutes made it difficult to evaluate the efficacy of the nitroglycerin in stopping the attacks. They were unaccompanied by digestive symptoms and apparently unrelated to body position. Past history included three operations—appendectomy (1917), left ovariectomy and right salpingectomy (1930), and the removal of fibroids with adhesions (1945). The family history was noncontributory.

Physical examination revealed a well developed, well nourished woman, experiencing repeatedly brief episodes of substernal oppression. Grade 1 to 2 basal and apical systolic murmurs were heard, the former transmitted to the neck. The blood pressure was 135 mm. of mercury systolic and 90 mm. diastolic.

Although the history appeared to be consistent with angina pectoris, she was able to climb two flights of stairs without the substernal choking, and the only objective abnormality was the depression of the *RS–T* segment in Leads 2, 3 and aV_F of the electrocardiogram taken on July 3. The possibility of a hiatus hernia was explored, but a gastrointestinal series revealed the esophagus, stomach and duodenum to be entirely normal. An exercise tolerance test was ordered for July 6, the results of which are demonstrated in Figure 269. It is of interest to note that the patient had shortness of breath, but no pain and no choking, after she had climbed twenty-eight steps. As the precordial leads of the *B* tracing were being recorded, she experienced mild distress with substernal choking.

COMMENT. This is an excellent illustration of a positive test of the effect of exercise on the electrocardiogram of a person with limited coronary blood supply, especially to the anterior wall of the heart. The greater value of the chest leads than of the limb leads in testing this case is well demonstrated in this record; such is in general a common experience.

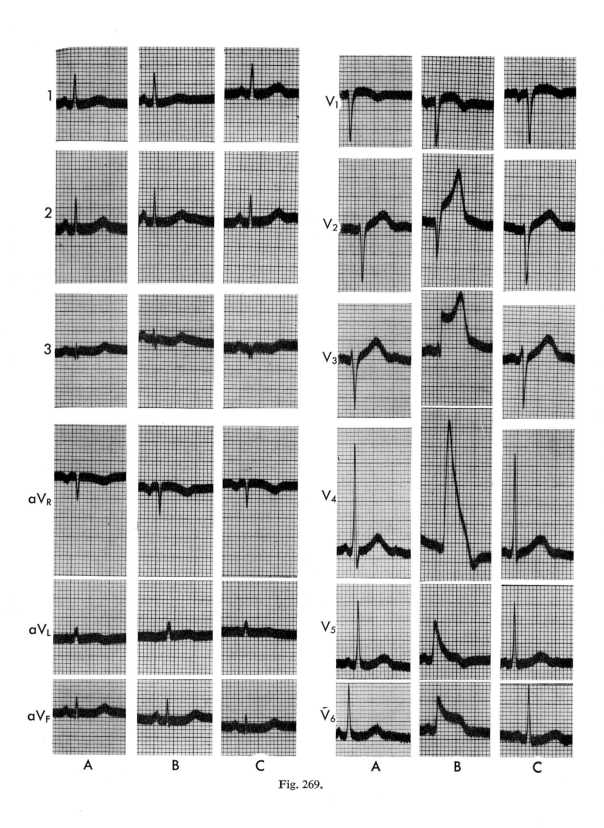

Fig. 269.

Fig. 270.

INTERPRETATION. Atrial fibrillation at a heart rate of about 65, with a few ventricular ectopic contractions, prominent Q waves in Leads 1 and aV$_L$, deep QS waves without R waves in Leads V$_2$ and V$_3$, probably absent R waves in Lead V$_4$, high R waves in Leads V$_5$ and V$_6$, and low to diphasic T waves throughout.

CLINICAL FINDINGS. V.C.H., a cryptographer of seventy-four years, entered the Emergency Ward on October 3, 1949. His chief complaint was pronounced difficulty in breathing. For ten years he had noticed easy fatigability, and over the past two years there had developed in addition orthopnea and frequent episodes of paroxysmal nocturnal dyspnea. Exertion and emotional stress tended to bring on brief pressure sensations in his left chest which disappeared with rest. Irregularity of the heart had been observed at the time of a physical check-up three years before. At the onset of the more pressing symptoms in 1947 he went to his local doctor, who placed him on digitoxin and a low-salt diet, with a resultant diuresis and improvement in his symptoms. Since that time he had been taking digitoxin, 0.1 mg. daily. However, there had been gradual increase in both dyspnea and edema, until in the fall of 1949 he sought advice at our medical clinic, where an electrocardiogram showed atrial fibrillation with multiple ventricular premature beats and left ventricular hypertrophy. An increase in digitoxin to 0.2 mg. a day was prescribed, but after three days on this regimen he felt no better and was admitted to the hospital for diuresis and further control of his digitalization.

Physical examination revealed a thin man breathing with difficulty. The neck veins were distended, rales were heard at both bases, and there was slight ankle edema. The heart rhythm was grossly irregular, with a pulse deficit of 10, at a rate of approximately 80. The heart was enlarged. There was a Grade 4, harsh systolic murmur at the apex. The blood pressure was 130 mm. of mercury systolic and 80 mm. diastolic. Laboratory studies showed a hemoglobin of 16 gm., a white blood cell count of 7500 per cu. mm., with a normal differential count. Subsequent electrocardiograms demonstrated no striking changes from the one obtained four days before his admission. The tracing shown here was taken on October 10. An x-ray film of the chest repeated on that day showed slight improvement over a previous film, in that there appeared to be less congestion and a minimal amount of pulmonary edema. The finding of pulmonary edema on entry had led to the diagnosis of acute myocardial infarction as a precipitating cause, but it was believed that there was no evidence to substantiate this diagnosis.

The patient improved on administration of tourniquets, oxygen, aminophylline and morphine. Digitalis and diuretics cleared the congestion, and he was discharged home on October 17, with the diagnoses of coronary heart disease and acute pulmonary edema.

COMMENT. The record gives evidence of marked left ventricular enlargement and irritability of the heart, and probably an old anterior myocardial infarct.

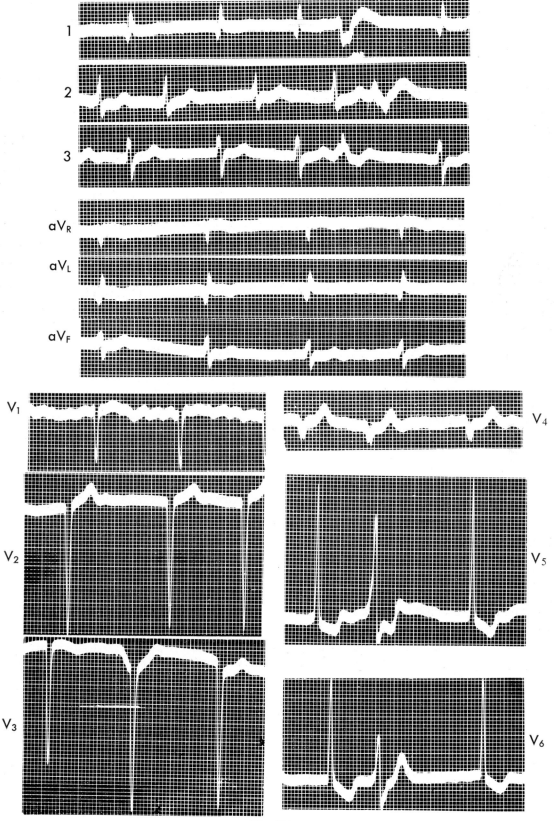

Fig. 270.

Fig. 271.

INTERPRETATION. Normal rhythm, rate 85, interrupted in Lead V_3 by paroxysmal ventricular tachycardia, rate 150, consisting of short runs of abnormal ventricular complexes of two types, first, five beats of W-shape and then, six beats of unidirectional inverted type. There is also absence of R waves in Leads V_1, V_2, V_3 and V_4, with much depression of the $S–T$ segments in Lead 2.

CLINICAL FINDINGS. R.S., an obese widow of sixty-eight years, was admitted to the hospital on December 13, 1949, complaining of persistent and severe chest pain. For the past three years she had experienced substernal tightness and oppression on effort, relieved by rest. Her doctor had prescribed a diet for the high blood pressure, angina pectoris, and "kidney troubles" from which she had suffered during this period. The present episode had its onset at 9 P.M. on December 12, with severe but intermittent substernal pain. At six o'clock the next morning the pain caused her to waken and was described as "tearing;" this time it radiated to both shoulders and to the left upper arm. She broke out in a cold sweat and called the doctor, who gave her nitroglycerin with some relief. The pain recurred, however, and after the administration of atropine and morphine sulfate she was sent to the hospital.

On entry, physical examination revealed an obese woman in no acute distress, with a blood pressure of 150 mm. of mercury systolic and 95 mm. diastolic. The white blood cell count was 10,150 per cu. mm. The heart rhythm was normal at a rate of about 76. An electrocardiogram taken shortly thereafter is shown here.

COMMENT. This electrocardiogram confirms the clinical diagnosis of coronary heart disease with myocardial infarction and dangerous cardiac irritability demanding the use of quinidine. She recovered from this attack. Subsequent tracings continued to show the myocardial scarring due to anterior infarction.

Fig. 272.

INTERPRETATION. Normal rhythm at a rate of 100, with wide QRS waves in all twelve leads, measuring 0.15 second. In the limb leads left axis deviation is predominant, with diphasic to upright T waves in Lead 1, but in the precordial leads over the right ventricle there are notched, mainly upright QRS waves, with deep wide S waves over the left ventricle, which combination of findings is diagnostic of right bundle branch block.

CLINICAL FINDINGS. J.A., a fat young man of thirty-seven, had been seen first in 1933, when he was nineteen years old, and the diagnoses of rheumatic heart disease, aortic regurgitation, (?) slight mitral stenosis, and cardiac neurosis had been made. Bundle branch block was an electrocardiographic finding first noted in 1947 upon the occasion of his second examination, at which time a further diagnosis of gross obesity was made. He was seen thereafter once or twice a year until the present examination in February, 1951. Earlier in the winter he had had rheumatism in the knees and ankles for several weeks, accompanied by a throbbing pain, but without swelling. Heat and medicine had cleared this. He complained of some dyspnea on stooping, but no chest pain.

Upon physical examination he looked enormous and weighed 277 pounds. The pulse was regular at 78. His blood pressure was 135 mm. of mercury systolic and 65 mm. diastolic. There was no edema. The heart sounds were good. Grade 2 aortic systolic and diastolic murmurs were present, as in previous examinations. By fluoroscopy the heart was found to be moderately large and round in shape.

It was recommended that this patient lose 50 pounds before reporting in six months for a check-up.

COMMENT. Unusual transverse position of the heart due to great obesity, with high diaphragm, doubtless explains this confusing picture. Rheumatic heart disease with aortic valve involvement is the explanation for the physical findings.

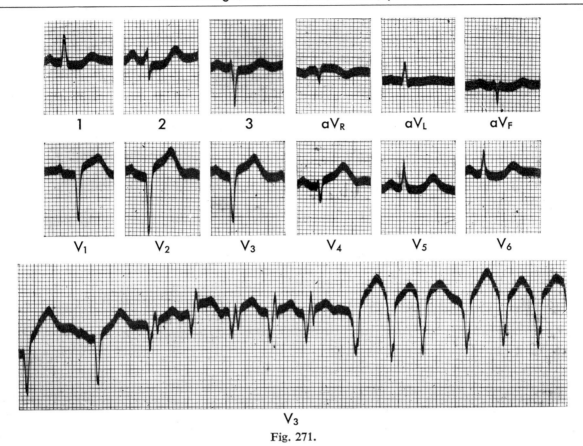

1 2 3 aV_R aV_L aV_F

V₁ V₂ V₃ V₄ V₅ V₆

V₃

Fig. 271.

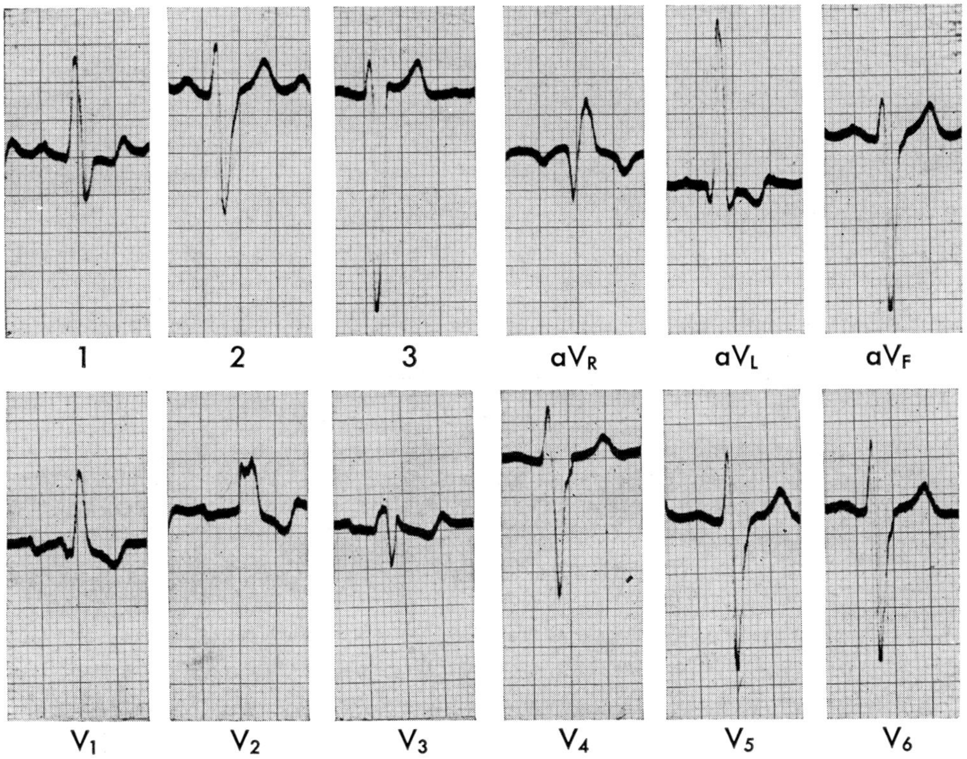

1 2 3 aV_R aV_L aV_F

V₁ V₂ V₃ V₄ V₅ V₆

Fig. 272.

Fig. 273.

INTERPRETATION. Sinus bradycardia and arrhythmia at a rate of 40 to 60, atrial premature beats followed for the most part by aberrant ventricular responses, a possible ventricular premature beat in Lead V_2, and a short $P–R$ interval at the second complex in Lead V_2, due probably to ventricular escape, which is also evident in the first and last complexes of Lead V_4 and in the next to the last complex in Lead V_5.

CLINICAL FINDINGS. J.B., a fifty year old Polish cook, entered the hospital on November 13 after an episode of weakness and nausea which came on after eating and was accompanied by generalized abdominal pain and pain in the shoulders and scapulae. He had vomited several times, and the "small white pills" prescribed by his doctor had afforded no relief of the pain. There had been no previous attacks of this nature, and there was no history of dyspnea, chest pain, orthopnea, cyanosis or edema. A white blood cell count of 17,000 per cu. mm. subsided after admission, and an electrocardiogram demonstrated no diagnostic changes, although there was some slurring and widening of the QRS complexes. Upon a restricted diet he improved. His amylase test showed 15 units, and a diagnosis of cholecystitis was made, though with a question of recent myocardial infarction.

A chest x-ray film the day after admission revealed increased density of the right lower lung lobe, and fluoroscopy of the chest on November 16 showed linear areas of atelectasis in both lower lung fields. The left diaphragm was slightly higher than normal, and at the right apex there were fibrotic areas and possibly emphysematous blebs.

Upon cardiac examination on November 16 he complained of feeling "hot" and appeared uncomfortable. The blood pressure was 110 mm. of mercury systolic and 60 mm. diastolic. There was no pulsation of the cervical veins. Rales were heard at the right lung base. P_2 was greater than A_2, and there were no murmurs. The heart was not enlarged. The rhythm was grossly irregular at a rate of 175, and an electrocardiogram confirmed the impression of "rapid heart rate in auricular fibrillation." There was no enlargement of the liver and no edema, nor were there any signs of thrombophlebitis.

He was given cedilanid (1.2 mg. and 0.4 mg.) on November 17, with daily doses of digalen, 1 cat unit intramuscularly, thereafter until, by November 22, he was fully digitalized. He was afebrile. However, a white blood cell count on this date was 26,000 per cu. mm. On cardiac consultation the following day no symptoms of myocardial infarction were elicited. There was a soft pulmonary systolic murmur. The rhythm appeared basically regular with many premature beats and some "dropped beats." There was slight tenderness deep in the right calf, but no swelling. The electrocardiogram of November 23 is shown here.

By November 28 the rhythm was entirely regular. An x-ray examination of the chest on this date showed little change except possibly for slightly more prominent linear densities in the left lower lung field. The x-ray changes were considered suggestive of multiple pulmonary infarcts, and it was believed that the cardiac arrhythmia might well have been precipitated by small pulmonary emboli or digitalis, or both.

COMMENT. This curious arrhythmia, consisting of sinoatrial bradycardia, arrhythmia, and block, of ventricular escape secondary thereto, and of extrasystoles, is most readily explained by the excessive effect of digitalis in a person who is sick, though not necessarily a cardiac patient (except for what seems to have been a complication of paroxysmal atrial fibrillation with rapid heart rate).

Fig. 274.

INTERPRETATION. Normal rhythm at a rate of 110 to 120, with marked right axis deviation, as shown in the limb leads, and prominent R waves in precordial leads V_1, V_2, V_3, especially in the first-named, over the right ventricle.

CLINICAL FINDINGS. J.R., a little boy two and a half years old, was first admitted to the hospital in 1947 at the age of sixteen months, after an episode of cerebral thrombosis believed to be secondary to polycythemia.

On physical examination the baby was slightly cyanotic: he had been "blue" from birth. The neck veins were not remarkable. The heart did not appear to be enlarged. The rhythm was regular at about 120. A Grade 4 systolic murmur was heard, loudest in the third and fourth interspaces along the left sternal border without a definite thrill; it was widely transmitted anteriorly and posteriorly over the chest. There were no diastolic murmurs. The liver and spleen were not palpable. There were good femoral pulsations. The extremities demonstrated definite clubbing. An x-ray film of the chest at this time showed great cardiac enlargement, chiefly ventricular. The great vessels could not be clearly traced, and it was thought that a shadow in the right superior mediastinum might possibly be an anomalous great vessel. The lung roots were somewhat engorged. The electrocardiogram shown here was taken on July 29, 1948.

Clinically, the diagnosis of tetralogy of Fallot seemed most likely, but later x-ray examination raised the question of a possible transposition of the great vessels, and it was decided that operation was indicated. A Blalock procedure was carried out in December, 1948, at which time the tetralogy was believed to be present, and a right-sided end-to-side anastomosis between the right subclavian artery and the right pulmonary artery was done.

COMMENT. This record is characteristic of considerable preponderant enlargement of the right ventricle, such as is always found with the tetralogy of Fallot. Other conditions, congenital and acquired, can also produce the pattern of right ventricular enlargement. The clinical history and physical examination are the clues to the probable diagnosis. The electrocardiogram is not specific.

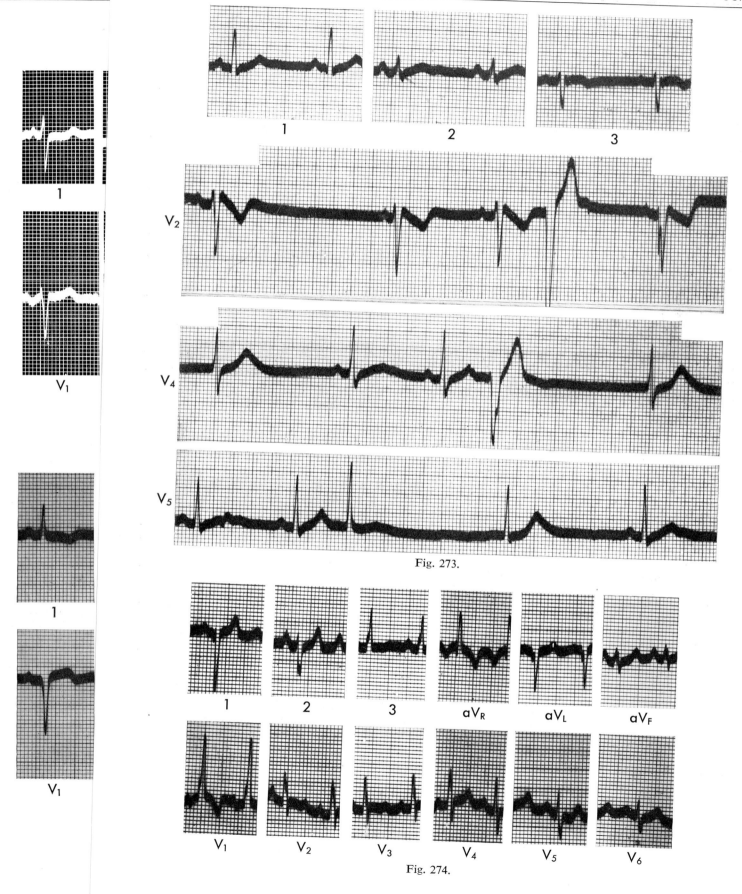

Fig. 273.

Fig. 274.

INTERPRETATION. I
Leads V$_2$, V$_3$ and V$_4$

CLINICAL FINDING
referred to the medi
the draft board beca
he had first noticed

X-ray examinatio
right ventricle appea
and probably left p
pericarditis.

Because of seriou
for study and treati
time was 210 mm. c
response, and becau
lumbodorsal sympa
removed from D 2 t
operation on the le
operation.

COMMENT. It is di
of the heart, but su
chronic calcareous
tions from what mi

INTERPRETATION
inverted T waves i
Lead V$_6$.

CLINICAL FINDI
had controlled by
five minutes of sul
pain of the same l
his being taken as
to be 250 mg. per
in an oxygen tent
but he was kept in
October 13, ten w

On physical exa
were distant. The
mercury systolic a
full left ventricle.

COMMENT. This
doubtless occurre

Fig. 277.

INTERPRETATION. Atrial paroxysmal tachycardia, rate 180, interrupted by a few ventricular premature beats and attended by depression of the S–T segments throughout.

CLINICAL FINDINGS. B.P., a woman of fifty-eight, came in for her annual check-up on December 5, 1949. She had first been examined at the clinic twenty-one years before, when a diagnosis was made of an irritable heart. On subsequent examinations cardiac irritability had persisted, as evidenced by palpitation and the presence of occasional extrasystoles and paroxysmal tachycardia. Quinidine proved successful in controlling these, and she continued well in other respects. Her life was active, and the cardiac arrhythmia was more bothersome when she was fatigued. Her electrocardiogram had shown for many years, in addition to moderate left axis deviation, the short P–R interval and slurred QRS complexes characteristic of the Wolff-Parkinson-White syndrome. In the fall of 1949 her palpitation had increased somewhat; she had not been taking quinidine.

On physical examination she looked well. The sounds were of good quality. There was a slight aortic systolic murmur which had been present before. Several times in the course of the examination she experienced palpitation, at a heart rate of approximately 160. The blood pressure was 150 mm. of mercury systolic and 70 mm. diastolic. On fluoroscopy the heart was found to be of normal size. The electrocardiogram shown here was taken upon this occasion and demonstrates the irritability, for which quinidine sulfate, 3 grains, was prescribed three times a day. Twelve years before, she had had a mastectomy for a benign breast tumor. During subsequent years chest films were obtained every two to three years as a precautionary measure.

At the time of her last visit, in December, 1949, an x-ray film of the chest revealed "a rounded, rather sharply defined density in the left chest just below the tip of the third rib," measuring approximately 2 cm. in diameter, not present in previous films taken in 1947. Cancer seemed the most likely explanation, and the patient was accordingly hospitalized for further study. In January the upper lobe of the left lung was removed. Upon pathologic examination the nodule was identified as a Grade 2 adenocarcinoma, presumed to be primary in the lung. With the aid of a restricted salt regimen and protective doses of quinidine she stood the operation well, was ambulatory on the third day, and her postoperative course was uneventful except for a brief episode of rapid heart action on the fifth day, lasting ten minutes.

COMMENT. The paroxysmal tachycardia demonstrated by this record can be accounted for by the usual tendency of persons with the Wolff-Parkinson-White syndrome to show such a disturbance or by the irritating pulmonary disease present here, or by both factors. An unusual phenomenon consists of the odd ventricular contractions which are premature rather than aberrant.

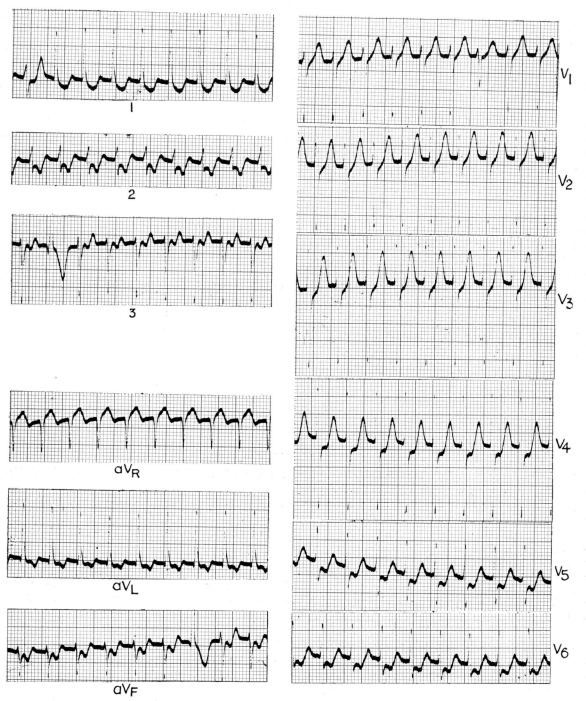

Fig. 277.

Fig. 278.

INTERPRETATION. Normal rhythm, rate 100, slight left axis deviation, normal complexes and time intervals throughout.

CLINICAL FINDINGS. M.S., an eighteen year old college girl, came into the hospital on October 26, 1949, with the diagnosis of subacute bacterial endocarditis. She had had chills, fever and general malaise of one month's duration. Because she had always been known to have a "machinery" murmur in her chest, she had led a protected and sedentary life, without symptoms other than slight exertional dyspnea. There had been no cyanosis.

Physical examination on admission revealed a thin, pale young girl, acutely ill, with a temperature of 100° F. There were no petechiae. P_2 was accentuated, and a continuous thrill was felt in the pulmonic area where a loud "Grade 4" continuous murmur was heard. There was a third sound at the apex. Examination of the abdomen demonstrated tenderness in the area of the spleen, which could not at this time be felt, and tenderness in the right renal area.

An x-ray film of the chest the day after admission revealed prominent vascular markings on the right. The heart appeared to be somewhat enlarged in a transverse direction, and the undivided portion of the pulmonary artery was prominent. The cardiothoracic ratio was 11.5/26 cm. An electrocardiogram taken on the same day is shown here.

Diagnoses of patent ductus arteriosus, subacute bacterial endarteritis and secondary anemia were made. Blood cultures established the presence of the subacute bacterial endarteritis, which responded to penicillin therapy, although a small pulmonary infarct on November 13 complicated her course. On stopping the penicillin, the temperature again became elevated, and it was believed that the ductus should be ligated. Blood transfusions were given, and the operation was successfully undertaken on December 6. The postoperative course was uneventful, and the patient recovered completely.

COMMENT. The majority of cases of patency of the ductus arteriosus show normal electrocardiograms, even though there is on occasion some cardiac enlargement. When, however, there is marked left ventricular strain, this may be manifested by the electrocardiographic pattern resulting therefrom. Although in this case there were prominent R waves throughout the precordial leads, and in V_1 to V_3 prominent S waves also, it is probable that the thinness of the chest wall with close proximity of the electrodes to the heart was the chief cause thereof, rather than ventricular enlargement alone.

Fig. 279.

INTERPRETATION. Normal rhythm at a rate of 85, with low T waves in the limb leads and unusually high S–T segments and T waves in chest leads V_2 to V_4 inclusive.

CLINICAL FINDINGS. A.F., a sixty-six year old Italian housewife, was admitted to the hospital with the complaint of intermittent chest pain for five days, which had culminated on the evening of entry in an episode of similar but severe pain in the anterior chest, radiating to both shoulders, down the left arm to the fingers, and to the right scapula; this was accompanied by sweating and shortness of breath. Demerol and morphine sulfate had been administered. Her past history included hypertension for many years and diabetes not requiring insulin, but there had been no cardiac signs or symptoms prior to this time.

Physical examination revealed an obese woman lying quietly in bed. Her blood pressure was 190 mm. of mercury systolic and 90 mm. diastolic; there was no cyanosis or edema, and the neck veins were not distended. There were no murmurs, gallop or friction rub. The electrocardiogram shown here was taken shortly after entry.

The patient's course was uneventful.

COMMENT. This record clearly demonstrates an early anterior myocardial infarct or at least a highly anoxic state of the heart muscle in that region before scarring has developed. It is of particular interest that the limb leads, although not fully normal, are far less useful in the diagnosis of the condition than the precordial leads, which give the answer at once. Subsequent tracings demonstrated a return of the S–T segments to the baseline with inversion of T's in Leads 1, 2, aV_L and throughout the precordial leads, characteristic of the evolution of anterior myocardial infarction.

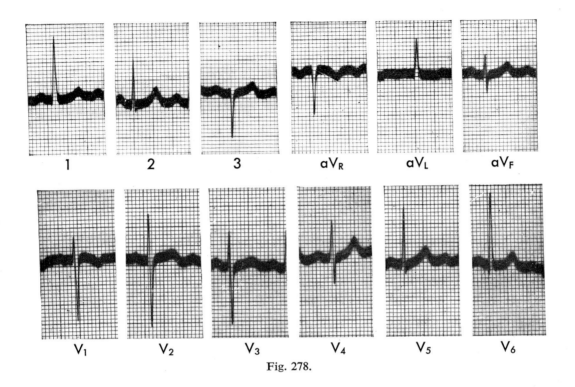

Fig. 278.

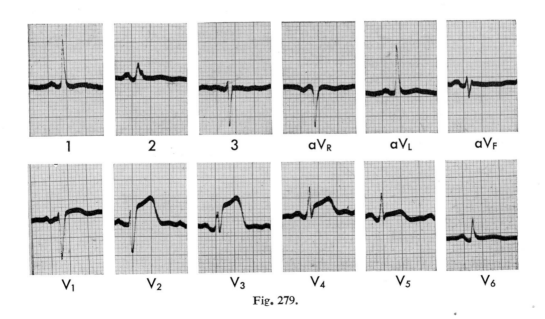

Fig. 279.

Fig. 280.

INTERPRETATION. Atrial fibrillation with heart rate of 70, occasional ectopic ventricular contractions, left axis deviation with inversion of T_1, upright T waves in Lead aV_R, deep S waves in Leads V_1, V_2, V_3 and V_4, and high R waves with inverted T waves in Leads V_4, V_5 and V_6.

CLINICAL FINDINGS. K.N., a seventy year old retired laborer, was admitted to the hospital on May 19, 1949, for treatment of congestive heart failure. For three years he had had known hypertension, and for two years had experienced easy fatigue, dyspnea on exertion, paroxysmal nocturnal dyspnea, and orthopnea. Exertion had also tended to produce precordial pain without radiation, relieved by rest. One year previously he had been admitted to a hospital because of his increasing dyspnea and had been told that "one of the arteries of the heart was blocked." He had been hospitalized for ten days and discharged with instructions to remain in bed for a few weeks and to take small white pills three times daily. This he had done, but he had continued to have dyspnea on exertion and occasional precordial pain, with considerable increase in these symptoms over the past three weeks.

Physical examination revealed a well developed, well nourished man, who was comfortable in the sitting position. The neck veins were full, but not pulsating. The breath sounds were diminished, as was tactile fremitus, and there were moist rales at both lung bases and in the axillae. The blood pressure was 240 mm. of mercury systolic and 130 mm. diastolic. The heart was enlarged to the anterior axillary line, with the rhythm totally irregular at a rate of 120 (pulse deficit 15). P_2 was greater than A_2, and both were accentuated. There were no murmurs. The liver edge descended two fingerbreadths below the costal margin and was tender to percussion. There was Grade 3 to 4 pitting edema of the legs to the knees and of the sacrum.

Laboratory studies showed a hemoglobin of 16.5 gm., white blood cell count of 10,100 per cu. mm., with normal smear and differential. Examination of the urine on admission revealed a specific gravity of 1.010, with 3 plus albumin, and two to three red cells, three to five white cells, many hyalin and occasional granular casts per high-powered field in the sediment. By x-ray film the heart appeared to be greatly enlarged, with pulmonary congestion and fluid in both pleural cavities. An electrocardiogram on the day of admission showed atrial fibrillation at a ventricular rate of 115 and low T waves, without evidence of myocardial infarction. The tracing shown here was taken six days later, after control of the heart rate by digoxin and digitoxin.

Mercurial diuretics and ammonium chloride resulted in improvement of his symptoms, a weight loss of 15 pounds, and the disappearance of his peripheral edema and liver congestion. He was discharged home on May 28, with the diagnosis of hypertensive heart disease with congestive failure.

COMMENT. This record is quite typical of that of a large, irritable hypertensive heart with atrial fibrillation and ventricular rate well controlled by digitalis. There is no need on electrocardiographic evidence to diagnose coronary heart disease in addition, although the clinical story suggests the possibility that he might have had also some effort angina pectoris.

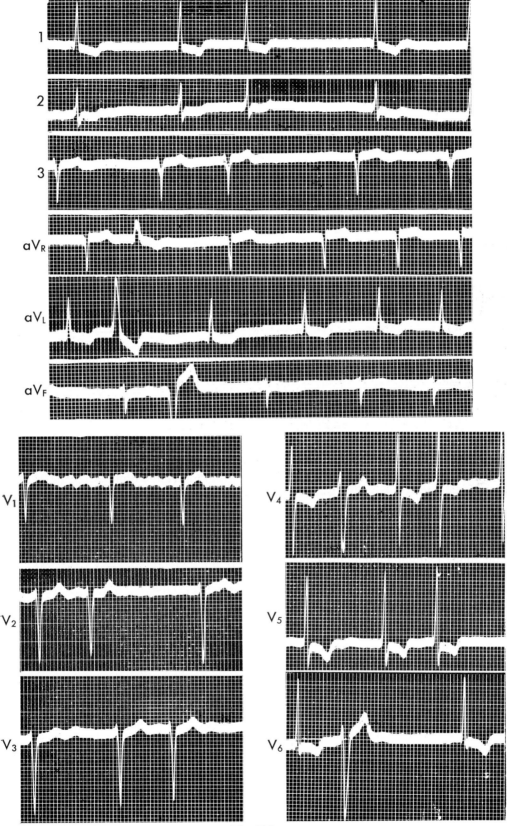

Fig. 280.

Fig. 281.

INTERPRETATION. *A*, Normal rhythm, rate approximately 100, with short *P–R* intervals and wide *QRS* waves (Wolff-Parkinson-White syndrome).

B, Normal rhythm with short *P–R* intervals, wide *QRS* waves (Wolff-Parkinson-White syndrome) and some changes in the *S–T* segments and *T* waves (higher in Leads 1 and 2; *R* waves higher in Leads V_4 and V_5).

C, Normal rhythm with normal *P–R* intervals and much narrower *QRS* waves. Slight residual *S–T* segment and *T* wave changes, but these are slight. R_4 is high in both *B* and *C*.

CLINICAL FINDINGS. E.G., a fifty-five year old supervisor of a rubber factory, was first examined by us on September 20, 1950. About four years earlier he had had an all-night episode of severe, squeezing, pressure-like pain in the substernal region. An electrocardiogram taken in a local hospital at that time had shown "left bundle branch block." About three years later he had begun to have pain in the left shoulder which was brought on by the effort of walking and disappeared with rest. He had also experienced a dull pain in the left shoulder while sitting quietly in a chair; it lasted only a short time and was relieved by nitroglycerin. The episode was followed by the occurrence of epigastric pressure about one half hour after meals. For the week prior to examination he had been awakened every morning at four o'clock with pain in the left shoulder, lasting up to one half hour.

On physical examination the pulse rate was found to be 75, and the blood pressure 140 mm. of mercury systolic and 70 mm. diastolic. The heart by fluoroscopy was of normal size and shape, with good pulsations. An electrocardiogram (found later to resemble closely the one taken four years before) is shown in *A*.

Because of his apparent acute coronary insufficiency, the patient was admitted to the hospital on September 22. He was uncomfortable most of this night, with substernal pain in spite of morphine. The electrocardiogram in *B* was taken on September 23.

C, Record obtained September 25, on which day he appeared to be feeling fairly well. That evening he seemed to have no pain and was talking with his doctor when suddenly he had a convulsion and died, despite the injection of epinephrine directly into the heart. Among the findings disclosed at autopsy were coronary sclerosis, old focal myocardial infarction, and (?) recent infarction at the apex of the interventricular septum.

COMMENT. An interesting example of the coincidental occurrence of acute and chronic coronary heart disease and the so-called Wolff-Parkinson-White syndrome, probably unrelated to each other, and of a moderately common change, under observation, from the short *P–R* interval and wide *QRS* wave to normal *P–R* and *QRS* durations. There is no reason why a good many persons with the Wolff-Parkinson-White syndrome in youth should not eventually, like many of their fellow citizens, coincidentally suffer hypertension or coronary insufficiency.

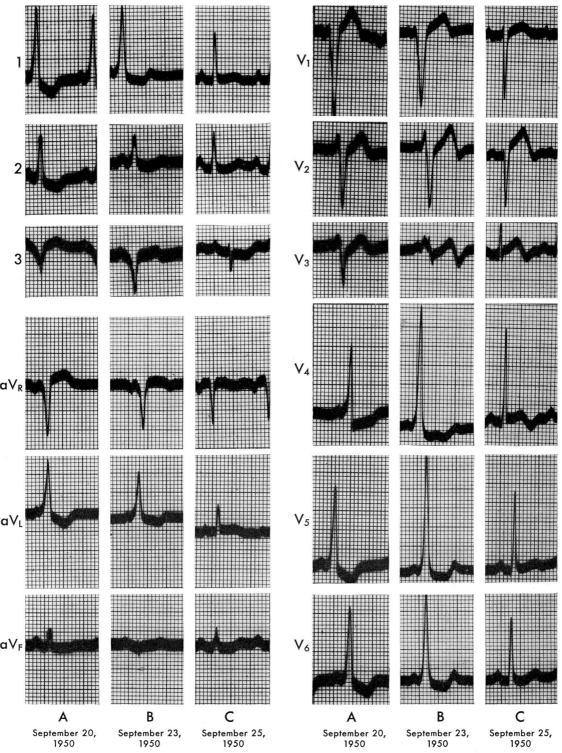

Fig. 281.

Fig. 282.

INTERPRETATION. Marked sinus bradycardia with slight arrhythmia (atrial rate 30 to 35) and ventricular escape, giving a ventricular rate of 50 to 60. The $S-T$ segments are depressed and the T waves decreased in Leads 1, 2, V_4 and V_5, suggesting a digitalis effect. There is a variable and coincidental bigeminy due to the occurrence of the P waves shortly after the T waves, permitting ventricular response. The prolonged $Q-T$ duration (0.42 second) is in keeping with the considerable bradycardia.

CLINICAL FINDINGS. R.T., a fifty-five year old housewife, entered the hospital on September 10, 1948, with complaints of precordial distress in the form of "heavy" pain across the upper sternum and disturbance of heart rhythm. The pain lasted for hours at a time, radiated through to the back, and was unaffected by exertion, position or emotion. Nine years before, a systolic hypertension had been discovered. Six years before, about the time of the menopause, she had first observed forceful, irregular heart action, most noticeable on excitement, after meals, and at night, and unrelated to effort. The heart action was usually slow during these episodes, with occasional rapid beating for periods of a few seconds. Trials of thyroid, belladonna, atropine and digitoxin had no appreciable effect. For the few months prior to admission she had been taking thyroid, 30 mg. daily, and digitoxin, and had restricted moderately the salt in her diet.

Past history had been negative for diphtheria, rheumatic fever, influenza, typhoid fever and meningitis, had included scarlet fever at the age of five (without known sequelae), tonsillitis, recurrent boils and abscesses, and a dental infection which had subsided with sulfanilamide therapy. Her father had had pulmonary tuberculosis, but died of coronary heart disease, and a brother was being treated for angina pectoris.

On physical examination she appeared to be under nervous tension, but looked well. The heart rhythm was irregular at a rate of approximately 56. There was a Grade 1 to 2 soft systolic murmur heard at the apex and in the aortic area. P_2 was plus and greater than A_2. The blood pressure varied from 200 to 190 mm. of mercury systolic and 80 to 90 mm. diastolic. Examination of the abdomen showed nothing amiss. There was slight edema of the extremities over the ankles and shins, and the left leg appeared slightly larger than the right.

An x-ray film of the chest on September 14 showed the heart to be prominent in the region of the left ventricle, with a cardiothoracic ratio of 14:27. There was no evidence of calcium in the pericardium or within the heart. No active disease was observed in the lung parenchyma, and the linear markings were not increased significantly.

An electrocardiogram taken the day after admission is shown here.

On September 14 the digitoxin and thyroid were discontinued, and over the course of the next few days atropine and epinephrine tests were made, without sufficiently favorable effects, however, to warrant their use in therapy. The patient was discharged on September 18 on a program which omitted the digitalis but included thyroid, moderate physical exertion with the avoidance of undue fatigue and strain, phenobarbital when needed for nervous stress, and a possible trial later of stilbesterol.

COMMENT. This is a rather bizarre arrhythmia, interesting but relatively unimportant, not indicative of myocardial disease per se, but in all probability a manifestation of the effect of digitalis in a sensitive heart.

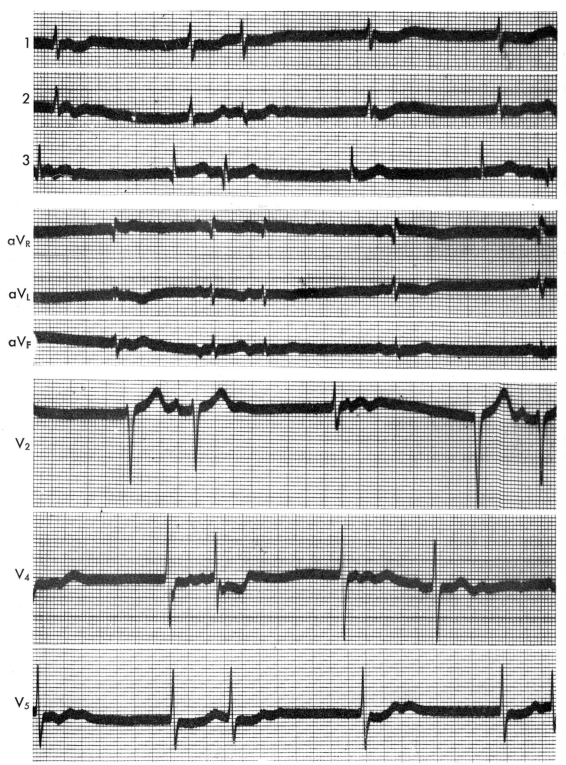

Fig. 282.

Fig. 283.

INTERPRETATION. Normal rhythm at a rate of 86, with delayed atrioventricular conduction ($P-R$ interval 0.28 second), left bundle branch block, and slight elevation of the $S-T$ segments in Leads 2, 3, aV_R, aV_F, V_1, V_2 and V_3.

CLINICAL FINDINGS. D.A., an eighty-five year old former housepainter, married within eight months for the third time, re-entered the hospital three weeks after his first discharge. He had previously been treated for bronchopneumonia, bronchiectasis, coronary heart disease and congestive heart failure. He had had successful diuresis with mercuhydrin and had been taking digitoxin, 0.1 mg. daily. His present complaint was shortness of breath progressing over the past five days to great respiratory distress, much coughing, some left chest discomfort with radiation to the back, and considerable orthopnea. On the day of admission the chest pain had increased and the cough was productive of a frothy, blood-tinged sputum.

On physical examination he was in acute respiratory distress. There were bubbling rales in the chest and an expiratory wheeze. The heart was enlarged to the left. There was a Grade 3, blowing aortic systolic murmur widely transmitted. No diastolic murmurs or gallop were present. The blood pressure was 105 mm. of mercury systolic and 70 mm. diastolic. The abdomen was slightly full, but there were no masses and no right upper quadrant tenderness. There was Grade 3 pitting edema of the extremities.

An x-ray examination on the day of admission showed the heart to be considerably enlarged. The findings were compatible with congestive failure, pulmonary edema and right hydrothorax. The electrocardiogram taken on the same day is shown here.

COMMENT. The electrocardiogram does not adequately reflect the seriousness of this man's heart disease and failure and so is an example of the need of surveying the total clinical picture in addition to the electrocardiogram. This record does show, however, the presence of scarring (doubtless due to coronary atherosclerosis) in the region of the bundle of His and of its left branch, and the elevated $S-T$ segments may be due to the presence of a cardiac aneurysm.

Fig. 284.

INTERPRETATION. Normal rhythm, rate 105, wide P waves in Leads 1, V_4, V_5 and V_6, right ventricular preponderance ($S_1 > R_1$, small R waves without S waves in Leads V_1, V_2 and V_3, and prominent S waves in Leads V_4, V_5 and V_6), slight sagging of the $S-T$ segments in Leads 1, 2 and V_2 to V_6 inclusive.

CLINICAL FINDINGS. C.B., a forty-nine year old schoolmistress, came in for examination on March 31, 1950. At the age of six she had had St. Vitus' dance, but not until 1944, when she was forty-three, was she told that she had heart disease. At that time she was given digitalis for symptoms of dyspnea and cough. In 1948 she had pneumonia, with congestion of the lungs and slight hemoptysis, and the following year an attack of rheumatic fever, with pneumonia again in October, 1949. The present complaints of dyspnea, cough and rapid heart action had persisted since that time. Pain in the left chest led her to be hospitalized for a week in February, 1950, but without relief of her discomfort and with continued loss of appetite, tendency to nausea, and sore liver. Her treatment up to this time had consisted of premarin for one month, digalen daily, and nembutal.

On physical examination she appeared somewhat frail and weighed 105 pounds. In the sitting position slight pulsations of the cervical veins were visible. The heart was considerably enlarged. There was at the apex a diastolic thrill corresponding to a loud, Grade 4 mitral diastolic roll which ended abruptly in a loud first sound, and over the body of the heart there was a slight, Grade 2 systolic murmur. The pulmonary second sound was accentuated. Her heart rhythm was normal at a rate of 90, with an occasional premature beat. Blood pressure was 140 mm. of mercury systolic and 90 mm. diastolic. There were a few rales at the lung bases, and the liver was slightly tender.

X-ray examination of the heart revealed it to be moderately enlarged, with prominence of the left upper border. The left atrium was found to be enlarged in the oblique view. The transverse diameter of the heart was 12.2 cm., and the internal diameter of the chest 24 cm. The lung root shadows were congested.

The electrocardiogram shown here was taken at this time.

COMMENT. This record in itself suggests mitral stenosis because of the unusual P waves superimposed on the evidence of right ventricular enlargement. It is, however, unusual for normal rhythm to persist in the presence of such a high degree of mitral stenosis at this age of forty-nine years. Ordinarily one would find atrial fibrillation in such a case. The sagging of the $S-T$ segments suggests a definite digitalis effect.

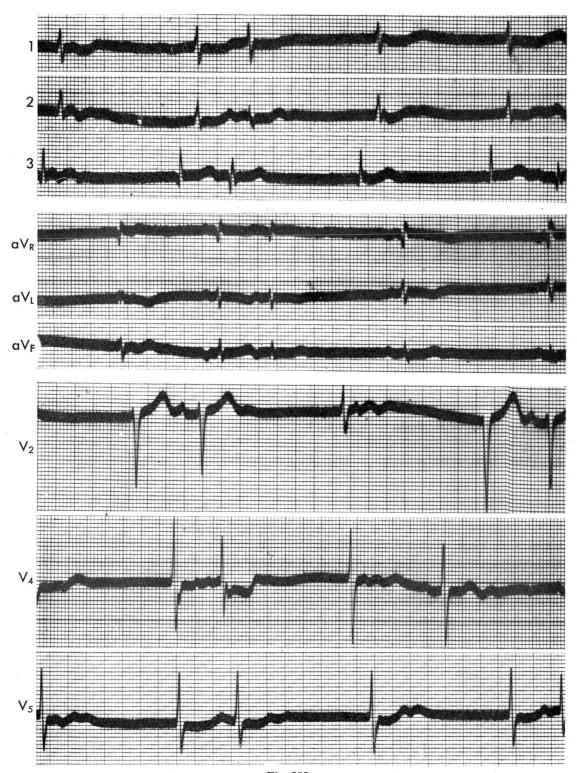

Fig. 282.

Fig. 283.

INTERPRETATION. Normal rhythm at a rate of 86, with delayed atrioventricular conduction (*P–R* interval 0.28 second), left bundle branch block, and slight elevation of the *S–T* segments in Leads 2, 3, aV_R, aV_F, V_1, V_2 and V_3.

CLINICAL FINDINGS. D.A., an eighty-five year old former housepainter, married within eight months for the third time, re-entered the hospital three weeks after his first discharge. He had previously been treated for bronchopneumonia, bronchiectasis, coronary heart disease and congestive heart failure. He had had successful diuresis with mercuhydrin and had been taking digitoxin, 0.1 mg. daily. His present complaint was shortness of breath progressing over the past five days to great respiratory distress, much coughing, some left chest discomfort with radiation to the back, and considerable orthopnea. On the day of admission the chest pain had increased and the cough was productive of a frothy, blood-tinged sputum.

On physical examination he was in acute respiratory distress. There were bubbling rales in the chest and an expiratory wheeze. The heart was enlarged to the left. There was a Grade 3, blowing aortic systolic murmur widely transmitted. No diastolic murmurs or gallop were present. The blood pressure was 105 mm. of mercury systolic and 70 mm. diastolic. The abdomen was slightly full, but there were no masses and no right upper quadrant tenderness. There was Grade 3 pitting edema of the extremities.

An x-ray examination on the day of admission showed the heart to be considerably enlarged. The findings were compatible with congestive failure, pulmonary edema and right hydrothorax. The electrocardiogram taken on the same day is shown here.

COMMENT. The electrocardiogram does not adequately reflect the seriousness of this man's heart disease and failure and so is an example of the need of surveying the total clinical picture in addition to the electrocardiogram. This record does show, however, the presence of scarring (doubtless due to coronary atherosclerosis) in the region of the bundle of His and of its left branch, and the elevated *S–T* segments may be due to the presence of a cardiac aneurysm.

Fig. 284.

INTERPRETATION. Normal rhythm, rate 105, wide *P* waves in Leads 1, V_4, V_5 and V_6, right ventricular preponderance ($S_1 > R_1$, small *R* waves without *S* waves in Leads V_1, V_2 and V_3, and prominent *S* waves in Leads V_4, V_5 and V_6), slight sagging of the *S–T* segments in Leads 1, 2 and V_2 to V_6 inclusive.

CLINICAL FINDINGS. C.B., a forty-nine year old schoolmistress, came in for examination on March 31, 1950. At the age of six she had had St. Vitus' dance, but not until 1944, when she was forty-three, was she told that she had heart disease. At that time she was given digitalis for symptoms of dyspnea and cough. In 1948 she had pneumonia, with congestion of the lungs and slight hemoptysis, and the following year an attack of rheumatic fever, with pneumonia again in October, 1949. The present complaints of dyspnea, cough and rapid heart action had persisted since that time. Pain in the left chest led her to be hospitalized for a week in February, 1950, but without relief of her discomfort and with continued loss of appetite, tendency to nausea, and sore liver. Her treatment up to this time had consisted of premarin for one month, digalen daily, and nembutal.

On physical examination she appeared somewhat frail and weighed 105 pounds. In the sitting position slight pulsations of the cervical veins were visible. The heart was considerably enlarged. There was at the apex a diastolic thrill corresponding to a loud, Grade 4 mitral diastolic roll which ended abruptly in a loud first sound, and over the body of the heart there was a slight, Grade 2 systolic murmur. The pulmonary second sound was accentuated. Her heart rhythm was normal at a rate of 90, with an occasional premature beat. Blood pressure was 140 mm. of mercury systolic and 90 mm. diastolic. There were a few rales at the lung bases, and the liver was slightly tender.

X-ray examination of the heart revealed it to be moderately enlarged, with prominence of the left upper border. The left atrium was found to be enlarged in the oblique view. The transverse diameter of the heart was 12.2 cm., and the internal diameter of the chest 24 cm. The lung root shadows were congested.

The electrocardiogram shown here was taken at this time.

COMMENT. This record in itself suggests mitral stenosis because of the unusual *P* waves superimposed on the evidence of right ventricular enlargement. It is, however, unusual for normal rhythm to persist in the presence of such a high degree of mitral stenosis at this age of forty-nine years. Ordinarily one would find atrial fibrillation in such a case. The sagging of the *S–T* segments suggests a definite digitalis effect.

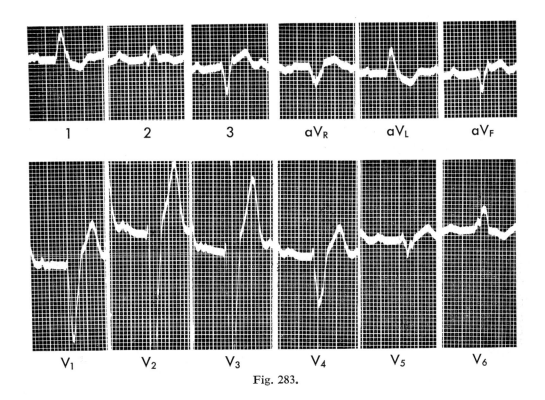

Fig. 283.

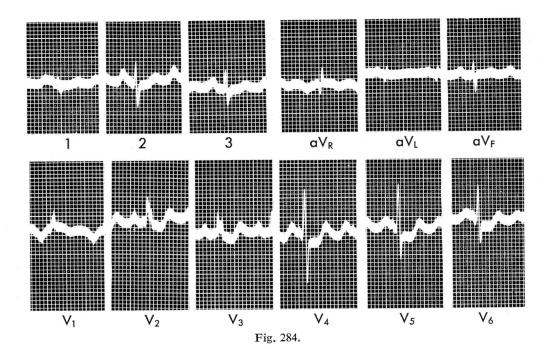

Fig. 284.

Fig. 285.

INTERPRETATION. Sinus tachycardia at a rate of 150, with normal complexes and time intervals throughout except for unusually high R waves in precordial leads V_2 and V_4 and deep S waves in Leads V_4 and V_5.

CLINICAL FINDINGS. D.M., a male infant of four months, had had constant cyanosis from birth, after which he had not developed normally. He had had frequent convulsive episodes lasting several minutes.

Upon physical examination the heart rhythm was regular, at a rate varying from 120 to 140. There was moderate cardiac enlargement, and Grade 2 to 3 systolic murmurs were heard to the left of the sternum. There were no definite diastolic murmurs, and no thrills. The liver edge was 3.5 cm. below the costal margin. The tetralogy of Fallot was considered at this time to be the most likely explanation for these findings.

An x-ray film of the chest revealed enlargement of the heart in the region of both ventricles. There was definite pulsation of the hilar shadows and some dilatation of the vascular shadows of both lung fields. The aorta did not push the esophagus to the left, and there was no evidence of dilatation of the superior vena cava. The aortic arch appeared to be on the left.

A cardiac consultation favored the diagnosis of transposition of the great vessels. However, in view of the obviously poor prognosis and the possibility of relief, should a tetralogy of Fallot be present, it was decided to attempt an exploratory operation. A Potts anastomosis of the left pulmonary artery to the descending aorta was performed. The infant survived this procedure, which was done from the left side. However, the postoperative course was stormy, and he died in pulmonary edema on the sixth postoperative day.

COMMENT. There is an indication from the precordial leads of enlargement of both ventricles, but this pattern is not diagnostic, and other methods of examination are of greater importance. In the course of the operative procedure, the great vessels were found to be transposed. Transposition of the great arteries, requiring for survival defects or absence of the septum, is best shown by the roentgenogram, with narrow vascular pedicle of the heart in the antero-posterior view, one great vessel overlying the other, and wide pedicle in the oblique views.

Fig. 286.

INTERPRETATION. Normal rhythm, rate 85 to 95, marked right axis deviation indicated by the limb leads, but with left ventricular enlargement shown by the precordial leads (deep S waves in Leads V_1, V_2 and V_3 and prominent R waves with inverted T waves in Leads V_4, V_5 and V_6.

CLINICAL FINDINGS. M.R., a woman of seventy-one years, was admitted to the hospital for treatment of acute glaucoma of ten weeks' duration. One and a half years previously she had experienced temporary left-sided paralysis. Her blood pressure had been known to be high for many years. She had been taking digitalis to control edema of the ankles.

On physical examination the blood pressure was found to be 250 mm. of mercury systolic and 105 mm. diastolic. There was a Grade 2 harsh systolic murmur in the aortic area, which was transmitted to the neck. The heart rhythm was normal except for interruption by frequent premature beats. There was no edema of the extremities.

A diagnosis of hypertensive heart disease with cardiac enlargement and calcareous aortic stenosis was made. There were no signs of congestive failure at this time. The electrocardiogram shown here was taken a few days after admission, because of frequent premature beats, which raised the question of digitalis intoxication.

COMMENT. The inconsistency of the limb and precordial lead findings in this case is quickly resolved if we consider the possibility of an error of technique consisting in a reversal of the wires connecting the right and left arms to the galvanometer. Both the clinical evidence of hypertension of long standing and the precordial leads, which are unlikely to be wrongly recorded, point to this technical error. Lead aV_R confirms this impression, which became a certainty upon inspection of a corrected record taken four days later as a check upon the artifact.

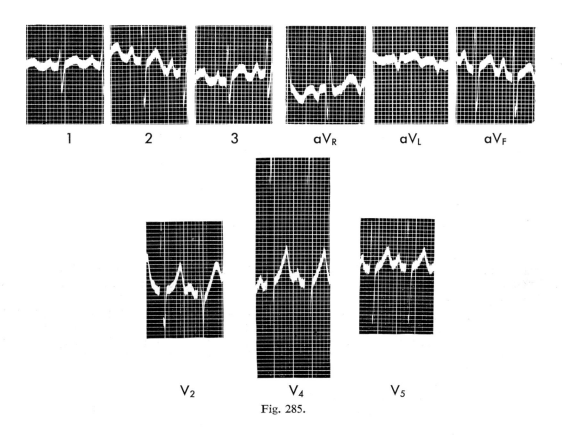

Fig. 285.

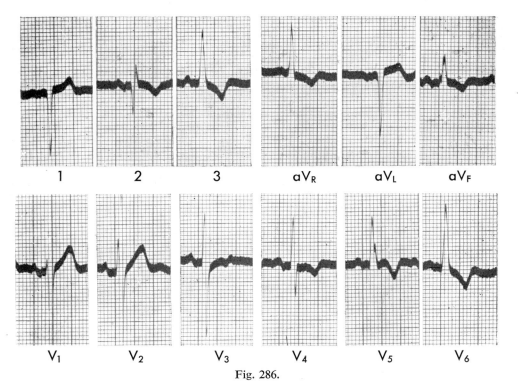

Fig. 286.

Fig. 287.

INTERPRETATION. Sinus rhythm at a rate of 95, with *P–R* interval of 0.24 second. The *T* waves are high with a narrow base. The *QRS* complexes appear normal. The *Q–T* duration measures 0.36 second (upper limit of normal for this heart rate = 0.35 second).

CLINICAL FINDINGS. W.M., a forty-two year old loom fixer, was admitted to the hospital on May 19, 1951, four weeks after the onset of his terminal illness, which had begun with a sore throat. At the onset he was treated with sulfadiazine, but this was not continued for more than a few days. Two weeks before admission he stopped work and complained of weakness and puffiness of the face, and for several days he had had severe oliguria.

Physical examination showed a moderately ill man with deep respirations, a dry mouth and slight pitting edema. His blood pressure was 150 mm. of mercury systolic and 90 mm. diastolic. Examination of the urine revealed a specific gravity of 1.020, 4 plus albumin, 200 red blood cells and 25 white blood cells per high-powered field, and waxy cellular and granular casts. Blood chemical studies done on the day of admission were reported as follows: nonprotein nitrogen, 265 mg. per cent; sodium, 137.4 milliequivalents per liter; potassium, 7.5 milliequivalents per liter; chlorides, 92 milliequivalents per liter; and carbon dioxide, 14 milliequivalents per liter. The electrocardiogram shown here was taken on May 25.

After treatment with low potassium fluids and ACTH there was a slight improvement in urinary output, but this never exceeded 400 cc. per day, and on the tenth hospital day the patient died. There was no evidence of respiratory paralysis in the terminal phase of the illness. Permission for a postmortem examination was refused.

COMMENT. This patient suffered acute nephritis following a respiratory infection. Renal failure may have been complicated by the administration of sulfadiazine at the onset of the illness. Cystoscopic examination on the day of admission revealed no blockage of pelves or ureters and no evidence of sulfadiazine sediment. The chief factor in the production of high levels of serum potassium in this case was renal failure with oliguria. Potassium intake was kept low during the hospital admission. The electrocardiogram obtained when the serum potassium level was 7.5 milliequivalents per liter shows partial atrioventricular block and the characteristic contour of the *T* waves in hyperkalemia, with high peaking. The *QRS* complexes are normal in duration and in contour.

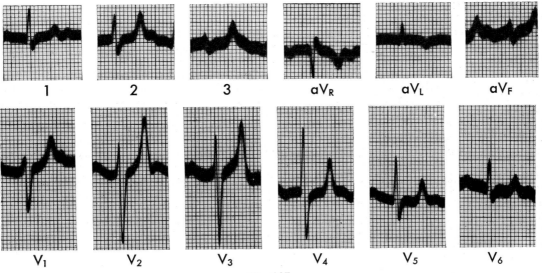

Fig. 287.

Fig. 288.

INTERPRETATION. Normal sinus rhythm, rate 75 to 85, interrupted by many atrial premature beats, some of which are attended by delay in atrioventricular conduction (*P–R* interval equal to 0.25 to 0.30 second), some completely blocked, and still others associated with aberrant ventricular contractions, that is, intraventricular or bundle branch block of the right branch type (M-shaped in precordial leads V_1 and V_2). The record is otherwise within normal limits.

CLINICAL FINDINGS. A.S., a sixty-four year old housewife, entered the hospital for treatment of a left saphenous thrombophlebitis. She had previously been followed in the clinic for a period of six years, with the diagnoses of myasthenia gravis, nontoxic nodular goiter and bilateral varicose veins. The myasthenia gravis had been well controlled by prostigmine, the goiter had been asymptomatic over a fifteen-year period, and the varicose veins had caused no difficulty until three weeks prior to the present admission.

Physical examination revealed a well developed and well nourished woman in no acute distress. There was considerable ptosis of the right eyelid. The left main saphenous trunk showed old and fresh areas of superficial thrombophlebitis. The blood pressure was 180 mm. of mercury systolic and 120 mm. diastolic. Heart size was at the upper limit of normal, and the rhythm was irregular at a rate of approximately 96.

The irregularity of heart rhythm was confirmed by an electrocardiogram taken on the day of admission and shown here. Quinidine (0.15 gm. subcutaneously) and prostigmine (15 mg. orally) were administered at once, with subsidence of the gross irregularity, although multiple atrial premature beats continued to occur. It was considered that these were related to the patient's state of nervous tension, inasmuch as they subsided when she was relaxed.

In this case the finding of a cardiac arrhythmia was incidental to the immediate problem of operation for thrombophlebitis. After the administration of quinidine on the day of hospital admission and ligation of the left saphenous vein under local anesthesia upon the following day, a cardiac consultation was requested. The patient was found to be comfortable with normal color, no orthopnea, and no venous pulsation in the neck. The lungs were clear. A heart rate of 120 and considerable cardiac irregularity at the time of this examination were attributed to the patient's nervous tension. The sounds were clear and of good quality, with no murmurs and no gallop. The liver was of normal size. Although hypertension was present, the cardiac consultant found the heart normal by history, physical examination and electrocardiogram, except for the frequently recurring premature beats. Because there was a possibility that quinidine sulfate would aggravate the myasthenia gravis, no attempt was made to prescribe for these. However, in the event of a striking recurrence of the arrhythmia in conjunction with symptoms such as dyspnea, chest pain or a drop in blood pressure, the use of quinidine lactate, 0.15 gm. intramuscularly, or slow administration of intravenous procaine, 50 mg., was advocated.

COMMENT. This electrocardiogram is indicative simply of considerable irritability of the heart in an older person with easily induced delay in conduction, but without evidence of intrinsic heart disease.

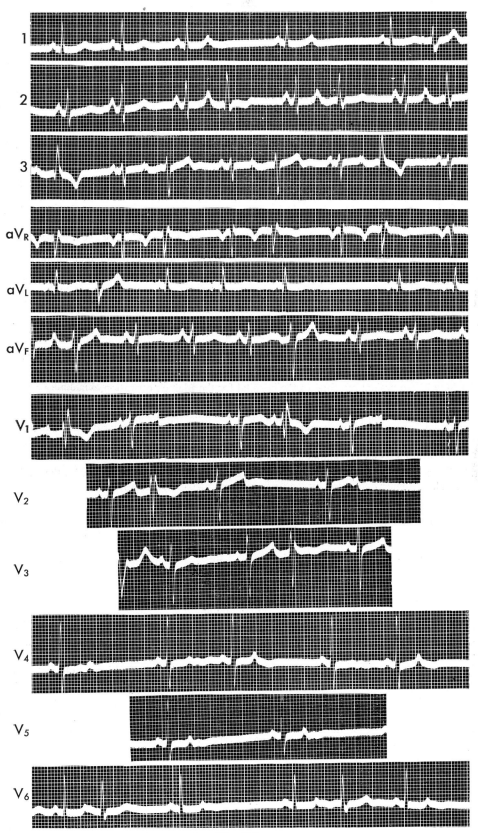

Fig. 288.

Fig. 289.

INTERPRETATION. Normal rhythm, rate 100, right axis deviation of moderate degree with high R waves in chest leads V_1 to V_4 inclusive. The T waves are all upright in the bipolar limb and unipolar chest leads.

CLINICAL FINDINGS. K.H., a girl of thirteen, was admitted to the hospital on April 7, 1950, for the study of her congenital heart disease. She had been cyanotic since birth, which occurred at full term and was preceded by an apparently normal pregnancy. Until she was six years old the patient had experienced almost daily "spells" in which she lost consciousness for two or three minutes; these occurred invariably after breakfast and, less frequently, after other meals. Ever since she had been able to walk she had found that she rested more comfortably when squatting. From the age of six she had learned to avoid the syncopal attacks by resting after meals and by eating lightly at breakfast. For the two years prior to this examination she had been unable to climb stairs without collapsing, and moderate physical incapacity in conjunction with extreme familial solicitude had restricted her activities to a bed-and-chair existence.

Physical examination revealed a well developed and well nourished young girl who was mentally alert and responsive. There were clubbing and cyanosis of the fingers and toes and slight cyanosis of the lips. The pulse rate was 108, the blood pressure 120 mm. of mercury systolic and 85 mm. diastolic. The heart sounds were of good quality. There was a harsh Grade 4 systolic murmur over the entire precordium, occupying all of systole, heard best at the left sternal border in the third interspace, and transmitted to the interscapular region and faintly to the neck. P_2 was loud but less than A_2. In the third interspace at the left sternal border a systolic thrill was palpable.

X-ray examination of the chest revealed somewhat sparse vascular markings and rather small pulmonary arteries, particularly the right. The heart size was within normal limits, with a cardiothoracic ratio of 11:25.5 cm. The aorta was on the left, possibly placed more medially than is usual; it displaced the esophagus only slightly. The combined shadow of the innominate artery and superior vena cava was rather prominent in the right superior paramediastinal area. The left subclavian artery was normal in size and in location. In the left anterior oblique and lateral views the right ventricle appeared somewhat prominent. The electrocardiogram shown here was taken seven weeks prior to the present examination.

Cardiac catheterization was performed on April 7, and the findings were indicative of pulmonary stenosis, right to left shunt (mild at rest), and right ventricular hypertension.

COURSE. On May 22 the patient returned to the hospital for the Blalock operation, which was attempted two days later. Unfortunately, in the course of anesthesia induction and during the first steps of this procedure she showed cardiac irregularity, with increased cyanosis, and by the time the areolar tissue had been cleared from the pulmonary arteries and separated from the pulmonary vein, frequent extrasystoles with short runs of ventricular tachycardia and a blood pressure drop to 60 mm. systolic and 40 mm. diastolic made it seem unwise to continue. On June 7, she was discharged home with her cardiac status unchanged.

COMMENT. This record is indicative of right ventricular enlargement and is consistent with the clinical diagnosis of the tetralogy of Fallot, further confirmed by the findings on cardiac catheterization.

Fig. 290.

INTERPRETATION. Normal rhythm at a rate of 95, with absence of R waves in Leads V_1, V_2 and V_3, presence of Q waves in V_4, inversion of T waves in Leads 1, 2, aV_F, V_3, V_4 and V_5. The T waves are upright in aV_R and diphasic in aV_L and V_6.

CLINICAL FINDINGS. S.L., a woman aged sixty-seven, had many complaints, of which the chief at the time of a clinic visit on August 3, 1949, was pain in the left upper anterior chest wall, beginning several months earlier and occurring almost daily until five days before, when it had lasted forty-eight hours. An electrocardiogram following that examination was consistent with the diagnosis of acute myocardial infarction. The record shown here was taken on August 17.

COMMENT. This record is characteristic of the presence of a large anterior myocardial infarct, doubtless involving the septum as well as almost the whole extent of the anterior wall.

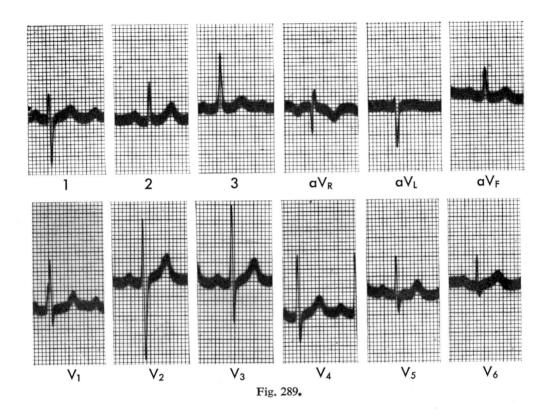

Fig. 289.

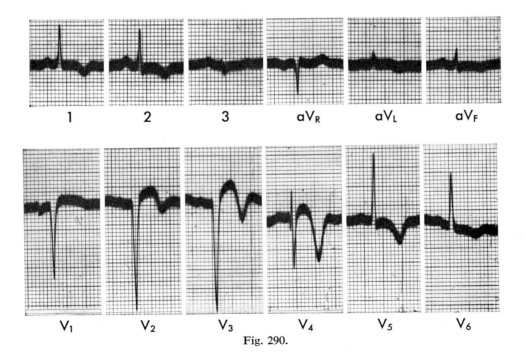

Fig. 290.

Fig. 291.

INTERPRETATION. Normal rhythm at a rate of 75, with deep S waves and small R waves in Leads V_1, V_2 and V_3, high R waves in Leads V_4, V_5 and V_6, inverted T waves in Leads 1, 2, 3, aV_F, V_5 and V_6, upright T waves in aV_R and diphasic T waves in Lead V_4.

CLINICAL FINDINGS. P.S., a man of forty-two years, was first examined by us in August, 1950. As a child and young adult he had experienced three bouts of active rheumatic fever, the last in 1935. Despite the diagnosis of rheumatic heart disease made at that time, he had continued to be active physically, and for the past seven years had been a stock clerk in a job which involved lifting and unloading of heavy cartons weighing up to 60 pounds. Over the year or two preceding this visit he had become increasingly short of breath, dyspneic upon two flights of stairs, and had required two pillows at night, with coughing and upon one occasion the production of a foamy pink material. He had noticed ankle edema at times and palpitation when he lay on his left side. Two weeks prior to this examination he had for the first time experienced substernal tightness across the anterior chest, lasting a few minutes, without radiation, and unrelated to exertion or emotion. There had been no symptoms of active rheumatic fever.

Upon physical examination he appeared slightly ill. His blood pressure was 170 mm. of mercury systolic and 70 mm. diastolic. There was slight cyanosis of the lips. The liver was just palpable but not tender. There were a few coarse wheezes at both lung bases. The heart rhythm was regular at a rate of 90, with a Corrigan pulse. Apical and aortic systolic murmurs of Grade 3 intensity were transmitted to the neck.

Fluoroscopic examination revealed a large heart, prominent in the regions of the left ventricle and the left atrium. An electrocardiogram at this time was similar to the one shown here.

The tracing in Figure 291 was taken almost one year later, in July, 1951, at which time, despite some cardiac irregularity, considerable heart consciousness, and apprehension, the patient was well stabilized upon a regimen including digitalis, ammonium chloride and a low sodium diet.

COMMENT. This record is clearly diagnostic of left ventricular enlargement, doubtless of considerable magnitude and here due, not to hypertension, the most usual cause, but to aortic stenosis and regurgitation.

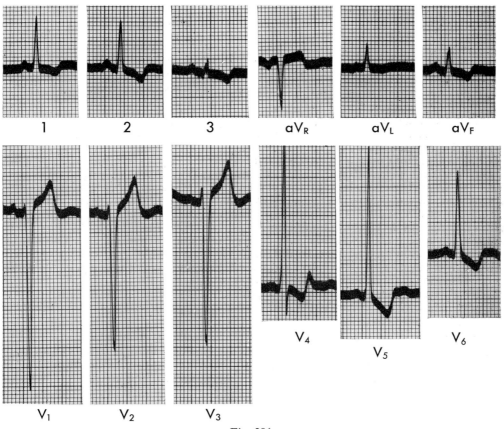

Fig. 291.

Fig. 293.

INTERPRETATION. Atrial fibrillation with occasional ectopic ventricular contractions at a heart rate averaging about 65. There is also slight right axis deviation, with high R waves in the precordial leads over the right ventricle, namely, V_1 to V_4, inclusive. The T waves are abnormal throughout, being slightly inverted in Leads 1, 2, V_2 to V_6, inclusive, and upright in aV_R.

CLINICAL FINDINGS. P.C., a man of forty-seven years, was examined in November, 1950, for consideration of a third operation for chronic constrictive pericarditis. In 1938 he had had his first pericardiolysis, with relief of symptoms for a period of eight years thereafter. In 1946 ascites again developed with cough and headaches, symptoms which persisted until May, 1949, when a second pericardial resection was performed. Despite an apparently good recovery initially, followed by a strict regimen of digitalis, ammonium chloride, mercurial diuretics and a low sodium diet, he failed to improve. The liver and spleen remained large, and symptoms of dyspnea and abdominal swelling with massive edema of the legs and scrotum persisted.

At this time of re-evaluation a year and a half after the second operation, it was believed that the accentuation of P_2 (2 plus), the deep systolic jugular pulse, and a shift of the electrical axis of the electrocardiogram toward the right were suggestive of an "external mitral stenosis" produced by constriction of the left atrioventricular groove or left atrium, and it was hoped that further resection of the pericardium, particularly over this region, might possibly be of benefit to this gravely handicapped patient. Cardiac catheterization was again unsuccessful, as it had been previously, in entering the right ventricle or pulmonary artery; the right atrial mean pressure was plus 15 mm. of mercury.

The electrocardiogram taken at this time is shown in Figure 293. Previous tracings had demonstrated atrial flutter and low voltage of QRS and T waves (1938) and subsequently (1946, 1948, 1949) atrial fibrillation and low voltage.

Upon x-ray examination of the chest free fluid was found in each pleural space with considerable pulmonary congestion and enlargement of the heart in all directions, particularly at the left atrium posteriorly. Calcification could still be seen around the anterior, inferior and left lateral aspects of the heart. Above the calcific pulsation at the apex there appeared to be relatively free pulsation, which was diminished in the area where the calcification was present inferiorly.

COURSE. In December, 1950, a third attempt to remove the pericardial constriction failed; the patient died on the operating table in cardiac arrest. The findings at autopsy included severe constrictive pericarditis over the left heart chambers, with fibrosis and calcification, generalized severe cardiac hypertrophy and dilatation, focal mitral and tricuspid insufficiency, focal calcification of the mitral valve, myocardial fibrosis of the anterolateral portion of the left ventricle, terminal focal myocardial hemorrhage, minimal coronary sclerosis, cirrhosis of the liver (cardiac type) and congestive splenomegaly.

COMMENT. This record suggests at first the problem of the presence of mitral stenosis causing right ventricular enlargement, with heart rate clinically controlled by digitalis, which could be responsible for the ectopic ventricular contractions. However, in this case, in contrast to that illustrated in Figure 292, the cause was not mitral stenosis, but chronic constrictive pericarditis involving particularly the left heart chambers. The T wave abnormalities somewhat suggest this possibility.

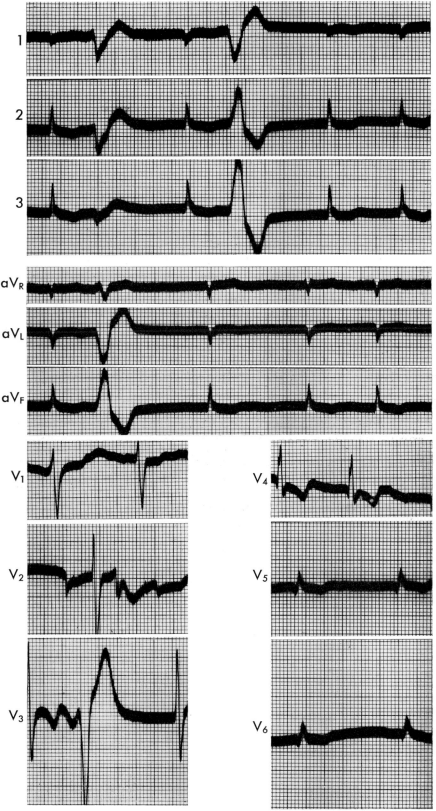

Fig. 293.

Fig. 294.

INTERPRETATION. *A* (May 12, 1951). Normal rhythm at a rate of 75. Normal complexes and time intervals except for prominence of the *Q* waves in Leads 1, V$_4$, V$_5$ and V$_6$ and the slightly elevated *S–T* segments in Lead V$_6$.

B (May 24, 1951). Normal rhythm at a rate of 75. Here there has been a distinct change in *T* waves without appreciable alterations of the *QRS* complexes. The *T* waves have become inverted in Leads 1, aV$_L$, V$_5$, and V$_6$, flat in Lead 2, and upright instead of inverted in aV$_R$. Also the *T* waves have become considerably higher in Leads V$_1$ and V$_2$.

C (May 29, 1951). Normal rhythm at a rate of 60. The changes noted in *B* have persisted, with slight increase in the abnormality of the *T* waves.

CLINICAL FINDINGS. A.K., a forty-six year old salesman, without previous history of cardiac disease, had his first acute attack of substernal pain on May 11, one day prior to hospitalization and to the electrocardiogram shown in *A*. The *B* tracing was taken on May 24. Five days later, on May 29, he experienced a recurrence of moderately severe anterior chest pain without dyspnea. The blood pressure at this time was 90 mm. of mercury systolic and 60 mm. diastolic. The heart sounds were of good quality, and there was no gallop rhythm. After the administration of morphine, 13 mg. subcutaneously, he felt better. The electrocardiogram taken upon this occasion is demonstrated in *C*.

COMMENT. These serial changes in the electrocardiogram are corroborative of the development under observation of anterolateral infarction of the left ventricle.

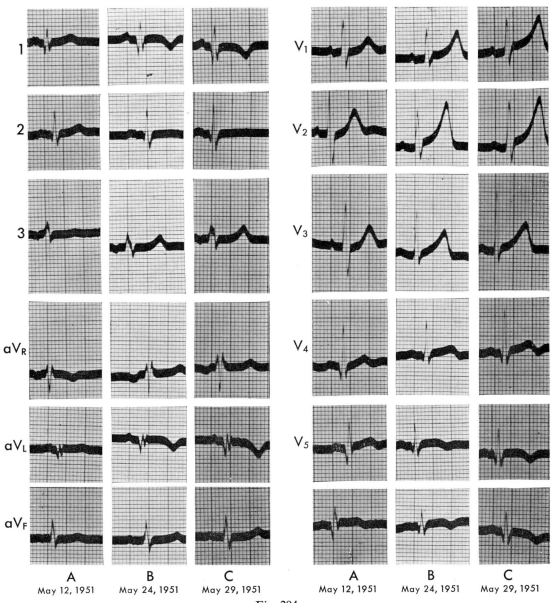

Fig. 294.

Index